Talking About Psychiat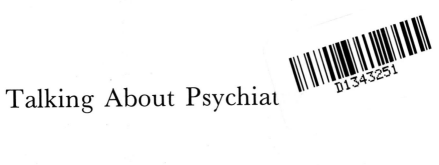

Edited by

GREG WILKINSON

Talking About Psychiatry

GASKELL

Gaskell is an imprint of the Royal College of Psychiatrists,
17 Belgrave Square, London SW1X 8PG

British Library Cataloguing-in-Publication Data
A catalogue record for this
book is available from the British Library

ISBN 0-902241-56-7

Distributed in North America
by American Psychiatric Press, Inc.
ISBN 0-88048-621-X

Phototypeset by Dobbie Typesetting Limited, Tavistock, Devon
Printed in Great Britain by Bell and Bain Ltd., Glasgow

For Professor Hugh Freeman,
on the occasion of his retirement as Editor of the
British Journal of Psychiatry (1983–93)

The Editor

Greg Wilkinson is Professor of Psychiatry at the London Hospital Medical College, and Editor of the *British Journal of Psychiatry*

Contents

Acknowledgements

My chief acknowledgement is to the subjects and interviewers whose work has been edited for publication in this book. The majority of these interviews were undertaken by Dr Brian Barraclough and Professor Hugh Freeman, who deserve great credit.

Professor Michael Shepherd provided me with the stimulus to undertake the task.

The work was undertaken during my tenure as Professor of Psychiatry, King Khalid University Hospital College of Medicine, King Saud University, Riyadh, Saudi Arabia, in the autumn of 1992. I thank the Dean, Professor Mansour M. Al-Nozha, and Drs A. Alhamad and F. El Aleem M. Abdul Rahim for their kindness and help.

Preface

This book tells the story of the recent evolution of British psychiatry. It represents an oral history, dealing with the period from before World War II until the present, and comprises a selection of interviews with prominent psychiatrists and policy makers, published in the *Psychiatric Bulletin* of the Royal College of Psychiatrists from 1981 onwards.

Talking About Psychiatry provides a unique perspective on British psychiatry. The interviews reveal personal and contrasting accounts of significant figures, institutions, practices, and historical developments. What emerges is a vivid account of a series of clinical and professional transitions characterised, at different times, by poverty of service provision, institutional decline, therapeutic and educational optimism and progress, and the establishment of professional standards in psychiatric training and practice – given impetus by the establishment of the Royal College of Psychiatrists in 1971.

Talking About Psychiatry offers an insight into the background, motivation and achievement of some of the foremost participants in this period of British psychiatry. Their testimony is a counterpoint to both the orthodox history of psychiatry and radical critiques of the subject.

Psychiatry remains, as ever, in the public domain. Amid the clamour, the Royal College of Psychiatrists has provided much of the stimulus towards improving the treatment and care of people with mental illness. Collectively, these accounts clearly show how humanity and wisdom, combined with leadership and vision, have transformed British psychiatry within a generation.

Greg Wilkinson

1 Eliot Slater, CBE

Interviewed by BRIAN BARRACLOUGH (1981)

Dr Eliot Slater, CBE, MA, MD Cantab, FRCP, FRCPsych 1971, FRCPsych (Hon) 1973. Dr Slater, formerly Honorary Lecturer, Institute of Psychiatry, was born in 1904 and died in 1983. From 1931–39 he was a Medical Officer at The Maudsley Hospital. He was Clinical Director of Sutton Emergency Hospital from 1939–45 and Physician in Psychological Medicine, National Hospital, Queen Square, WC1 from 1946–64. Dr Slater was Editor in Chief of the *British Journal of Psychiatry* from 1961–72. He was co-author of *Physical Methods of Treatment in Psychiatry* (with William Sargant), *Clinical Psychiatry* (with W. Mayer-Gross and Martin Roth) and *The Genetics of Mental Disorder* (with Valerie Cowie). In his 76th year he was awarded his PhD for a thesis devoted to a statistical word study of a play, *Edward III*.

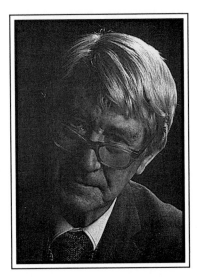

BMB We might start with your editorship of the British Journal of Psychiatry

ES   I was elected at the Annual General Meeting of the RMPA in 1961. Fleming, who was the existing Editor, was in bad health and wasn't able to carry on with the work. I don't quite know how my name came up. Somebody approached me and I was very pleased to do it because I felt it was something I would very greatly enjoy. I felt that it was something I could do.

BMB Had you any previous experience as an editor?

ES   None. I remember discussing the job of an editor with Arnold Carmichael, who was the Editor of the 'green rag', the *Journal of Neurology & Psychiatry*. It later changed its name to the *Journal of Neurology, Neurosurgery & Psychiatry*.

I said my idea was to get a lot of helpers, let them do what they liked to do, and just collate it and gather the threads. There should be many advisers, so you could always have a paper vetted by somebody in whose field it lay. Carmichael said 'Oh no, that isn't the way to do it. What you want to do is to have two good friends and the three of you decide everything.' But I thought that isn't the way I'd do it.

BMB And what about the Journal's name?

ES   The *Journal of Mental Science* had already taken on a subtitle, *The British Journal of Psychiatry*, thereby pre-empting it from being gobbled up as a title for any new psychiatric journal by the Tavistock Square publishing house. When they published a psychiatric journal of their own, it couldn't take that name.

In due course, I went down to Fleming's house in Gloucester with a suitcase and took the papers that he hadn't been able to deal with. Then I got on with the job of going through the pile, and started to think of people who could be invited to come in as assessors.

BMB *What was the standing of the Journal of Mental Science then?*

ES   Pretty low, but like the famous plum pudding, it did have the odd plum. Good papers got published now and again, even if it published a lot of rubbish. By getting a lot of help, we raised the standard. Assessors only got half a dozen or so papers in the course of a year, or if they were lucky up to a dozen, and this wasn't impossible for anybody. And people liked doing it. One or two said 'sorry' after a couple of years, 'I have had enough' or 'I'm getting too busy'. But as a rule, they like to go on for the term.

BMB *What journals published psychiatry then?*

ES   Well, one didn't try to go to American journals, like the *American Journal of Psychiatry*. I don't think you would have got much chance of being accepted if you did, but the *Lancet* and *BMJ* took the odd paper, so did the *Journal of Neurology & Psychiatry*.

BMB *How do you explain the success of the British Journal of Psychiatry?*

ES   I suppose it filled a vacuum. I think you are right in thinking there wasn't a lot of space to get your papers published. But also people weren't writing for publication much. The idea of writing papers for the young man who is building a career is modern, I think.

BMB *How often did the Journal come out?*

ES   At first, two-monthly, six issues a year. It was a big adventure to go into monthly publication. That was possible because the readership went up so much; the subscriptions from overseas increased no end. And there was plenty of stuff coming in too.

BMB *For how long were you Editor?*

ES   A bit over eleven years. I took it up in the middle of 1961 and I finished at the end of 1972. I went on as acting Editor when the College was formed because I was ineligible to be Editor. I was too old.

BMB *Would you like to say anything about your time as Editor?*

ES   I enjoyed it no end. I loved the work, and it was never difficult for me. Edward Hare followed me and did it very conscientiously, but he never enjoyed it like I did. I regard myself as a bad organiser, but there was no trouble about organising that show as far as I was concerned.

BMB *You concerned yourself with the papers published in the Journal rather than the general production?*

ES   I paid attention to the production, in the sense of what kind of printing we were getting, what kind of paper we should use, what our format should be, the wonderful new golden cover that was going to attract attention in all the scientific libraries, and how the advertisement income was organised, and so forth. I wasn't as enthusiastic about that, but I covered it more or less. I put any sticky things to the Journal Committee.

The thing that interested me was the stuff that came in and how it could be produced, and how people could be encouraged and not squashed. I remember one young man sending a paper in. He got an awful brush off from the assessor, who said 'No, this is unacceptable; he doesn't know how to write a paper'.

I was all in favour of open editing. The style in those years was 'we regret we are unable to accept your paper for publication'; no more, no explanation, nothing. I thought 'this isn't the way to do things' and I nearly always sent a copy of the report of the assessor to the author. Sometimes a piece would be cut out if it was too painful or rude, but as a rule, the author got an unvarnished opinion.

Anyway, on this occasion, I sent back the report from the assessor complete. It may not have been unkind, but it was quite annihilating. The wretched young man from a provincial hospital wrote back to say that he was greatly obliged to have this report because he realised now that writing papers was not for him and he would never try it again. And I said 'My God, that's not the way to do things!'

BMB *Was the colour of the cover your idea?*

ES   I can't say, but I fell for it. The idea was that if you went into a library, and instead of all the dull grey and brown you saw this golden yellow thing staring at you, you'd have to pick it up.

BMB *Do you think of any papers published during your editorship as being especially remarkable?*

ES   I remember a long paper that came from America. It was about monozygotic twins who had been specially selected as discordant in respect of the American diagnosis of schizophrenia and were taken in under observation in the National Institute of Mental Health. A huge amount of work was done on them.

I thought the selection was illegitimate. The twins were picked to be discordant. They weren't from any known or limited population. It was anybody the authors could find in the whole of America whose parents were willing for their offspring to come under observation in the research centre. But one couldn't suppress the data; I accepted this paper for publication, but I wrote to the authors and pointed out the defects in selection.

Another thing I think of is the work by my colleagues at the National Hospital on the schizophrenia-like psychoses of epilepsy. I was determined to publish the whole of this, however egoistic it looked, and it took up 70 pages of the *Journal* to put it all out in grand array – total lack of false modesty.

BMB *Well, you had a good time with the Journal.*

ES   I did indeed.

BMB *And thought you achieved something?*

ES   Well, the *Journal* improved in quality and status in my time; I think it was partly because of what I did, but very largely because of what all the other chaps did. A lot of people worked on it. It was a big cooperative effort of British psychiatrists.

BMB   Let's continue on publishing and talk about the two books you are so well known for.

ES   Those I wrote with Willi Mayer-Gross and Martin Roth on the one hand and Will Sargant on the other hand.

BMB   Which would you like to start on?

ES   The one with Will Sargant was the one to get off the ground first, in 1944. This was built up on his experience of active treatment, and what some people would call an adventurous approach to treatment in psychiatry. I liked this approach. I liked his way of working with patients.

He and I got to be very friendly. He would come to me with problems about how to make his points, or for criticism of points he wanted to make, and I collaborated with him. But he was the leading spirit. He was always thinking of new ways of treating people. When I first went to the Maudsley, there was, practically speaking, no treatment at all.

BMB   You are talking now of before the war?

ES   Yes. I went to the Maudsley in 1931. The most appalling thing was the chronic melancholics, often people of most excellent personality, sunk deep in a depression which nothing could move. People have no idea now of what that illness could be. It never gets anywhere near that stage now. But then there was absolutely nothing.

BMB   It would be worthwhile if you could recall the features of the chronic melancholic before ECT.

ES   The involutional melancholic would be a thin, elderly man or woman, inert, with the head lifted up off the pillow. There were some sort of Parkinsonian-like qualities, mask-like face sunk deep in misery, and speaking in a retarded way. If you could get them to say anything, it would be something about how hopeless things were, how they were wicked, doomed to disease, death, and a terrible afterlife, if there was one.

And there wasn't anything you could do, except to try to make them sleep, try to get them to take some food, tube-feed them if they were refusing food, which happened frequently. If they were very retarded and inert, then they were reasonably safe from a suicide attempt. If they began to improve, or were at an early stage of the illness, you had the risk of a desperate suicidal attempt.

A lot of the patients who came into the hospital were in that condition, and quickly went on to suicidal caution. Even then, we had suicides. I remember a man in the male acute ward, with its own enclosed garden, who was found to be dying. His stomach at postmortem was full of yew leaves. The beds were wheeled out into the garden, and his bed had come under a yew tree. He had assiduously chewed up these leaves and swallowed them. None of us knew the yew is poisonous. Its alkaloid (Taxine) killed him all right.

Poor Edward Mapother, our Medical Superintendent, went into a panic about this getting into the newspapers, and getting to County Hall. Staff were sent next thing to cut that tree down. It was a very handsome yew tree, which shouldn't have been there, admittedly.

The pleasanter sort of case, of course, was the manic or hypomanic, where you could get some rapport. The schizophrenics would go into any kind of state. We might give them some form of sedation. We tried out the Swiss treatment of continuous narcosis for a week or fortnight. This is a dangerous treatment if it's done really properly, with 16 hours of deep sleep a day.

We didn't have any short-acting barbiturates then. We had phenobarbitone and medinal; but they were long-acting, and in a heavy dosage, as for continuous narcosis, they were dangerous. Bromides, paraldehyde and, by injection, morphine and hyoscine – we had to do our best with them, and with physical measures such as the continuous bath. Sulfosin was tried out in schizophrenics, but with no good results.

Then, before the war, along came first convulsive therapy with cardiazol and then insulin treatment. Both of them, of course, have achieved a bad name. But there was absolutely no question in my mind that insulin coma therapy would produce a remarkable remission in acute schizophrenics who, in the ordinary way, one couldn't expect to do anything but go bad.

Will Sargant was an enthusiast, and he and Russell Fraser, who went off into general medicine, managed the Villa as an acute treatment centre. What happened there was most encouraging; it was really quite wonderful.

Then came Cerletti and Bini and electroshock; and then electroshock under sedation; then under anaesthesia with an antispasmodic, and the modern form of treatment. There was absolutely no question about the revolution in treatment. A few cardiazol epileptic fits are horrible to witness, but for the involutional melancholics, the response was almost miraculous.

So I arrived in psychiatry at a time when one was quite hopeless and helpless, practically speaking. Before these advances, the only treatment where you could really do something was the malarial treatment of general paresis. A breed of mosquitoes was kept at Horton Hospital and they were brought around if you got a GPI. I saw quite a few GPIs in my early days, but you don't see them now; penicillin has done its work.

With the neurotics, one did the sort of psychotherapy that suited one's personality. Quite a few people, of course, went and got some sort of analytic training, but there wasn't much of a move towards psychoanalysis at that stage. The big surge towards psychoanalysis came after the war.

BMB   *What kind of psychotherapy suited you?*

ES   Perhaps what you might call commonsense psychotherapy, trying to find out what was hurting this individual and how it could be influenced by persuasion, by making some intervention or suggesting some intervention. I was never a depth explorer.

BMB   *Shall we get back to how Sargant & Slater got written.*

ES   Sargant said 'Come on you, you must write the introductory chapter and the section on psychotherapy in conjunction with physical treatment.' He would write everything else, and I would have to take it and see what his line of thought was and improve it in logical progression and coherence. When he first started to write, his English was not good. He went on writing, and got to be a good writer in the end. His paperback books are very good.

BMB   *When did it first come out?*

ES   Before the end of the war, in 1944. Will was very keen that it should be on the market soon. He wanted it priced low, so that his big message should get to the world. As he saw it, this was a very big message. He is the son of a Methodist minister and he is an evangelist for the good way of doing things. He would sacrifice himself to help his patients. He is one of the few people who really would do almost anything to help the patients he thought could be helped.

I once talked to him about this and asked him if there were any limits to this. He said 'Oh yes, indeed, if I come to the conclusion that I can't help somebody, then that's that. I have to go on to someone else whom I can help.' So he keeps things within a reasonable measure. But he is a great enthusiast. He got this book published quickly and it was of course very influential. I always feel it was because of the popularisation of physical methods of treatment in psychiatry that Britain was saved from following America down the psychoanalytic path.

An Introduction to Physical Methods we called it. It contained every item of knowledge that we had. But an 'introduction' it was; things have gone on a very long way since then. When physical treatments started, it was purely a guess. Somebody tried it – malaria, cardiazol, insulin. The convulsive treatment of mental illness was started because Meduna thought that epileptics didn't get schizophrenia.

Sakel was allowed to try insulin coma at the Vienna clinic. I saw insulin coma there before it was being done anywhere else. I thought to myself – this is a lot of poppycock. Because they discovered that malaria cured GPI, they think they can do another miracle cure. I regarded the whole issue with contempt. But I changed my mind when Will Sargant and Russell Fraser took it up.

BMB *Do you still believe insulin is a useful treatment in schizophrenia?*

ES   There is no point in giving it because there are other treatments.

BMB *I was thinking of the controlled trial of barbiturates and insulin.*

ES   I could never quite believe that trial because deep sleep therapy had not proved successful in schizophrenia. But insulin therapy was replaced by phenothiazines. They proved to be the effective treatment.

BMB *But I thought that controlled trial of insulin coma and barbiturate coma which was published by Brian Ackner put a finish to the use of insulin.*

ES   I wouldn't say that's all wrong, but I'm doubtful about it. Nobody's gone on to give barbiturate coma to schizophrenic patients as a systematic treatment, so in a way he was comparing insulin coma therapy with non-therapy, and I am firmly convinced that insulin coma therapy was quite remarkably successful in cases which would have been utterly hopeless in the pre-treatment era.

Good clinical judges thought so. Mayer-Gross was a superb clinician. He had absolutely no doubt about what he was seeing. When you see things happen under your eyes, it is very difficult to say it's all chance.

BMB *I suppose that applies particularly now, with ECT being under such heavy criticism as being a useless treatment and investigations to find out whether it is the anaesthetic or the convulsion which causes the improvement. What you are saying is that people were so ill in the '30s and were not going to get better.*

ES   The involutional melancholics I was talking about might take six months and then start getting better in 12 or 15 months. If they went on much longer than that, they went into a chronic depressive state which was immovable. I think that in the mental hospitals, they did take electroshock into the wards for people who had been certified as suffering from chronic melancholia for years, and still got results.

I think the anti-ECT campaign is ideologically directed in the main; that is to say, it is by people who believe that psychic illness is the product of psychic causes, so that to intervene along a physical line is a form of assault, and they are not going to believe it does any good. There have recently been controlled trials on ECT which show it does have an effect. Anyway, the way it is done now is pretty harmless.

BMB *You mention William Mayer-Gross.*

ES   Willi Mayer-Gross was one of three German Jewish refugees who came to us about 1934, when things were getting impossible for the Jews in Germany. Mapother organised it with Rockefeller's help. It was one of the most far-sighted things he ever did; and it has made a historic difference to British psychiatry.

The other two were Eric Guttmann and Alfred Meyer, who was – and still is – a world-famous neuropathologist. Mayer-Gross was rather short, powerfully built, very extraverted, a ball of energy. Eric was long and thin, elegant, aquiline. Freddie Meyer was the most slightly built. He was sensitive and retiring, one of the kindest and gentlest souls I ever met. Freddie went upstairs to work in Golla's laboratory; the other two were with us in the wards. All three would come to lunch with us. They were an immense addition to our society, which was a warm, intimate one in the years before the war.

Mayer-Gross was greatly respected as a clinician of the German phenomenological school. The idea was that if one couldn't do anything to cure schizophrenia, at least let us study it. What is the form of thought disorder, what kind of ways does a delusional idea appear in the mind of a schizophrenic, and so on. And that was one way to save one's soul, because it was soul-destroying not to be able to do anything for patients.

Mayer-Gross came with a whole world of subtle clinical observations to instruct us in, and taught us above all to talk to our patients in an attempt at getting an understanding of the way their minds were working. I got on very well with him, and with the other two as well. Eric Guttmann gave me endless help in my own work. But Willi Mayer-Gross said 'Come on, let's write a textbook of psychiatry for England, for the British'.

BMB *That was before the war.*

ES   It can't have been. During the war, Mayer-Gross went to the Crichton at Dumfries.

BMB *Why did he do that – an extraordinary thing to leave London?*

ES   Because he had to find a job. And he was offered one there. The hospital was keen and progressive, and he would have his own house and a reasonable income to live on. I don't think he was at all keen to leave London itself, but he adjusted himself to it very well. The fact is there weren't a tremendous number of jobs going around. Why, for instance, didn't I become a professor?

BMB *Yes, I have wondered that.*

ES   Because there weren't any professorships worth having. There was one in Edinburgh and one in London. When other chairs did come along eventually,

I found they were terrible jobs organising psychiatry in new towns, so to speak, where nobody cared about psychiatry and you would have to fight tooth and nail for everything. You would have to be an empire builder. It wasn't my line at all.

Freddie Meyer had to go for a time to Barnwood House in Gloucester with Fleming. Eric Guttmann was actually interned for a time. The Maudsley closed down. It just became Mill Hill and Sutton.

Anyway, after the war, Mayer-Gross and I proceeded to write this book. He wrote most of it. I had to turn his Germanic English into English. I wrote chapters of my own, some of which were an awful sweat; the chapter on law, for instance, was a frightful toil. We both began to get stale and thought we really must have more help, and we asked Martin Roth to come in and write the organic stuff. It worked very well indeed and the book came out in 1954.

BMB   Were there any competitors for it at the time?

ES   The textbooks available at that time were either not very comprehensive or not all that good. The American ones were mainly full of Freud, or Adolf Meyer's psychobiology. Henderson & Gillespie was rather an old-stager. Curran & Guttmann had come out in 1949, but was meant principally for beginners.

The best textbooks available were in German, especially Bleuler and Bumke. I believe there were excellent textbooks in French, for instance by Henri Ey; but I could never read French psychiatry.

BMB   Do you think they were an influence for the good?

ES   The Mayer-Gross–Guttman–Meyer influence was, as far as I am concerned, profoundly to the good. I think it enlarged the vision of British psychiatry tremendously. It gave a lot of people a lot more to think about. It taught them to pay close attention to their patients, to sift, to discriminate.

BMB   Was it only the subject matter of research or a new approach?

ES   I think the effect of these Germans upon me and some others was to promote enthusiasm. You really became enthusiastic about the subject in which you spent your every day. In point of fact, that degree of acute interest antedated their arrival. I can remember first arriving at the Maudsley Hospital and being completely overwhelmed with curiosity by a young nurse from one of the mental hospitals who was possessed with the Devil.

The Devil compelled her to write screeds of stuff and then God would stop the Devil, and there was a sort of colloquy between God, the Devil and her going on. It was, of course, a lot of hysteria, but some of the ideas coming out were very strange. I was completely fascinated by it, I was staying there up on the ward, writing it all down, up to 10 o'clock at night before going home.

I remember we had a very high-level Jesuit priest, tormented by obsessions. This was in Aubrey Lewis's ward. Aubrey spent hours, and hours and hours talking to this priest. They shared a common fund of arcane knowledge, because Aubrey himself had been brought up in a Jesuit school; he knew all the Jesuitical ways of looking at things, and he could talk to this Jesuit fine.

The Jesuit eventually left the hospital just as obsessional as ever. It was a big change from the absolute apathy in the county mental hospital I had come from to the enthusiasm I found at the Maudsley. I must not put it all down to the Germans, but they provided a whole lot of new outlooks.

BMB *How did the Maudsley become so lively a place; was it a German influence at second-hand, because people had been there?*

ES   No, it was Edward Mapother looking around for the brightest young people he could find in British medicine, and inviting and persuading them to come there. He made a great effort to get Desmond Curran to come.

When Aubrey Lewis turned up from Australia on an anthropological study year, Mapother was very struck, as of course one would be, by his intellectual abilities. Mapother got him to go over to America and spend time with Adolf Meyer, and then come back to the Maudsley. He was later made its Clinical Director. Before I ever came near the Maudsley, I was told that in psychiatry, the Maudsley was a place where one wouldn't be ashamed to go.

I originally wanted to be a neurologist. I had seen wonderful demonstrations by James Collier at St George's Hospital, and I was fascinated by the crossword-like accuracy with which one could pinpoint lesions. So I tried to train myself into neurology and to get to Queen Square, but Queen Square wouldn't have me. They looked at me the first time I applied for a house physician job, but said 'Come again another day'.

Then I thought I would go and get some psychiatry; I went to see Mapother, who said 'Sorry, we haven't got anything at this time, but keep in touch'. So I took a job in a provincial mental hospital and got a princely salary of £350 a year and keep, which was very worth having.

From there, I tried for a second time at Queen Square; but now, of course, I was tarred with a dirty brush, and they wouldn't look at me. After six months, I couldn't stand it any longer and felt I must leave, for the sake of my soul.

I wrote to Mapother, and he took me on as a locum. That is how I came to the Maudsley and that is how he picked up people. He collected people who had a good record in medicine. He loved to have people who had the MRCP. He wanted to make his staff respectable in the eyes of medical teaching in London. And he succeeded.

BMB *Did you go there to do research?*

ES   I don't know, I must have had some sort of idea about doing research, because when I wrote to Mapother, I said 'there's no research going on here'. And he thought this was super, I suppose. Here was a young man who wanted to do research, and at the Maudsley he had this fellow Lewis, who was telling everybody 'Come on now, you have got to do a bit of research'. Everybody had to do something.

We had Tuesday evening meetings after the day's work was over, and you would stay and have an evening meal and then you'd go and sit in Lewis's room. It was Lewis who said I must provide something interesting for one of these meetings, and suggested hypnagogic hallucinations as a subject: How many people have them? What are they like?

I proceeded to make an enquiry among the patients about whether they had any hypnagogic hallucinations. And after this, the more I did of delving and researching, the more I liked that kind of activity.

BMB *So Lewis was the main influence, at least to begin with, in directing your attention to research?*

ES Yes, he was emphatically. We must give him that credit very much. Eventually, though, he had a devastating effect on enquiring minds. In the early years of his professorship at the Maudsley, he was found quite crushing by some of the registrars when they presented cases at his conference.

I don't think that considering what they had in the way of bright people, the Maudsley research record is very good, at any rate in the early years. I wouldn't like to say what it's like now. But in Lewis's early years, the post-war years, there wasn't a lot of new thought going on. It wasn't that Lewis wasn't stimulating, but he was so sceptical. If you thought up any idea, he would find reasons for debunking it. You can't go on researching if you are just debunked.

BMB *What about other influences in the '30s on your developing interest in research?*

ES Well, I suppose the critical thing for me was finding I liked playing with numbers. And then going and getting myself a statistical training.

BMB *Where did you get that?*

ES At the School of Hygiene & Tropical Medicine. I only had about six weeks of it, but I learned a lot of stuff. There was a lot of work on incidences and prevalences, on birth rates, death rates, national statistics. But they also gave you a training in small sample statistics. It was that, of course, that was invaluable in psychiatry. They used to give us lectures and then set exercises and we would sit at a desk, about a dozen or fifteen of us, with a little mechanical calculator in front of us, and work out tables and come to results and they would be checked.

My great teacher was R. A. Fisher. I absorbed his book *Statistical Methods for Research Workers*, and when problems came up which I didn't know how to handle, I would write to him at his journal office – he was Editor of the *Annals of Eugenics*. He was always helpful. He was a great saint in my mind.

BMB *I once remember reading a paper you had written, about admission rates or discharge rates in British mental hospitals that you had got from the Board of Control, and you ended up . . .*

ES 'These statistics are not absolutely useless.' The journal was the *Annals of Eugenics*. When Lionel Penrose took over the editorship, he disliked the term 'eugenics' – Galton's idea – so much that he got it changed to *Annals of Human Genetics*. The article was published there. It was great fun.

Lewis said to me, 'Why not try to duplicate the work that has been done in Germany': finding out what the risks are for members of the general population to get this, that, and the other psychiatric disorder.

I got permission to go into the medical and surgical wards at King's and obtained information from people having their appendix out or having a hernia done. But this was a biased population too. Lots of these people were neurotics and only in hospital because of neurosis. The incidence of psychiatric disorder in their relatives was much too high. Then it occurred to me that one could make use of the Board of Control data, the central statistics, and I got permission to see them. But of course, the official diagnoses were out of date: primary dementia, systematised and non-systematised delusion insanity, etc. But I suppose it was the first big thing I wrote. It started off with an idea of Lewis's, not of mine.

BMB *What happened next in your research career?*

ES I went to Germany on a Rockefeller fellowship. After that, I went up to the Medical Research Council and said what about doing research on twins. They said 'Yes'. They gave me a grant and I spent a couple of years or so going around the London County Council mental hospitals, collecting twin cases. If a patient was reported to be one of twins, I had to go into the case in depth, which meant going off and doing the fieldwork myself. Very laborious and taxing.

When the war came, this work hadn't been completed, but after the war, the MRC agreed that I finish it off and polish it up. I got James Shields to come and do it. It was such a relief that he could visit the relatives instead of me, and knock on their doors and get them to answer questions, rather like being a politician, worming your way into people's homes.

BMB *Where did the idea for the twin method come from?*

ES It was around. When I went to Germany, I spent a year at Munich and met Klaus Conrad. He did a wonderful piece of research into the monozygotic and dizygotic twins of epileptics. It was a model of perfection technically. You could say I took the twin idea from the *Forschungsanstalt für Psychiatrie* in Munich. I made a very good friend there, Bruno Schulz, who taught me a lot on genetic methods in psychiatry.

When I came back, I got the MRC grant and did the twin job, and then came the war. I went to Sutton and started doing things on the soldier population there: patterns of marriage with Moya Woodside, and fascinating things like that. And then picking and delving became something that had to be part of my life wherever I went.

When I went to Queen Square as psychiatrist to the National Hospital, I was keen to pursue research there, which wasn't so easy. They didn't like it there. They wanted good clinical work and top-level teaching. I started off at Queen Square with every sort of encouragement from people like Carmichael.

Gradually things went wrong. I got at cross-purposes with my colleagues. Looking back, I can't blame them. For instance, I refused the job of Dean. Of course, that was very bad. If you are on board a ship and the captain says you will be the officer who will receive the guests when we have our great gala day, you are then the officer who receives the guests; there is no help for it. I wasn't playing fair by the chaps.

Lectures on psychiatry struck me as a ghastly thing to have to do. What I really enjoyed was having teaching rounds or conferences on my own patients.

The young housemen – not all that young, some of them were getting on – were wonderful people to teach, and be taught by. The interesting thing was that the really brightest of the bright were the young house physicians who were going to be accomplished general physicians. These young people told me about everything that was going on in medicine, and were constantly keeping me up to the mark.

What happened eventually was a sad story. The Mental Health Research Fund had some money with which they wanted to endow an academic unit at one of the hospitals. I put in an application which they agreed. It was going to be an appointment for a senior lecturer, working in my department.

It would have been the top of my ambition to make a small academic psychiatric unit at the National Hospital. This was battled in the hospital's Medical Committee for about a year, and they turned it down. I felt that was too much for me and I sent in my resignation. But I think if I hadn't blotted my copybook, neurologically speaking, I might have got their support.

BMB   Do you think their refusal was a personal matter?

ES   In a way, I think. We were such different sorts of people, the more senior physicians and I. Another thing which must have irritated them very much was when I did a follow-up study on National Hospital cases diagnosed as hysteria and found that a big loading of organic disease had been missed. It was not a good thing.

BMB   I don't suppose it could have been entirely personal, or there would now be a larger psychiatric component at Queen Square.

ES   When I left the National, I asked the MRC to give me another couple of sessions in the Genetics Unit, and they kindly agreed. Jerry Shields was very active, though he was confined to a wheel-chair after an attack of polio. I was collaborating with him, and with Valerie Cowie on mental subnormality. We had guest workers from America, Australia, and the Far East. Ming-Tso Tsuang took a PhD with us.

Our biggest acquisition was Irving Gottesman, who brought outstanding ability, new ideas, technical aids, and finance into a most productive collaboration with Jerry Shields. They took up twin work where I had left it off.

When I was approaching retirement, the MRC had to consider what to do with the Unit. They decided it must be closed down, but also that the twin work under Shields should go on. So Jerry was transferred to the Institute, with MRC support, and Irv Gottesman came over regularly from the USA to continue work with him.

BMB   Do you think that psychiatry will disappear as a speciality, one part being taken up by the neurologists or physicians and the other by psychologists and social workers?

ES   No, I don't. Perhaps it is because I have always thought of myself as a psychiatrist, I haven't thought of myself as being a geneticist or an MRC man, and it seems to me such a fascinating field. You can approach it from physical medicine with human and humane interest, and find such an enormous lot to do.

I can't think that the psychologists are as well placed, and certainly not the sociologists. A lot of them are totally misled by bogus ideas. The psychologists are better than the sociologists, who get their ideas from social knowledge which is knowledge about societies and groups, not about individuals. And I think they go completely adrift when they come up against individuals. They have these dogmas – that a child's best place is with his mother, for instance. Even when the child is with his mother, for instance. Even when the child is running away at every possible opportunity they still send him back.

As for the neurologists, I have no hope for them at all. I think they could only advance if they really became neuropsychiatrists. If you are interested in brain function, you must pay attention to the top-level functions of the brain – to speech, emotional reaction, and communication with other people at the highest level.

2 Max Hamilton

Interviewed by **BRIAN BARRACLOUGH (1982)**

Professor Max Hamilton, MB BS 1937, DPM Eng 1946, MD Lond 1950, FRCP Lond 1970, FRCPsych 1971, FRCPsych (Hon) 1982. Professor Hamilton was born in Offenbach, near Frankfurt, Germany in 1912 and when he was 3 years old accompanied his parents to England. He died in 1988. He qualified from University College Hospital, London in 1934 and joined the RAF as a medical officer in 1939. He served as senior hospital medical officer to Tooting Bec Hospital and moved to Leeds in 1953 as senior lecturer in psychiatry. His rating scale was published in 1960 in the *Journal of Neurology, Neurosurgery and Psychiatry*. He was appointed to the Nuffield Chair of Psychiatry, Leeds University in 1963 and retired in 1977 (Emeritus). Professor Hamilton was the foundation President of the British Association of Psychopharmacology.

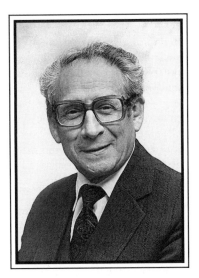

BB   Where did you go to school?

MH   At the Central Foundation School in London. I now realise what a remarkably far-seeing and modern headmaster we had. He had grasped the fundamental points about teaching mathematics; that it is not an easy subject and you must devote time to it. In my matriculation year, out of 35 lessons a week, 18 were on mathematical subjects. Most of the boys who left that school had one characteristic which I also had: I wasn't a mathematician, but I wasn't afraid of it. Most people tremble when they sit in front of a page of maths – it doesn't worry me. I know it is going to take time, but if I go at it long enough, I can understand it.

I was keen on science and took up medicine as the most practical aspect, but once I got into clinical teaching at University College, I found it dull. The teaching was *obiter dictum*. They laid down the law. These are the signs and symptoms, this is the diagnosis and this is the treatment. I took little interest and as a result I claim, I will not say I boast, that I have failed in more examinations than most people have taken. As I took one half of my MB, I failed in one subject and the next time I took it I failed in the other.

I went eventually in 1936 to work in Mile End Hospital and became District Medical Officer – a sort of GP to old age pensioners and the unemployed. I used the opportunity to try and do some worthwhile work. One of the first things I discovered was that my diabetics never stuck to their diet; they were a menace because they were likely to go into hypoglycaemia. I slowly cottoned on to the fact that they weren't on a diet because it was expensive and too complicated.

Some patients had high blood pressure, so I decided to do research on the subject. Before I started trying to treat them, I considered the placebo effect, which I had heard of vaguely. Medicines in those days were always 'one tablespoon three times a day'. So I put in a trace of quinine which made it nice and bitter, put them all on it and as the weeks went by, their blood pressure came down.

BB   What about the war?

MH   I joined the RAF when the war broke out and as I had worked in general medicine, I became a station medical officer in an engineering unit. Our job was to pick up crashed aircraft, repair what was reparable, and cannibalise what wasn't. But because it was a back unit, we had a lot of people who had been downgraded from the fighting units on psychiatric grounds. I had an opportunity of meeting them, not only as patients but also as officers and colleagues, and it was very obvious that there was real suffering. There was no question that one could dismiss it, as was traditional in medicine, as just 'neurotic'.

BB   Was this your first encounter with mental illness?

MH   I had been presented with the usual array of 'freaks' as a student, and I had been at Bernard Hart's clinic, the first English psychiatric out-patient unit at a teaching hospital, but it all rather passed over me. By 1943, I saw the war was going to end; I had to make up my mind what to do. I could continue in general medicine, but with great difficulty because I had been out of touch with hospital medicine. General practice in a military unit is a cinch – at one time, it was less than half an hour's work a day. There wasn't enough experience there to cope with Membership. To go into psychiatry, I would have to take the DPM. That was in two parts, so I thought here's something practical I can do, and that is what started the whole thing.

The first part of the DPM was neuroanatomy, neurophysiology, and psychology – just reading. I decided to work for it and joined a postal course. When I started to read books on psychology, Woodworth's *Introduction to Psychology* was the one I got hold of. It was a revelation, one of the great experiences of my life. For the first time, I met serious discussion of fundamental problems. What is science? What's the difference between scientific theory and non-scientific theory? What is an experiment? How do you draw conclusions from an experiment? How do you experiment on the mind?

What is the difference between scientific theory and non-scientific theory? My favourite example is: the moon is made of green cheese and that all the troubles of the world are due to the machinations of the Communists. The first statement is a scientific theory because you can test it – either it is made of green cheese or it is not, but the other one is not, because you can interpret everything that way.

For the first time, I met somebody dealing with important things in a sophisticated way. That decided me. I was definitely going to do psychiatry. Time came to take the DPM. I sat down seriously to decide what sort of things I was likely to be asked. For the first time, I grasped that there are important things which examiners ask and there are unimportant ones they don't. The result was that of the nine odd questions I had to answer, I had got seven at my fingertips. I never had had such an easy examination in life. I had my *viva* on D-Day! I put on my best RAF uniform, nice two stripes of a flight lieutenant to impress the examiners. I came to the exam and there was Desmond Curran of St George's, in naval uniform with gold rings all the way up to his shoulders. 'Now', they said, 'what are the characteristics of reflex action?' I was staggered. This was a question I had answered, and as I had memorised them and written them all down, it was the perfect answer. I asked, 'All of them?' 'Yes, of course.' So I took a deep breath and started. I was stopped after the first four. I had never had such an amusing exam in my life.

After that, I was stuck. You couldn't get the DPM without experience and I was in general medical work. There was not much point in reading psychiatry without seeing patients, but I could read more psychology. I am the only person who has read through Pavlov's book three times. And Lashley. Have you ever heard of Lashley? He is the man who dug bits out of rats' brains. By this time, I was beginning to get some understanding of what I wanted to do. I would have to learn statistics and psychometrics. I left the RAF at the end of 1945 and joined the Maudsley. I had an interview with Aubrey Lewis and talked him into taking me on.

BB *Did you interview Aubrey Lewis?*

MH   If you like. I wrote and sought an interview. I explained that I had become interested because of my experience and reading and I wanted a proper training. He immediately fired, 'Ah yes, have you read so and so?' Well, I was able to say yes. This was a characteristic of Aubrey, he always had to be one up on you. 'Have you read Lashley?' 'Oh yes Sir, I have read K. S. Lashley.'

Once at the Maudsley, I worked under Eric Guttman. He was brilliant clinically, worldly-wise and sophisticated. When you think he was an immigrant, the subtlety of his knowledge of the English social scene was extraordinary. He could tell you the difference between the social flavour of West Kensington and South Kensington. I went to the Department of Psychology, then run by Hans Eysenck. He had psychologists there working for their PhDs and he organised a course in factor analysis. This was just what I wanted. At first it was difficult, but when it got on to factor analysis I suddenly thought, 'This is what I did at school – co-ordinate geometry'. After that, I sat back and enjoyed it.

Soon, Aubrey Lewis took a dislike to me. When he looked at me with those rather prominent eyes of his, I trembled. Instead of doing an ordinary ward-round, he went through every one of my patients in detail. He was gunning for me. Why he did it, I don't know. I got three months' notice.

BB *That must have been a disappointment.*

MH   A great shock. But I rushed around saying 'I am going to do something' and finally I got hold of Dr Moody, head of the Department of Psychological Medicine at University College Hospital, and told him that I would like to work at UCH because of the opportunity to learn psychology. At first, they didn't know what to do with me. After a while, I managed to establish a job in liaison psychiatry – having been called once to Casualty and once to the Obstetric Department, word got around that somebody was available.

I did a good deal of psychotherapy under supervision, but there was plenty of time to spare and all of it was in the Psychology Department.

BB   Who was the Professor?

MH   Sir Cyril Burt. I saw a fair amount of him. He was always kind, very friendly, and had endless patience – if you went in with a problem or difficulty, he would sit down and discuss it with you. He had a 'thing' about doctors and was delighted I was coming to his department. Remember he was a clinical psychologist. When he was first given a part-time job as psychologist to the London County Council, mental subnormality was diagnosed by the school medical officers by putting a tape around the children's heads. His inquiry on the young delinquent is a classical work. His lectures were superb; my lecture notes are 39 years old now, but are still good. He was a statistical psychologist of the highest order; we didn't know he was doing a little faking. What staggers me is that he faked it so badly.

I also met his postgraduates – 70, from all over the world; most have become eminent professors in psychology. They had been in five or six years of war, and were mature and well selected. So for the first time, I was mixing with a group of highly intelligent people, all doing research and wanting to learn about research – Egyptians, Indians, New Zealanders, Australians, Canadians, Americans. That was a halcyon period for me. I was doing my work during the day, popping over to the Department and meeting these people and listening to their ideas. I don't suppose I went to bed before 2.00 for three or four years. Within a couple of years, I was probably the only psychiatrist in the country who knew psychometrics, rating scales, and theories of measurement.

When I decided to do an MD, I thought I would study a psychosomatic problem – gastric and duodenal ulcer – and use my knowledge of psychometrics. I had also got a letter out of the blue asking me if I would like to write a short book on psychosomatics, offering me £20 down. £20 was a lot of money then, especially for a poor registrar, and I agreed. That hung over me for years, and a number of times I would have given it up, if only I had had £20 to give back. Anyway, I did write it and it was a classic in its way – a small book, *Psychosomatics*, but compared to other books in the field, it was different in approach.

BB   Did you have an objective in view at this point – that you wanted to be something?

MH   No. Although I was in my 30s, I was naive. Nobody ever suggested to me, for instance, that I should join the Royal Medico-Psychological Association, though I had joined the British Psychological Society. I was engrossed and fascinated by new sciences – psychology, neurophysiology, mathematics, statistics, psychometrics – worlds of ideas were opening up to me. Cyril Burt was the first teacher I had had who took notice of me. He set high standards, and I would sweat blood to meet them.

My chiefs in the Department of Psychological Medicine at UCH obviously thought me mildly crazy. What's he doing with all these figures? How do you experiment in psychiatry? I tried to explain to them; they listened very patiently, but whether or not they understood, I don't know. It was exciting and fascinating and this was what I was going to do one day. Science, scientific method – that is the thing to do in psychiatry.

BB *Apply the scientific method to mental illness. Do you think the Maudsley had any influence on you in this way?*

MH　Eric Guttmann had the German phenomenological approach and his ability to describe a patient, the personality, symptoms, and behaviour, fascinated me, and I have always tried to follow that. Aubrey Lewis was stimulating in many ways. He was critical and would think about ideas – not just repeating what was in textbooks. I had never had that before in medical teaching. His lectures on classification convinced me, for example, that the distinction between psychotic and neurotic is absurd. In the same way, organic and functional has little meaning now. One sees this vividly in discussions on neurotic versus psychotic depression. In other ways, it was surprising how little the Maudsley touched me.

BB *Getting back to UCH . . .*

MH　By 1950, I had been a registrar at UCH for four years and they had made several attempts to eject me. Finally, they said: 'Out, no more'. Of course, I could have got a job as senior registrar, but not at UCH; so I went to Cane Hill.

BB *That must have been a contrast.*

MH　It was fascinating. I was put in charge of chronic wards and I started to go through them systematically. I was meeting clinical material found in textbooks which I hadn't seen before. I enjoyed it immensely. Alexander Walk was the superintendent. He was nice – a wise bird. Very old-fashioned, insisted on the office meeting every morning, which everybody grumbled at, but I didn't because I had seen what it was like in the RAF. In my first Unit, the CO had insisted there was a dinner for all the officers once a month, but at the other units they didn't. I noticed the difference. In the first place, I had got to know everybody. If everybody meets in the morning for coffee and talk – you get to know your colleagues.

I left to become senior registrar at King's; back to Denmark Hill, but on the other side of the road. That was 1950–1. I worked there under Denis Hill, the departmental head. It was amusing because I was two years his senior. It was a clinical job; a department based on out-patient psychotherapy and a consultation service, but we did have ECT.

I did one piece of research which I never published. In fact, I did two. My medical colleagues said we took so much time with patients. I thought I would check on this. I took all new patients for three months, and a year afterwards, and found out how much time had been spent with them. Of the hundred patients, only three or four were still having psychotherapy: an average of three hours had been spent on a patient. That compares favourably with what other patients in other specialities get. People always think that medical and surgical patients don't require much time, but when you work it out, it is not like that at all. Take the shortest case you can possibly think of – acute appendicitis. The patient will be seen by the casualty officer and by the surgical registrar: about three-quarters of an hour altogether. He goes into the wards, is interviewed by the anaesthetist and then has the operation which takes 20 minutes, but there are three people there, so that is an hour. There is already an hour beforehand, so that's two hours. He will be seen at least once or twice by the houseman, and the registrar, and the consultant will perhaps have a word with him before his discharge; that is nearly three hours and that's the shortest surgical case one can think of. The patient with duodenal ulcer will be seen in out-patients, if he is going to have surgery, by the registrar, he will come in, there will be a case conference on him, radiology, barium meal, that's a radiologist's time, operation, follow-up, perhaps transfusions – the amount of time they pile up is quite high. They don't realise it because several people are doing it and not anyone does much. It is a delusion that psychiatric patients take a long time.

BB   Did you publish that?

MH   No.

BB   Wasn't that part of the ethos then, to publish?

MH   I published my MD thesis.[1] That was a piece of research, but it never struck me these other things should be published. It was just a 'cases I have cured' paper. Most papers were of that type in those days. Look at the *Journal of Mental Science* for 1950.

After King's, I got a job as senior hospital medical officer at Springfield. I picked on that because my home was near the hospital. I didn't appreciate that an SHMO post was regarded as a dead-end job. To me, it was a rise in income and it was working in a hospital.

Dr Beccles was the superintendent. It was said of him that he knew the first and surname of every patient in the hospital and their relatives – could speak to every one personally. He checked on everything I did. I was in charge of an acute admission ward with ten new cases a week, and I had four chronic wards with 70 patients each. I am proud of that job. I think I am the only professor who has been a SHMO, who knew the routine grind of the mental hospital. It has stood me in good stead.

BB   What was it like working in a mental hospital in 1950?

MH   You had ECT, unmodified at first. There were sedatives, barbiturates, and, at a pinch, morphine if a patient was very disturbed, but experienced nurses could talk them down. The conditions were appalling. Patients were locked in. They looked like chronic patients in their old, dilapidated clothes; they sat and did little. But I never knew that they were bullied or ill-treated.

Each morning, I worked in the acute ward, and every afternoon in the chronic wards. The nurses presented me with prescription cards to sign, as they had at Cane Hill. I wouldn't do it. I insisted on seeing the patients, wondering what these prescriptions were for. It was very hard work at first. I had to do one ward at a time. (At Cane Hill, I had found a patient who had been on weekly liver extract in enormous doses (this is in the days before Vitamin B12) for five years. The prescription derived from a single blood test, which had shown a hyperchromic count). I did that with all the wards, cutting down on sedatives and hypnotics.

---

1. The personality of dyspeptics with special reference to gastric and duodenal ulcer. *British Journal of Medical Psychology*, **23**, 182–198.

In the acute ward, I devised a little board. Every patient had a tag which was hung on a hook and arranged so that the patient who had been in the ward the longest was on the top left and the newest patient was added in at the bottom right. Every morning, I said to the ward sister: 'What are these patients at the top doing here? What are we going to do about it?' And we would go through them systematically.

As for the chronic patients, Beccles insisted they were to be examined twice a year instead of the statutory once, and so I brought along a sphygmomamometer and ophthalmoscope, which apparently had not been seen there before. Looking at fundi of a chronic schizophrenic is not so much a science as a sport. You have to wait to get a glimpse of it as it flicks past. I found fascinating neurological conditions. I remember vividly one Parkinsonian patient who had had a hemiplegia and it had gone on the hemiplegic side. You read about that in books, but I saw it. I had cards, one for each patient, to enable me to remember who they were, such as, 'This is the one who calls me bastard every time I walk into the ward'.

I remember Denis Hill coming up to me once and saying: 'How much work do you do, Max? How many patients have you got to look after?' I took out my pack of cards and counted them. Here are the patients I see once a week, these once a fortnight, these once a month and so on. He went away with a dazed look in his eyes!

I was later given a senile ward. I went through those patients to see how many were depressed and thought, 'Now's my chance, I'm going to give them ECT.' Muscle relaxants had just arrived. The nurses said 'Poor old things, haven't they got the right to be left alone and pass away in peace?' But we found a few who improved. Several were transferred to ordinary wards and we even discharged one patient. I never thought of writing that up.

BB *You would have anticipated Martin Roth.*

MH I think he was doing it at the same time. As soon as the relaxants arrived, it was obvious you could give ECT to patients to whom previously you couldn't. But he had the wit to realise that that was publishable. One thing they said, though, was that you could now give ECT to patients with hypertension because you wouldn't have the physical effort increasing the high blood pressure. So I measured the patient's blood pressure before and after the ECT to see whether it did rise.

I discovered the 'Hamilton manoeuvre', the trick of closing off the circulation to the other arm before injecting the muscle relaxant; then you could see if the patient had a convulsion by observing that arm. I published that.

I looked at another problem. We had a part-timer who did the insulin therapy. I passed on schizophrenics to him. Some he accepted and some he refused. I had to treat them as best I could – some with ECT – and I realised I could look at this. I had two series of patients. I couldn't tell why he rejected some. I looked through all my data and carefully collated it, and I got the Regional research prize. Whether they had insulin or ECT made no difference. He turned down the older patients. But I correlated age with symptoms and history, and it didn't make any difference.

MH No, because it wasn't a properly randomised trial. From Springfield I went to a Senior Lectureship at Leeds, in 1953, under Professor McCalman. The foundation professor had been Henry Dicks, but he had left after 18 months, in about 1948. I think the official reason was that his wife didn't like being in Leeds and wanted to get back to London, but there is no question that he had an awful lot of difficulties. Leeds had a surgical tradition; Moynihan was the great god. Not even a medical tradition! Psychiatry would never have got in unless the Nuffield Foundation had offered the money.

When I got there, McCalman had been trying to do a drug trial. I left Springfield just before May & Baker asked us: 'Would you do a trial of chlorpromazine for us?' I could never decide whether that was good luck or bad. Chlorpromazine was first tried out in Springfield, but there was no control, no assessment, no analysis. If I had remained there, it would have been done. At Leeds, McCalman was comparing chlorpromazine, reserpine, and placebo, and he had tried to produce assessment forms. It was coming to its end, unfortunately, when he asked me to give a hand. I looked at the data sheets and things went dark.

In 1953, when chlorpromazine was introduced, there were probably only two psychiatrists capable of doing a controlled trial – Linford Rees and myself, and there was one capable of devising a rating scale – myself. Perhaps Linford Rees could have done, but I had certainly gone through the grind.

McCalman was ill with severe rheumatoid arthritis and high blood pressure, and eventually had to go part-time. Professor Hargreaves arrived on the scene with a dowry: two big boxes, one containing a new anxiolytic, the other placebo. Miltown (meprobamate) had just been discovered. He said: 'Max, organise a clinical trial.' First, I looked through rating scales of symptoms: none were any good for my purpose. So I devised an anxiety scale.

There were two other nice things in that trial. One was finding how important suggestibility is and how patients respond to comfort and reassurance. I ensured that the patients were suffering from an anxiety neurosis. They had the pills and were seen every week. But for the first fortnight they were all on placebo, which we knew, but they didn't. One patient said: 'I can't stand the strain of this terrible drug', and had to go out. After two weeks, half were randomly changed to the active drug. We followed them up for three weeks. I had my rating scale. I also used an analogue scale and found it gave me exactly the same answers as the other rating scale, so I didn't bother with it again. If I had had any sense I would have done. But an analogue scale was old hat; they were invented before World War I.

I had to analyse two treatments, in a two-way factorial design with unequal numbers in the cells. I think it was the first time in psychiatry. The assessment was from week 2 to week 5. The patients who were on placebo for five weeks continued to improve. I suggested in the paper that patients with anxiety ought to be four weeks on placebo before anxiolytics. Somebody rediscovered that a few years ago.

The trial was over. We still had the patients, we still had to see and treat them. Then something profoundly interesting happened. Two or three of these patients, carefully selected and diagnosed as anxiety states, became severely depressed and had to be given ECT, and responded very well. That set me thinking. About this time, I got fed up with a heavy clinical load. I had gone to an academic department to do research. I had got a taste of it and wanted to do more, but Hargreaves said I couldn't be relieved of any duties. I managed to get a part-time grant and he collected further money so I could do a full-time research job for a couple of years. But the University said, according to him, they could not let me off because they would not be able to get a temporary replacement. I was faced with a dilemma and resigned to take the research job.

BB　*How old were you?*

MH　45.

BB　*An adventurous thing to do?*

MH　I suppose so, but I always felt that if the worst came to the worst, I could get an NHS consultant job. I got Jack White at Stanley Royd Hospital to co-operate with me. I devised a rating scale for depression, played around with it, tested it out, and then started work. The depression rating scale came after the anxiety scale, and is much better.

Both scales have deficiencies, but they were carefully designed, and sophisticated, even though I say it myself. You see, a scale must not be too long. The Wittenborn scales have 150–250 items: that is ridiculous, useless. But it mustn't be too short or it loses reliability. The ideal number of items is somewhere between 10 and 20. With all-purpose scales, most items are inapplicable. They waste time and are a source of error because of the temptation to put something in if in doubt.

I devised these scales specifically – one for anxiety, one for depression – and I didn't deal with any other symptoms. I devised them so they would be easy to use, and they were about clinical matters which clinicians were interested in, and that is why they endure. If you have a clinical interview with a patient, you can fill it in. It doesn't take any time; it's not complicated. Americans say there are too many somatic symptoms and not enough psychological ones. My answer to that is 'That's what my patients are complaining about – that's what they are suffering from, that is what is a burden on them, and that is what I am measuring – the burden of illness.'

BB　*Do you know how many times it has been cited?*

MH　About 700 in 20 years, according to Science Citation Index, an incredible figure. It has now reached the point where people refer to the Hamilton scale without giving the reference. Now there's glory for you.

BB　*What do you think of the PSE?*

MH　It's magnificent as a research instrument, but it's not practical. It can be used only by a research unit. It is superb if you want to do something on schizophrenia, but the PSE cannot be used by practising clinicians and that's its disadvantage.

BB　*Do you think it would be possible to have a scale for schizophrenia of the kind that you devised for depression?*

MH　While I had this research job, I compared chlorpromazine with placebo. I also crossed it with extra occupational work and social rehabilitation against none of these. I was looking for the interaction between psychological and drug factors – the first time anyone had done this in a planned trial. I started with the hypothesis that the drug facilitated the patient's response to social influences. It doesn't. I found that patients improved with the drug, and they improved if you gave them extra social therapy. But both together didn't have any additional effect. If anything, the drug seemed to inhibit the effect of social influences.

For that trial, I picked out a set of items which were applicable for chronic schizophrenics from the Lorr scale. There were about 20. I have used that scale on two or three occasions since then; it's effective enough for chronic schizophrenia. It is a set of items on hallucinations, delusions, autism, things like that and a bit about mood. It is not good, but it does the job.

BB   *What followed the two years of research?*

MH   When it was coming to an end, Hargreaves got me a job for a year in the NIMH Clinical Neuropsychopharmacology Research Centre in Washington. It had begun to get around America that there were new drugs coming from Europe. The people who gave funds to the NIMH wanted to set up a clinical research unit. They looked around for somebody to head it and got Elkes from England. He was in difficulty when he wanted someone to do clinical research because he couldn't find any clinicians in the USA – and that's how I got the job. I was in charge of a unit at St Elizabeth's Hospital.

BB   *What did you do there?*

MH   That's a tale in itself. I found half a dozen people who were officially doing clinical research. A medical man conscripted into the army (there was still conscription then) can go into public service as an alternative. For psychiatrists, this meant St Elizabeth's. Most were busy getting psychoanalysed and preparing for private practice, so their research projects . . . you can imagine what they were like.

Elkes said: 'Find out what everybody's doing, take your time, and then organise things.' They were all busy on the most dreadful things. There was I, responsible, but he hadn't given me authority. He hadn't told anybody that when Max says jump, you jump! I was in the situation where nobody was going to take any notice of this damned Englishman, and he wasn't even an analyst; he was an 'administrator'. They divided psychiatrists into therapists and administrators. It soon became fairly obvious that nothing was going to come of it.

At this point, I said: 'Look, if you just change it round and do it this way we can get a job done'; I elaborated my previous trial of drugs against placebo on the one hand and rehabilitation and non-rehabilitation on the other.

BB   *Did you get much done?*

MH   I got that trial done, essentially. I was also interviewing people about my depression scale and trying to see if I could get some work going on depression. I went around with my scale and it created a tremendous wave of apathy. They all thought I was a bit mad. Eventually, I got it published in the *Journal of Neurology, Neurosurgery & Psychiatry*. It was the only one that would take it. Now, everyone tells me the scale is wonderful, but I always remember when it had a different reception. This makes sure I don't get a swollen head.

I should mention that fundamentally, my interest is as a clinician. Long ago, I came to the conclusion that ultimately, the discoveries in psychiatry were going to be made by biochemists. Before World War II, it was the biochemistry of urine; after the War, it has been the biochemistry of blood and CSF. But until we get down to the biochemistry of neurones, we are not going to get anywhere. That is what we *are* doing now.

I was faced with the fact that if I wanted to do research, biochemistry was the thing. But I wasn't a biochemist. Yet without the clinician, the biochemist is blind. Unless they can link their work up to clinical phenomena, it doesn't mean a thing. So the clinician is still critical. He is the man who leads the biochemist through the jungle. Systematic and subtle clinical studies must underlie all biochemical research. That is one reason why such wonderful biochemical research in America is nullified by inadequate clinical work.

BB *On your return, you had a job at Leeds as MRC External Scientific Staff?*

MH   Yes, officially attached to the Department of Psychiatry, but for clinical work to Stanley Royd Hospital, Wakefield. I had worked with one of the previous consultants, but things had changed and it wasn't possible to return to the previous collaboration. I was stuck with the problem of getting clinical work. The local out-patients and domiciliaries were all buttoned up, so I came back to Leeds to start an out-patient session. I worked away, but it was very unsatisfactory. I was the new consultant who comes in and everybody has to make room. If they are unwilling, he doesn't get patients and has a bad time. I managed to get some work done, but it was slow and difficult.

After I had collected data on 50-odd patients, I went to the computing laboratory and asked could it be analysed. They said, 'Yes, of course'. 'How do I get it done?' 'If you just study this book on how to write programmes, we will teach you how to punch them onto tape and how to use the computer.'

It is amazing what you can do when you have to. I had to learn to write and test programmes and do my own computing. And that was a profoundly significant experience for me. I had always tried to think clearly because, being an obsessional, uncertainty was difficult. But here, for the first time I came up against a situation where clarity and precision of thinking are absolutely necessary.

I had learned in 1943 that an experiment is not done by going around with a vague question mark, looking at the world. You have to have a definite hypothesis and an experiment that will get an answer. But when writing programmes, I had a new order of clarity and precision. For the first time, I looked critically at the way people were arguing, and realised how vague were people's ideas, how discussions are often beside the point. I was surprised. Now, when I listen to arguments about politics or religion, they seem a waste of time.

In psychiatry, there are no clearly defined entities. We can't talk about schizophrenia, or depression, or anxiety states as if you can define them clearly. This is the trouble of attempting to apply mathematical logic to the real world. That does not mean that you can't have clear thinking. Even if there is vagueness, your thinking can still be clear. It is like Fisher's remark about experimental results – you can never prove anything absolutely; there is always uncertainty, but you can specify the uncertainty.

BB *How many years did you work for the MRC?*

MH   From 1960 to 1963 – three years.

BB *What did you achieve?*

MH   Damned little. I didn't have enough patients, and I hadn't got very far, and I didn't publish much in that time. However, I had laid the foundations for the work, so when the Chair came up, I applied. I didn't think I would get it because Leeds Infirmary was notoriously anti-Semitic. I remember McCalman said he had heard one consultant boast he had never had a Jew higher than a houseman. But it was in the hands of the University as well as the Infirmary. Compared with the other two candidates, I had a better research record. The other two candidates, incidentally, were Frank Fish who got Liverpool and John Hinton, who went to the Middlesex. I got the job and thought that now I had a department with beds, research should be much easier; in some ways it was and in some it wasn't. Now I was involved in organising an undergraduate department with minimal staff and no funds, without a research tradition and with all sorts of restrictions. But I managed something.

In 1963, Leeds was second-bottom in the percentage of medical students who took up psychiatry. When I left, it was third from the top. And I think this was the result of my policy. Very few medical students are going to become psychiatrists; therefore it is no good teaching them psychiatrists' psychiatry. You have to teach the psychiatry of the general practitioner and the general physician and surgeon.

We taught them about the common disorders. By the time they finished, they were running out of their ears with depressions and anxiety states – the way psychiatry impinges on you in practical life. I always gave the introductory lecture and pointed out that as medical undergraduates, most of their time was spent learning how to make a diagnosis. But one of the facts to be faced was that whether they were in general practice or hospital medicine, diagnosis became a trivial problem because most of their patients had been diagnosed anything from two weeks to twenty years before, and of those who had not been diagnosed, the majority were straightforward.

All the fuss is on a tiny percentage of cases, and between you, me and the postman, it generally doesn't make much difference either. Most doctors in the past have had to spend much of their time with patients for whom they could do little. (Big smile from the students.) What is more, they still do. (Smile is a little less.) What is more important, they always will. (And that wiped the smile off their faces.) Once medicine solves the problem, it doesn't occupy our time. So what is your time occupied with? The patients for whom you can do little or nothing. And that is what your job is and that is what you are going to spend your life doing. It shakes them. And we are going to teach you about the problems of patient management. That is what we taught.

We also took them for a short period into mental hospitals, where they had more contact with patients than at any other time in their medical career. And I said to them, 'You are going there, not because I want you to learn psychiatrists' psychiatry, but because everybody should know what goes on in a mental hospital. You are going to be asked about this by patients and their relatives. I don't do surgery, but it is important that I should know what goes on in an operating theatre. That became the most popular part of the course, and I think the reason why we went up from the bottom to near the top.

BB *What about postgraduate responsibilities?*

MH   Henry Dicks had started a DPM, which ran every two years – a two-year course. This was obviously useless. We had to run a course every year, which meant doubling the work. In a provincial medical school and in provincial hospitals up north, you have to attract trainees or they will not come. Having been a mental hospital doctor, I still felt part of that community; my attitude was that the Department of Psychiatry will always be regarded as an ivory tower, so it is important to have strong links with the mental hospitals because that is where the patients are! I saw my position as a focal point for the psychiatry of the Region. Our job was to provide training which would attract staff to the hospitals. They had the patients, and I therefore wanted all my staff to have honorary attachments, so they would have access to patients by right. In exchange, I offered consultants an opportunity to work in the University department and to teach students.

We started an MSc course, which included research methodology, for psychiatric social workers; even when everybody said the PSW is out, old-fashioned, we kept the course going. I also said to the Department of Psychology: 'Let's offer jointly an MSc in clinical psychology.' Eventually, we were the biggest postgraduate department in the medical school, with students in clinical psychology, psychiatric social work, and postgraduate psychiatry – roughly 20 in each.

BB *And what about research in this busy life?*

MH   That was done in the interstices. I encouraged other people to do things and a small amount of work came out of the department every so often.

BB *What was the theme?*

MH   There wasn't one in that sense. If you haven't full-time people and equipment, you have to use ingenuity. My example of a simple ingenious idea which yields dividends is the one that Clive Tonks had. The majority of the parasuicides were young women. He asked them the time during the menstrual period they had made their attempt. Those who did not have pre-menstrual tension had a preponderance of attempted suicide a week before the menstrual period – the opposite of what you would have expected. A research fellow (Stephen Tyrer) compared the psychological aspects of women who have hysterectomy for cancer with those who have it for functional disorders. He produced a questionnaire under my guidance and collected the information and got a nice paper out of it.

BB *You have always been interested in psychology and were made President of the British Psychological Society.*

MH   I had a greater reputation in psychology than in psychiatry, until recently. I joined the BPS during the war. I kept up my contacts and almost all the work I have done has required methodology developed by psychologists. I argued that psychologists have something to contribute to psychiatry. That is why, for example, one of our registrars was one of the first psychiatrists to try out behaviour therapy.

Psychology is a basic science for psychiatry. Psychologists have a sophistication in research and in theorising which is lacking in our subject. When I started to read clinical psychiatry, the stuff in the textbooks had an extraordinarily old-fashioned air about it. We have disorders of affect and the schizophrenias, which are primarily disorders of thinking. What about disorders of will? They are the psychopaths. Here are the three faculties – all the way from Aristotle. But even within one illness, what do we say about the symptoms of depression or mania? There are disturbances of affect, of thought, and of behaviour. Here are the old Aristotelian faculties still present and we still think in these terms. The psychology of psychiatry is antediluvian – very odd. The psychologists have been looking at faculty theory for a long time, very carefully, and we ought to take account of them.

BB   Why haven't they made more impact?

MH   Let me give you an analogy. I once picked up an early issue of the *Lancet*, and noted an editorial introducing a new series of articles: doctors ought to know something about chemistry, so they were going to provide a series of articles. And do you know what the first one was? How to make oxygen from potassium chlorate! Now I think you will agree that the physician practising at that time would have looked at it and thought 'what a lot of nonsense'. It has taken time, but now you can't study medicine without chemistry. A similar problem occurred when Harvey discovered the circulation of the blood. Since all the practitioners were worrying about the balance of the humours, would it matter whether the heart pumped or not? It was irrelevant. They didn't see the connection.

We have to recognise that psychologists tended to start on simple things like reaction times. Obviously of little relevance. By and large, it never had much impact. And when psychologists made contact with clinical work, psychiatrists thought of them the way they thought of clinical pathologists. Let's order a blood test or an intelligence test.

BB   Psychiatrists have adopted behaviour therapy techniques from psychologists because they are effective.

MH   But who developed them? Psychologists. And this was on the basis of learning theory and animal behaviour. The contribution, therefore, is in an outlook – the application of scientific method. The work, for example, that Robert Kendell has been doing on the classification of schizophrenia, is based on the psychometric approach. Who developed it? The psychologists. It is in the fields of methodology, theory, and sophisticated scientific outlook that the psychologists have important contributions to make.

BB   You have written six books?

MH   I have written two on my own – one on psychosomatics, the other on the methodology of clinical research.[2] It has always been regarded rather snootily by the College, since it came into competition with Peter Sainsbury's volume.

---

2. *Lectures on the Methodology of Clinical Research* (1974). Edinburgh: Churchill Livingstone.

BB　*What about the other four?*

MH　I edited *Readings in Abnormal Psychology*, where I dug out a series of papers which I thought formed an important background to our thinking. The most important thing now is to keep three out of four of Frank Fish's books going – *Clinical Psychopathology*, *Schizophrenia* and *An Outline of Psychiatry*. I got into that accidentally. We recommended them for our postgraduates, but they complained that they weren't available, so I wrote to the publishers, who asked me to prepare new editions. Since I knew Fish well, I was pleased to do so.

BB　*What do you think about the state of current psychiatric research?*

MH　It's active, alive and go ahead. The *British Journal of Psychiatry* and *Psychological Medicine* are so full of meat I can't glance through them and think, 'Well there's a couple of articles worth looking at'; there are so many that are so good. It is impressive. And the trends are interesting – there is so much work on classification of disorders, discriminant function, psychometric applications. What we are doing is worthwhile. Then the work in social psychiatry, on parasuicides by Kreitman, for example – characteristically British. We are doing biochemical research as well. We can't hope to compete with the Americans. Psychiatry in this country follows the British tradition; it has a good, sound clinical basis and it isn't rigid or limited. It is not middle of the road, but on a broad front, covering all fields. I believe the fundamental discoveries are going to come in biochemistry.

But it is a long way from the problem of management of patients; patients are human beings with human feelings, who live in a social environment with personal relationships, and all these have to be dealt with and taken into account. I will give you an example. I found I became successful clinically because early on, I cottoned on to the fact that it is not enough to see the patient; the relatives need treatment, comfort, reassurance, support, help, and I spend almost as much time with relatives as with my patient. It makes a lot of difference. The result is that my patients take their drugs and come for follow-up. If they don't turn up, I send a postcard: 'Sorry you couldn't turn up – I am going to be there tomorrow' – and I go round to the home the next day. I used to be afraid that I would have the door slammed in my face. Nothing of the sort – I was invited in and offered tea and cake. My capacity for follow-up depends on my capacity for tea and cake!

3 Sir William Trethowan

Interviewed by BRIAN BARRACLOUGH

Professor Sir William Trethowan, CBE, MA MB BChir (Cantab) 1943, FRCP 1963, FRACP 1961, FANZCP (Hon) 1965, FRCPsych 1971, FRCPsych (Hon) 1983. Sir William Trethowan was born in 1917. He was a student at Clare College, Cambridge and Guy's Hospital, London. In 1944 he joined the Royal Army Medical Corps, starting as a general duty medical officer and ending as a medical specialist. He was Professor of Psychiatry, University of Sydney, Australia from 1956–62; Dean of the Faculty of Medicine and Dentistry, University of Birmingham from 1962–74 and he was Professor of Psychiatry there from 1962–82. In 1975 he was asked to become Chairman of the Medical Academic Advisory Committee to set up a new medical school at Hong Kong University. He was knighted in 1980.

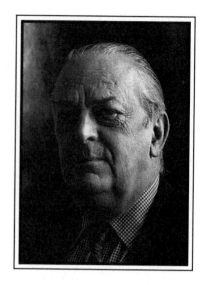

BB You had a medical family background.

WT My father was an orthopaedic surgeon at Guy's; my great grandfather on my mother's side was also a surgeon there; my younger brother became an ENT surgeon, and there were others. My mother actually qualified in medicine on the same day I did. When a child, she went to one of those schools where they taught deportment and dancing, but precious little else. So she first had to matriculate and then went to the Royal Free and did Conjoint.

BB What about your children?

WT My son is lecturer in occupational medicine at Birmingham.

BB Has there been a psychiatric interest in the family or were you the first to take it up?

WT No, I was the first and only.

BB You went to Clare College, Cambridge. Was there a psychological influence there when you were an undergraduate?

WT I don't think so. I was a dilatory student and spent most of my time making music. Blowing my own trumpet, actually!

BB And after Cambridge?

WT I went to Guy's – during the war – and qualified at the end of 1943, did a year's house jobs, and went into the RAMC. I started as a general duty medical officer and ended as a medical specialist having gone through training as a graded physician; I then went to India, where I was made a medical specialist and came out intending to be a physician. I went back to Guy's and did some postgraduate work and then got more and more interested in psychiatry.

BB *Why was that?*

WT All supernumerary registrars in those days were given their share of chronic medical out-patients, and I found myself seeing people with curious conditions about which nobody had taught me. I came to the conclusion that they were suffering from psychiatric disorders, so I bought a couple of books on the subject. One was Yellowlees'[1].

BB *That's the father of the last CMO?*

WT A rather colourful character. He wrote a highly entertaining book. And then I think that Stafford Clark had already brought out the first edition of his *Psychiatry Today*,[2] I read that and got interested in psychiatry, and decided to take it up.

BB *Was Stafford Clark at Guy's then?*

WT This was in the early post-war years and psychiatry hadn't returned to Guy's.

BB *Where had it gone to?*

WT At the beginning of the war Guy's, like other teaching hospitals evacuated, in this case to Kent – Orpington, Farnborough and Pembury. I had a job as house physician at the County Hospital, Farnborough, which included working with Felix Brown who was responsible for psychiatry then, and who undoubtedly influenced me.

When I decided to take up psychiatry, I rang him up. He said that I must go to the Maudsley. I told him I had been offered a job by Dr Leslie Cook at Bexley. I was going to take that, but both Felix and 'Bird' Partridge, whom I also consulted, said, 'No, you must go to the Maudsley'. An appointment was arranged for me by Felix, because 'Bird' was apparently *persona non grata* at the Maudsley at the time.

I went to see Aubrey Lewis. On the strength of having had experience as a physician and having the MRCP (on which Aubrey was very keen at the time), he took me on as a registrar. That was in 1948. I did about two years at the Maudsley and then went to the Massachusetts General for six months.

BB *What are your recollections of the Maudsley?*

WT It was very stimulating. There were some very considerable people working there – Clifford Scott, who later went to America, Emmanuel Miller, the father of Jonathan Miller, Eliot Slater, Aubrey Lewis, some of the greats of psychiatry of that period. However, the influence was very strongly Meyerian, which I never took to; I regarded it as a milk and water synthesis between psychoanalysis and phenomenology. I don't think it came off.

---

1. YELLOWLEES, H. (1932) *Clinical Lectures on Psychological Medicine*. London: J. and A. Churchill.
2. STAFFORD CLARK, D. (1952) *Psychiatry Today*. London: Penguin.

BB *Where did it come from?*

WT   It came from Lewis and several others who had gone to Baltimore and studied under Meyer at Johns Hopkins. Psychobiology was the order of the day, the great protagonists being Clifford Scott and Lewis himself.

BB *Who did you work for?*

WT   For Edward Anderson first of all, whom I later worked with in Manchester. Then I went to the children's department, where Kenneth Cameron and W. H. Gillespie were, and Wilfred Warren, of course. I was also in charge of the observation ward at St Francis for a short time as a locum. I learned a lot from that.

BB *People are interested in what the Maudsley was like in the period you were there.*

WT   One went there with no clear idea of what was in store. There was a training scheme, which included the possibility of gaining experience in child psychiatry and psychotherapy, but one never knew what was coming next.

D. L. Davies, who was the Dean, and for whom I later grew to have the greatest respect was, at that time, regarded by the registrars with considerable suspicion. He was seen very much as the servant of the master, in that he was Aubrey's 'hit man' and kept us in a state of constant suspense – you never knew where you were going next. Aubrey Lewis used to come round and hold seminars with the registrars. He would suddenly appear. This was anxiety-making because the first thing he did was to take the case-notes and thumb them through, while you found yourself presenting a patient to him quite unprepared. This was because you never knew when you would be called upon. He was highly critical and extremely searching. I remember an occasion when I presented two weeks running; this was because the other registrars in our group said they hadn't got an interesting patient and I had.

When Aubrey Lewis arrived, he was annoyed at finding me presenting once again. He said, 'Why are you presenting this case? You presented last week.' I replied, 'I'm the only one who has an interesting case'. He said to me, 'What sort of case is it?' I said, 'It's a case of depersonalisation.' So he said, 'What's interesting about that?' I said, 'It may not be interesting to you, but I have never seen one before, so it is interesting to me.' That shut him up and I presented the patient. I have seen him reduce house officers and registrars to tears because he could be so critical.

Apart from this, he had one of the finest minds I have ever met. Very impressive. I remember once seeing him interviewing a patient who mentioned an obscure author. Immediately, Aubrey entered into a dissertation on the works this author had written. The patient was an expert, but so, clearly, was Aubrey. It was difficult to find anything that he hadn't read.

BB *What do you think about his influence then?*

WT   It was considerable. We went in awe of him. He was an intellectual giant. With Aubrey, you could never get away with a loose statement. He would pick you up at once and ask what you meant. You had to justify it. If not, you might be severely castigated. He did have a sense of humour, however, and could be a very great friend when needed.

BB *After the war, you went to Boston. How did you come to go there?*

WT This was again due to Aubrey. The Maudsley had an arrangement with Stanley Cobb at the Massachusetts General under which selected registrars were sent out to do a six-month period. My immediate predecessor was Stafford Clark and I was followed by Bruce Sloane, now Professor in Los Angeles. About two weeks before Christmas, I received a summons from Miss Marshall, who was Aubrey's secretary. The Professor wished to see me at 4 o'clock that afternoon.

He said 'I want you to go to America on 1 January'. I was quite unprepared for this event; not that it mattered to Aubrey. I also had a wife and two children to consider. He said, 'I can get you a Fulbright Scholarship' – which he did. I went out there to the Massachusetts General as assistant resident, at the princely salary of $39.00 a month. My financial embarrassment was further compounded by currency control regulations at the time, preventing me from taking money out of the country.

BB *What was the point of the link?*

WT The Massachussetts General was a kind of finishing school. You learned there that they didn't know much more about psychiatry than we did, which was comforting. These were the great days of psychosomatic medicine, with Stanley Cobb, Eric Wittkower, and Franz Alexander. It was believed then that every psychosomatic disorder had a specific personality profile, but forty years have passed and shown that doctrine to be untrue. But it was interesting at the time. So was working at the MGH. They had a 17-bed psychiatric unit. We weren't allowed to use any drugs and no ECT, only psychotherapy, a salutary experience when you have all-comers to treat: alcoholics, depressives, some psychotic as well as neurotic patients. I don't think we were all that successful, mark you!

BB *What do you think Massachusetts General did for you?*

WT Gave me a little bit of polish. It was challenging. You might be asked by very senior and eminent people, quite suddenly on a ward round and without warning, what your opinion was. Not a thing that happened much in England. In America, they were more inquisitive of their juniors although always kind, polite, and interested.

BB *What about research?*

WT I wrote my first paper[3] in America on Cushing's syndrome. I saw five or six cases personally and Fuller Albright, the eminent American endocrinologist, made all his other cases available to me. I was then able to publish a description of the psychiatric aspects of 25 cases. If I am remembered for any research, I hope it will be that paper, because it was the first major description of the psychiatric aspects of Cushing's syndrome.

---

3. TRETHOWAN, W. H. & COBB S. (1952) Neuropsychiatric aspects of Cushing's syndrome. *A.M.A. Archives of Neurology and Psychiatry*, **67**, 283–309.

BB *What did you find?*

WT I found what had been reported in a small way before – that about two out of five cases of Cushing's syndrome were psychotic. The psychoses were affective, schizophrenic, or paranoid, but there were also some who had understandable neurotic reactions to the disfigurement of Cushing's. I have realised since then that psychiatric disorders in endocrine conditions have something to do with the rate of their onset. Where the rate of onset is rapid, there is more likely to be a psychiatric illness. This applies not only to Cushing's syndrome, but to other endocrine conditions such as thyrotoxicosis.

BB *How did you come upon the original observation?*

WT Patients with Cushing's syndrome suffering from severe mental illness were admitted to the psychiatric unit at the Massachusetts General.

BB *This has been an influence for most of your life, I suppose.*

WT My attitude towards psychiatry has always had a strong medical bias. I have tended to favour the medical model, although I have embraced others from time to time.

BB *What happened when you came back?*

WT I went to Manchester, where I was lecturer and then senior lecturer with E. W. Anderson. How I came to be there is interesting. Just before I went to America, I thought it was time I took the DPM, the only postgraduate exam for psychiatrists in those days – the London University DPM – so I took both parts at once and I got through before I went. I did the clinical at Atkinson Morley Hospital. The examiners were Edward Anderson and Bill Nichol (of Horton Hospital).

After presenting my case, a depressed Irish woman, extensively leucotomised and suffering from leucotomised depression, I was leaving the building when the registrar in charge of the exam came after me and said that the examiners wanted to see me again. Anderson then offered me a job in Manchester. I explained that I was going to America and asked if it would be all right if I didn't start until August, when I came back. I took up the job in September 1951, and I was there for five years until I went to Sydney.

BB *Anderson is thought by many to be a neglected figure in British psychiatry.*

WT He was an important figure – he had something which many others hadn't. As he was trained in Germany as a phenomenologist with Jaspers and Kleist, he brought to British psychiatry a solid basis of phenomenology. I sat at his feet at the Maudsley and again in Manchester.

BB *Why do you think phenomenology so important?*

WT Psychiatry lacks objectivity. Most psychiatric work is subjective. Nevertheless, it is vital to use the tool of subjectivity in such a way as to make it as objective as possible. Anderson was a skilled interviewer. He knew how to disentangle what patients said and make their descriptions of their symptoms as objective as possible, so that they could be compared with statements made by other patients. This kind of examination of minutiae has no substitute at present. A patient describes his symptoms and you evaluate them by asking yourself, 'How would I feel if I was this patient describing these symptoms?' Doing so allows you to go some way towards objectifying subjective data.

BB *What use, though, do you think phenomenology has?*

WT It makes diagnosis more accurate. In medicine, and psychiatry, diagnosis comes first, before treatment and prognosis.

BB *You spent five years in Manchester. What did you do?*

WT I virtually ran the department. Teddy Anderson was not a particularly active man; his working day was rather short. He left a great deal of the running of the department to me, and I was the only senior lecturer. We had a lecturer later on and a secretary. I was sought after considerably elsewhere in the hospital to give psychiatric opinions on other cases. In fact, although I hesitate to say this, one of the things my five years with Edward Anderson taught me was how not to run a department. Although not a good administrator, he was extremely kind to me. On the whole, he was somewhat of an absent Professor, partly due to illness.

BB *He has only recently died.*

WT Yes. He died tragically of Alzheimer's disease. I wrote several of his obituaries in which I said he was the founder of the Manchester school of psychiatry. He trained a lot of people, despite the fact that his was a small department, and to my mind, never properly established. Anderson was not a man who pushed himself forward. He wasn't a good lecturer either, and muttered into his notes. His presence was never fully felt and yet much of the material he produced was of great value.

BB *He was the first Professor in Manchester? When was he appointed?*

WT About 1948, from the Maudsley. He never liked Manchester and always longed to return south. When he retired, two years early, he reached for his hat, became a Lord Chancellor's Visitor, and went to live in Sussex.

BB *What kind of undergraduate teaching was there in Manchester then?*

WT Students got 20 lectures from me and a fortnight, half-time, of clinical experience.

BB *How many students were there?*

WT 120 – we had them in fortnightly lumps.

BB *In the general hospital or the mental hospital?*

WT In both. I used to demonstrate psychotic and florid cases at Crumpsall Hospital.

BB *Did you find time for research?*

WT I was interested, after my initial work on Cushing's syndrome, in psychoses due to cortisone and ACTH. I wrote a paper on that. Not much else. I didn't really have time, nor much in the way of material. It was such a small department.

BB *Then you went to Sydney. That must have surprised many people.*

WT   When I left London for Manchester, my friends thought I was mad; when I went from Manchester to Sydney, that confirmed it.

BB *How did you come to go there?*

WT   The job was advertised and I applied. I had applied, unsuccessfully, to go to Guy's. After three years at Manchester, Monro, who was at Guy's, went north, hankering for his native Scotland, and Stafford Clark moved up to the senior position. His job was advertised and I put in for it. I thought I couldn't fail. I had the Guy's tradition and the right sort of background. I was interviewed together with Fleminger. I interviewed appallingly. I didn't get the job, which put my nose considerably out of joint. But I was fortunate, because what happened subsequently would never have been possible if I had gone to Guy's then. The Sydney job came up and I was appointed – without interview. They didn't interview people in Sydney in those days, but they took considerable references. I went out there in April 1956.

BB *Was that the first Chair at Sydney?*

WT   The Chair had previously been held from 1927 to 1951 by W. S. Dawson, who may be remembered to older British psychiatrists as the man who wrote *Aids to Psychiatry*, a popular book among medical students and the book on which Anderson's *Psychiatry*, which I later took over, was founded.

The first Professor of Psychiatry at Sydney University was Sir John Macpherson, who was appointed at the age of 61 and occupied the Chair from 1922–26. Dawson was the second Professor, and when he and the University fell out in 1951, he retired. For five years before I was appointed, the Chair remained empty. During that time, psychiatry in Australia got itself into a pretty appalling state.

About 1953, the Federal Government asked Alan Stoller, a well known Victorian psychiatrist, and a psychologist, Arscott, to survey the psychiatric services in Australia. They produced what came to be known as the *Stoller Report*,[4] in which they said scathing things about Australian psychiatry, and in particular, about psychiatry in New South Wales. They didn't pull their punches.

BB *Was it about the services or academic psychiatry?*

WT   Services – there was no academic psychiatry. Dawson was the only Professor in Australia, except for John Bostock in Brisbane who was Professor of Experimental Psychology, without clinical facilities. When I went out there, I was the only Professor of Psychiatry in the whole of Australia. Things are very different now.

As a result of the *Stoller Report*, the Chairman, the late Mr Wallace Wurth of the New South Wales Public Service Board (an institution which then stood between the Treasury and the Ministries, which controlled the money, and was therefore the most powerful body in State politics) got together with the

---

4. STOLLER A. & ARSCOTT K. W. (1955). *Mental Health Facilities and Needs of Australia.* Canberra.

Vice-Chancellor of the University of Sydney, Stephen Roberts, and re-advertised the Chair, because they felt an academic presence might improve what was then an appalling situation.

BB *Appalling is a strong word.*

WT I can justify it. In Callan Park Hospital, the main mental hospital in the city of Sydney, there were 2000 patients. Every door was locked. The male patients, and the female for that matter, were kept in airing courts, places with large high wire fences, like you see in a zoo. The male patients had no belts or braces because a man can't fight if he has got to hold his trousers up, and no boot-laces. You can't run fast in bare feet or if your boots haven't any laces. The first time I went round the hospital, there were eleven patients in straitjackets (they called them 'camisoles'). I had never seen them used before. There were four doctors: the Medical Superintendent, suffering from a chronic illness and unfit for work most of the time; two Medical Officers, one of whom had never been taught any psychiatry and another who couldn't speak English; and the Deputy Medical Superintendent, Steve Sands, who was really running the hospital, looking after those 2000 patients. The nurses were 'bolshie', threatening to strike at any promised innovation. I felt I was looking at a mental hospital as it might have been in England about the time the County Asylums Act was passed, early in the nineteenth century. There were others no better.

My appointment to Sydney University was a particularly interesting one. Wurth and Roberts advertised the Chair in conjunction with an appointment as Adviser on Mental Health to the New South Wales Government. I was paid another £1000 a year for that.

BB *You mean an adviser about the clinical services provided by the State Government as well as an academic appointment? A powerful position.*

WT I was in an especially powerful position because Wurth and Roberts were sensible enough to ensure that my entire salary was paid through the University. The extra salary for being Adviser on Mental Health was not, therefore, paid directly to me by the State Government. So I was not a civil servant, and not bound by civil service regulations. This was important, because it gave me freedom of speech. I had to use it.

About the same time, an active New South Wales Association of Mental Health was formed, because people had such strong feelings about the appalling conditions under which the mentally ill were kept. It was a mixed body, with social workers, some doctors, and citizens of conscience. I was made its first President. It was a very active pressure group. At one stage, it even threatened to unseat the New South Wales Government on a mental health platform.

Those were exciting days. Virtually single-handed, I re-wrote the Mental Health Act for New South Wales. I cribbed a great deal of it from the 1959 Mental Health Act here and modified it for local conditions.

BB *What did you do there, besides what you have described?*

WT I found 180 students awaiting me. They had just sat their fifth year examination. I was handed all the examination papers, four essay questions each, and one of my first tasks was to mark them, single-handed, as I had no academic staff then to assist me. It took me a fortnight.

The teaching was rather limited. I used to give twenty lectures on psychiatry. We set up a unit at Broughton Hall Hospital, next to Callan Park, a very nice hospital, now closed down, which had some 200 beds; it was the only hospital in New South Wales which took voluntary patients.

I received a great deal of co-operation from the Medical Superintendent, Herbert Prior. We built up a very enthusiastic staff and ran a postgraduate teaching programme. I also used to give demonstrations to 180 undergraduates; I hope I never have to do that again. To demonstrate psychiatric cases to 180 students at one time is difficult, and hard both on the patient and the demonstrator. It wasn't even in a lecture theatre, but in the recreation hall of the hospital. I had a clinical appointment at the Royal Prince Alfred Hospital, one of the large teaching hospitals in Sydney, and also at the Royal North Shore Hospital.

Periodically, I visited the other mental hospitals in a very large parish, which covered all of New South Wales, where I would be invited to pronounce on difficult cases. But the main centre of teaching was the Royal Prince Alfred and Broughton Hall.

BB *How did you get a building up your department?*

WT   The department was always small; the University always impecunious. However, I had an outstanding Senior Lecturer, the late David Maddison, who died recently. He succeeded me and later became Dean, and then Dean at Newcastle, New South Wales, a new University. I also had some part-time lecturers, notably Dr John Ellard for instance, who is now a senior Sydney psychiatrist, and a full-time lecturer in psychiatric social work. That was it.

BB *You couldn't teach very much with that.*

WT   There were, of course, honorary hospital consultants and they had firms of students attached to them and did some teaching.

BB *What about research?*

WT   I produced a steady stream of rather second-rate papers on various subjects, largely clinical. Nothing that I could care to be remembered by.

BB *What would you care to be remembered by in Australia?*

WT   I hope I am remembered as an undergraduate teacher and I am certainly remembered in Australia as an entrepreneur. I did manage to get a good deal done in six years with, of course, the aid of a lot of other people.

BB *I am not clear what you mean by entrepreneur.*

WT   It's a kind of midwife, isn't it? You appraise a situation, which is pregnant, and then are responsible for delivering the baby.

BB *What did you deliver?*

WT   I delivered mental health care to New South Wales, which simply wasn't in existence. I was critical and not afraid of speaking my mind, which was effective. I managed to effect changes in the administration of the Mental Health Department and to arouse a forward-looking atmosphere which didn't exist before. A major building programme was started. At least in Australia, when they do decide to build something, they build it, and up it goes before your eyes. I was responsible for getting many of these schemes under way. I was also involved in much of their design and planning.

BB *What about the rest of Australia?*

WT   I learned early on that the way to get things done in Australia, was to play one State off against another. I played Victoria off against New South Wales. They were more advanced in Victoria because of Cunningham Dax.

BB *He was English, wasn't he?*

WT   Yes. He was Medical Superintendent of Netherne, and went out some years before me to become Director of Mental Health Services in Victoria. He did a lot. I held him up as an example to New South Wales of what could be done. This stimulated them. Inter-State rivalry is really something in Australia. Dax is still alive, living in Tasmania, he enormously improved the mental health services in Victoria.

BB *Had you anything to do with South Australia and Western Australia or New Zealand?*

WT   I was invited to go to them after I had become known in New South Wales. I went to Perth, Brisbane, and Adelaide to look at their facilities which, on the whole, weren't very good, nothing like Victoria. I well remember once visiting Toowoomba Hospital outside Brisbane. I was presented with a series of obscure inherited neurological disorders and expected to pronounce on them. None were worked up, but they all had gross physical signs. It was quite interesting. But I didn't get much time to visit other places, I was so busy in Sydney.

BB *Would you like to say something about the development of psychiatry during the later part of your stay and since you have been away from Australia?*

WT   This has been considerable. Apart from the improvement in the psychiatric facilities, there has been a large development of academic psychiatry. When I went to Sydney, I was the only Professor in Australia, a pretty daunting prospect. But now there are Chairs and Departments in Brisbane, two in Sydney, Sydney University and the University of New South Wales, Newcastle; Victoria – that was the next development after my Chair – at the University of Melbourne and Monash, in South Australia in Adelaide, and Flinders, at Perth and in Tasmania. Newcastle has appointed the first woman Professor of Psychiatry. The Royal Australian & New Zealand College of Psychiatrists has become a very thriving organization.

BB *What do you think of their membership exam? Ours is compared adversely with theirs.*

WT   This is because of misunderstanding. Private practice is much more advanced in Australia than here. Obtaining the Membership of the Royal Australian & New Zealand College of Psychiatrists shows that you are of consultant standard; it is a hallmark.

Here, the Membership of the Royal College of Psychiatrists only qualifies the successful candidate for further training as a senior registrar. The Australians found this difficult to understand, and complained about the relatively lower standard of our Membership, without realising that it is no more than a ticket for further training.

Here, but not in Australia, there is a further test, for to become a consultant psychiatrist, you have to obtain a National Health Service appointment in competition.

BB   *There are features of their examination which are good, aren't there?*

WT   It is more searching, more in accord with the American Boards. I was the first Senior Censor of the Royal Australian New College of Psychiatrists, but never conducted an examination. The failure rate was high and caused discontent.

BB   *Is the divide between the Royal Australasian College of Physicians and the Psychiatrists' College a big one?*

WT   I don't think so. They maintain friendly relations. There are senior Australian and New Zealand psychiatrists who are Members and Fellows of both. I am a Fellow of both Colleges, although I didn't take any examinations.

BB   *After you left Australia you came back, to Birmingham. How did that come about?*

WT   In 1961, I went to Montreal to the World Congress of Psychiatry. Since my fare was paid, not by the University of Sydney I might add, I decided that as I had not been to England for six years and had a few relatives remaining, it was time I looked in on them. So I decided to go right round the world. Doing better than Phileas Fogg, I went round in 23 days, including spending a week in England.

Birmingham were looking for someone to fill their first Chair of Clinical Psychiatry and I was invited to meet the Dean, the late Professor Pon d'Abreu. He showed me round the hospital. He seemed to be interested in me, but said the Vice-Chancellor wasn't there, and could I come back on Saturday. He asked me to stay with him at his house in Coughton Court. He, the Professor of Medicine, and the Vice-Chancellor offered me the Chair over the port. Now that's a civilised way to get a job.

BB   *What was psychiatry like in Birmingham then?*

WT   Such teaching as there was, was in the hands of two or three part-time consultants. There was a Chair in Experimental Psychiatry, which was really neuropharmacology and had been held by Joel Elkes, now Professor at Johns Hopkins.

BB   *Was that a personal appointment or an established Chair?*

WT   I believe Elkes's Chair was established. However, Birmingham is a conservative place, so that when the University first decided to embrace psychiatry, it wanted to make sure it was 'respectable'. Respectable psychiatry was to do with neuropharmacology in those days – maybe it still is! Elkes went to America about three years before I came, leaving the Chair to Philip Bradley, whose Department has since become Preclinical Pharmacology.

BB   *There is no longer a Chair of Experimental Psychiatry?*

WT   No. Mine was the first Chair of Clinical Psychiatry.

BB   *And how did you find things when you got here?*

WT   I was given a lot of promises. I was told there were funds and facilities to set-up an equivalent of the Maudsley in the Midlands. Of course, it never materialised. In fact, I never expected it to. But I was promised more facilities than I ever actually received. Within a year, I had a small allotment of beds and I finished, after 21 years, with the same small allotment of beds.

I looked at the existing facilities to see how they could be exploited. We set up a clinical tutors' scheme in the West Midlands, which was the first to be established and which was later widely copied. Every mental hospital had a clinical tutor with an official University appointment. Also, a scheme for rotating senior registrars, which was so successful we were allowed more senior registrars in psychiatry than any Region outside London. I think exploiting existing facilities is more likely to pay dividends than trying to set up something new and waiting hopelessly for money.

BB *What about your own department?*

WT   The department was always small.

BB *What was it when you arrived?*

WT   Just me! I insisted on a first assistant and senior lecturer. Nobody can operate in isolation, if only because of clinical commitments. When I retired last year, we had two senior lecturers in adult psychiatry, one senior lecturer in child psychiatry, a lecturer in psychiatry, and two in clinical psychology.

BB *Turning to undergraduate teaching, would you like to say something about objectives in training undergraduates?*

WT   I believe that the most important thing a university department of psychiatry can do is to train undergraduates; it is more important than postgraduate teaching.

When I came to Birmingham in 1962, undergraduates received an optional four weeks of psychiatry; fifty per cent of them elected to do it. Soon, the four weeks were made compulsory and increased to six, eight, and finally ten weeks, and psychiatry was made a final-year subject. In Birmingham, we place great emphasis on continuous assessment. The final year comprises five ten-week periods: senior medicine, senior surgery, obstetrics, paediatrics, and psychiatry. Batches of students come for ten weeks, full-time. At the end of the ten-week period, they are examined. If they pass, they are finally through as far as that subject is concerned. If they fail or are of distinction standard, they have another examination in June.

BB *What is the advantage of that?*

WT   When a student is doing psychiatry or any other final-year subject, he is doing that and nothing else. He is not swotting for a major final examination. In ten weeks, you can teach them a lot. The time to inculcate an interest in psychiatry is the undergraduate level. In a recent study[5] of interests shown by medical students on qualification which rated various specialities, Birmingham in 1961–65 was fifteenth for students taking up psychiatry. In 1971–75, Birmingham was fourth. I am told it may now be even higher. I am very proud of that.

---

5. BROOK P. (1983) Who's for psychiatry? United Kingdom medical schools and career choice of psychiatry, 1961–75. *British Journal of Psychiatry*, **142**, 361–5.

Also, since we have been teaching more psychiatry, young general practitioners and young house officers are picking up psychiatric patients and telling their chiefs: 'You have a psychiatric problem here and ought to refer it.' The letters we get from general practitioners are also much more insightful and more perceptive of psychiatric problems.

BB *What do you aim to teach undergraduates?*

WT   An overview of the range of psychiatric problems they are likely to encounter in general practice, or in a general hospital, or in some other kind of practice.

BB *By lectures?*

WT   I gave up lecturing years ago. That's not absolutely true. I do give the occasional (usually guest) lecture. But in teaching undergraduates, we tend to concentrate on small-group teaching – seminar teaching.

BB *Rather than case demonstrations?*

WT   Using patients or video-tapes – to teach awareness of psychiatric problems and to recognise those patients who need referral to a psychiatrist, and not to be contemptuous of psychiatric patients, like people in my student days used to be. The next thing is how to interview psychiatric patients. How do you get the information. I used to be appalled at the inability of the average doctor to get information from patients and understand it, even how to listen properly. These skills apply to all medical practice. How to do it quickly, without letting the patient waste your time, or wasting your own time. Simple psychiatric conditions can and are being treated adequately by general practitioners and non-psychiatrists.

There will never be enough psychiatrists to cope with psychiatric patients. Paradoxically, the more we teach undergraduates, the more difficult our clinical problems become.

BB *You were one of the first departments to take up television teaching?*

WT   I think we were the first department in this country to use a video-tape recorder. There was one at the Maudsley and one in Edinburgh, but we got ours unpacked first. It was a black and white reel to reel – and what a thing that was, I can remember the trouble we had.

BB *Was it any use?*

WT   It made an immediate impact. We progressed to the more sophisticated studio we have now, with cameras and colour. The advantage of video-tapes was to see what a psychiatrist does with his patient. At the Maudsley, many years ago, there was this mysterious thing called 'psychotherapy'. We all had to do it, but nobody ever taught us how; it was done behind closed doors and we wondered what it was that was going on. Now, you can see it all on a TV screen.

BB *What do you use it for in teaching undergraduates?*

WT   Teaching interviewing, so students can see themselves interviewing, and for showing interesting cases. In a small unit, there is always a shortage of patients and a video-recorder gives you a demonstration library of cases of mania, manic–depressive psychosis, schizophrenia, and so on.

BB *That's expensive on staff time.*

WT Luckily, members of my staff, particularly Tim Betts, were keen. In recent years, I dropped out because I felt they did it better. We also experimented with video as an examination medium, and the College paid for a research fellow. We concluded it was best used as a talking-point. Show a little bit of a video-tape and ask the candidate to comment, rather like a short case in a medical exam.

BB *With such a small department, how did you get on in research? Do you feel that undergraduate departments should do research?*

WT I felt it was my duty not so much to do research myself, but to find funds and facilities for younger members of the department to do research. This is a professor's job. After all, they are making their careers; it doesn't really matter to me whether I do any more research, or at least it didn't over the last few years. My reputation is already made – or broken.

BB *What happened in your department?*

WT I never believed in directing research. People should find their own research subjects and if they are good, I encourage them. I never believed one should say, 'Why don't you look into this?' I am rather against that. People must generate their own research ideas. Once they have them and say, 'Do you think this is a good idea?', then you are at liberty to criticise or say, 'Yes I do' or 'It's been done before; I don't think you will get much joy from it', or something of that kind. But I don't believe it is my duty to tell other people what they should research.

BB *I remember one paper[6] from your department about coal gas and the suicide rate in Birmingham. How did that come to be done?*

WT The Coroner wrote and said that suicide was dropping considerably and they did not know the reason for it. So Christine Hassall, senior research fellow in my department, and I looked at the coroner's record cards. Sure enough, the number of suicides in Birmingham had dropped in the most extraordinary way. There seemed no reason for it.

So I said to Christine, 'Let's go about it in the simplest way we can'. The Coroner kept cards which showed the name, sex, and age of the person, the verdict, and the method of suicide. So I said, 'We'll take these first' and divided them into active methods (cutting, self-hanging, jumping in the river, jumping in front of lorries), completely passive (taking pills of various kinds, overdoses) and an in-between group – coal gas – a sort of halfway between active and passive. We found that violent methods of suicide or active measures had risen slightly in males, while the number of passive suicides with pills had remained constant. But coal gas ones had greatly fallen. Birmingham was not on

6. HASSALL, C. & TRETHOWAN, W. H. (1972) Suicide in Birmingham. *British Medical Journal*, **1**, 717–8.

North Sea gas. So I wrote to the secretary of the Gas Board, who wrote back that they had detoxified the ordinary town gas from about 20% carbon monoxide to 2.5%.

He was also kind enough to enclose the figures for industrial accidents due to coal gas, which followed a similar curve to suicides. This finding has sometimes been passionately disputed at conferences I have attended, but it seems to me to be unchallengeable. The figures are absolutely plain.

BB   Sainsbury doesn't believe that the change in the toxicity of gas has reduced the national rates.

WT   What does he believe it is due to?

BB   He believes it is partly due to an improvement in treating depressive illness with antidepressant drugs.

WT   I don't think there is much evidence of that, otherwise the number of suicides with pills would have dropped over this period, and what's more, the decline in the number of coal gas suicides begins precisely at the point that it was detoxified. It seems to be inescapable.

BB   I agree with you. And the national rate has flattened out as the coal gas detoxification programme has been completed. Can we turn to your books? Did you co-author Anderson & Trethowan or just take it over?

WT   I co-authored the second edition.

BB   Did Anderson take it over from Dawson?

WT   Originally, it was *Aids to Psychiatry* by W. S. Dawson. Anderson took it over and wrote the first edition – considerably different from Dawson's; for the second edition, I became his co-author. I wrote about a third of it and re-wrote a lot of what he had written.

For the third edition, I became the principal author and he the sleeping partner. Anderson, whose psychiatry was German-based, also wrote English in a Teutonic style. His publishers said to me, 'For goodness sake, put some paragraphs in' (some of his paragraphs lasted several pages) – so I did. The book is more readable.

The fourth edition[7] I wrote completely by myself, as he had died.

The fifth edition, due to come out shortly, is being re-written with the help of Andrew Sims who, of course, shares my phenomenological interests. He can take it over for the sixth edition. The book has a life; it sells well. Over 3000 copies a year are sold now, almost 50% abroad, and the abroad sales are increasing.

BB   What do you aim to do in the book?

WT   To give an intelligible account of psychiatry, its possibilities, its limitations, in such a way that undergraduates and general practitioners will take an interest in the subject, and young graduates who wish to learn more can profit from it. The book is not intended for those training for psychiatry.

---

7. TRETHOWAN, W. H. (1979) *Psychiatry, 4th Edition*. London: Baillière Tindall.

BB *Your other book is* Uncommon Psychiatric Syndromes?[8] *How did you come to write that?*

WT I have always been interested in the byways of psychiatry and so has David Enoch, my co-author. He wrote papers on the Capgras syndrome and the Othello syndrome. I was interested in the other topics. We thought we would write a book on the more colourful aspects of psychiatry – nearly all of them paranoid states, incidentally. We collected historical and literary material, as well as clinical, which is the point of the book, not just unadorned clinical description. We wrote it for our own entertainment and hopefully for that of others. The second edition has certainly gone much better than the first, which was over-priced. There is also a Japanese edition.

BB *You came to Birmingham in 1962 and you were appointed Dean of the Medical School in 1968. It is unusual, I think, for the Professor of Psychiatry to become Dean.*

WT I was the first Professor of Psychiatry, south of the border, to become Dean of a Medical School. There was one in Scotland, Malcolm Millar, Dean of Aberdeen. Of course, there have been others since – Neil Kessel in Manchester, for example, and Arthur Crisp at St George's, representing London University.

BB *How do you think being Dean affected the development of psychiatry in the University. Were you able to give it a special force?*

WT One has to bend over backwards not to favour one's own department, to be neutral and be seen to be neutral. However, I did get another senior lecturer out of it – I had to, because I didn't wish the department to fall to pieces. The effect on the Department was on the negative side. Work that I would have done as Professor fell on the shoulders of others.

BB *Looking from the vantage point of Dean, did you think the Department of Psychiatry was receiving a fair crack of the whip?*

WT I never thought the Department of Psychiatry had a fair crack of the whip during my time in Birmingham. I was promised facilities, a new unit for psychiatry, none of which ever came to pass. I am not saying that psychiatry fared worse than other departments, but as usual, medicine and surgery reign supreme. In short, I don't think being Dean brought any advantage to the Department of Psychiatry.

I said to the Vice-Chancellor, 'Why do you want me to be Dean?' He said, 'I think it is a good thing to have a psychiatrist as Dean – they understand other people's motives!'

BB *Did his joke turn out to be true?*

WT Yes, I think so. Psychiatrists do understand other people's motives – we are trained to do so, but in respect primarily of patients. One has to be careful about bringing too much psychiatric understanding into dealings with people who are not, at least overtly, suffering from psychiatric illnes.

BB *Did you find the fact of being a psychiatrist and Dean led to your being treated by your admin colleagues as more respectable?*

WT I must have been regarded as respectable to be made Dean.

---

8. ENOCH, M. D. & TRETHOWAN, W. H. (1979) *Uncommon Psychiatric Syndromes*, 2nd Ed. Bristol: John Wright.

BB *It's a democratic decision?*

WT   It isn't entirely. The Dean is not elected at Birmingham. The Medical School existed long before the rest of the University and the Dean of the Medical School is appointed by the Council of the University on the recommendation of the Vice-Chancellor, who does, however, take soundings. Deans of other faculties are elected by their faculties.

BB *Can we turn to the Royal College of Psychiatrists? What are your views about the College being founded?*

WT   In the early days, I was against its foundation. When meetings took place at the Royal Society of Medicine, I, with other colleagues, opposed the foundation for a time.

BB *Why did you oppose it?*

WT   Because I felt we were multiplying Colleges needlessly. I felt there should be a closer affiliation between psychiatry and the Royal College of Physicians and was against the creation of yet another diploma, which would inevitably follow upon the foundation of the College.

BB *Who were the others who shared your view?*

WT   Sir Denis Hill felt the same way, and a lot of the senior people in psychiatry; also Desmond Curran, if I remember rightly.

BB *If the Physicians had been more accommodating, would an affiliation have been possible?*

WT   It is a big 'if' though, because that College has never shown itself to be particularly accommodating.

BB *Not since 1519?*

WT   I have great respect for the Royal College of Physicians, but if there is blame to be laid anywhere, I would put it at their feet. Some specialities had to form themselves into Colleges to shake off their shackles.

BB *Do you feel the Royal College of Surgeons has been more accommodating in the way they have coped with, say, the dentists?*

WT   On the surface, at least, yes. They are less involved and less threatened. The surgeons are a race apart, though, and they always were, having, to a certain extent, to defend themselves against the physicians, although that goes much further back into history. However, those of us who opposed the formation of the Royal College of Psychiatrists felt bound to give it our support when it was shown that the majority wanted it.

BB *Did you play a part in the formation of the Charter – all those long negotiations?*

WT   No, I played no part in that at all.

BB *But when the College was founded, you became the first Chief Examiner?*

WT   I became the first Chief Examiner, for my sins!

BB *Since you have mentioned sins, what were they in relation to that exam?*

WT   First of all, having an exam at all. You could say I connived, yet we are not at a stage where we can get away from exams.

BB *What would you have instead?*

WT   There is no substitute at the present time. One can't do without an exam, yet I am always hesitant to add another to the fate of the young postgraduate. At a time when a young man should be doing research, he is faced with an exam. But what's the alternative? It blocks his research; the College tried a research option without success.

BB *Why wasn't it a success? I did the Maudsley DPM. The compulsory research dissertation had a marked effect on my development and career, as I think it had with others like myself.*

WT   It's difficult to compare the Maudsley DPM, an internal examination which the training was geared to, with the Membership, and it was compulsory research. The College one was not.

BB *Why wasn't it?*

WT   One reason is that most people examined for the College diploma never write a research paper in their lives and are not capable of doing so. I am sure you know that's true.

BB *I'm not sure I do agree. I believed it was more because of the influence of the Privy Council and the Royal College of Physicians through the Privy Council.*

WT   If that's so, I have no direct knowledge of it.

BB *Anyway, you became Chief Examiner. Why did you?*

WT   I can't remember why I became Chief Examiner. I suppose I was fool enough to volunteer. I got landed with it for seven years and by that time, I had had enough.

BB *What did you try to do through the examination? It determined what young doctors did for some three years of their training.*

WT   The exam was a test of knowledge at a half-way point in a young man's career, which would determine whether it was worth his going on training.

BB *How did you decide what the test should be?*

WT   We had a committee – of course – to which people brought varying degrees of experience of examinations. How else can one do it? And out of the deliberations of this committee, the exam took the form which it more or less has at present – a multiple-choice exam, a clinical, and vivas. The College built in from the beginning an examination of the exam in statistical terms, which was far-sighted.

Christine Hassall, senior research fellow in my department, produced statistics to monitor the exam, and these were interesting. They told us about the abilities of candidates from different parts of the country and allowed inferences to be made about the quality of their training. The north of England candidates were less successful than those from the south, and overseas candidates were less successful than home ones. Of course, the exam was geared to British candidates.

It also showed, although we didn't publish this, some interesting things about examiners.

BB   What did it show?

WT   Tremendous variation in the ability of the examiners, and how some examiners were probably unqualified to examine.

BB   Were they removed?

WT   No, possibly because the statistics did not refer to them as individuals. The most interesting thing which I think the figures show incontrovertibly is that the clinical exam and the multiple-choice tests are the only worthwhile parts of the exam. Whatever rude things people say about multiple-choice tests, they are the best sort of screen.

I was appalled at the extraordinary differentials in the essay examiners' marking. When the College responded to this by producing model answers, it seemed not to make the slightest difference. Either the examiners didn't read the model answers, or, if they did, they disagreed with them, or for some other reason it made no difference – the discrepancies were just as bad. Although multiple-choice questions are tedious things and people say they only test the ability to do multiple-choice questions, they seem to correlate extremely highly with clinical ability. It makes you think.

BB   You have remained in the College even though you have stopped being Chief Examiner?

WT   Oh yes! I have not held any office for some time, but that's because of increasing age. You can only do so much.

BB   What do you think about the College at the present time?

WT   It is thriving. I was opposed to its formation, but I am happy about the way it has progressed, though I'm much more a University than a College man.

BB   Is there much difference?

WT   The great advantage of a University post, something I value greatly, is working in close association with people of varying interests, whereas the Royal College of Psychiatrists is virtually only concerned with psychiatry. It is the same in all Colleges. In universities, there is a cross-fertilisation of different disciplines. It makes life much more interesting.

BB   You were the Chairman of a DHSS committee which considered how psychologists were to be recruited and employed in the National Health Service. There was a report[9] which caused a bit of a stir when it first came out.

WT   Now this is interesting, because this was a sub-committee of the Standing Mental Health Advisory Committee at the Department of Health. I was Chairman of the Standing Mental Health Advisory Committee, as successor to Denis Hill. During the time I was Chairman, this sub-committee was set up to consider the role of psychologists in the Health Service and found itself without a parent, because the Standing Mental Health Advisory Committee got quangoed and abolished. The Department had an economy drive and decided to get rid of lots and lots of committees, including the Central Health Services Council, but the sub-committee continued in being.

---

9. DEPARTMENT OF HEALTH AND SOCIAL SECURITY (1977) *The Role of Psychologists in the Health Service.* HC (77) 14. London: HMSO.

BB *I suppose this happened because of the emergence of behaviour therapy as an effective treatment?*

WT Partly, but also because the role of the clinical psychologist in the National Health Service was under scrutiny. Behaviour therapy stimulated this further, but it was ripe anyway. This report has been favourably received by psychologists, if not by psychiatrists.

BB *What do you think it did for the clinical psychologist?*

WT The main recommendation was the setting up of an organised Area-based service and a structured career for clinical psychologists. In 1974, the National Health Service underwent an upheaval and Areas and Districts were born. A lot of people, particularly the paramedicals, felt themselves to be in limbo in this administrative structure.

BB *A proposal was made in that committee that psychologists should only accept patients who had first of all been vetted by psychiatrists. That was removed, wasn't it, later?*

WT I don't think it was ever officially removed, not as far as I can recollect.

BB *In practice, psychologists take referrals from anywhere?*

WT This was certainly not the recommendation made by my committee.

BB *What did your committee recommend then?*

WT Our committee was quite firm, and the psychologists on the committee themselves agreed, that medical responsibility as such should not be taken by psychologists; all cases should be screened by a psychiatrist, or other doctor, before referral to a psychologist.

BB *If we can turn now to the Worcester project.*

WT The Worcester project was set up to demonstrate that sufficient general hospital facilities and community services could cope with all the work which would normally be done by a mental hospital. The DHSS chose Powick Hospital, near Worcester, for this purpose because they felt Worcestershire was an area which represented both urban and rural mental health problems in reasonable proportions.

The DHSS came to me with a huge document and an offer of considerable facilities for a research project. These were on a grandiose scale. I was worried because I felt they were providing facilities to see what they wanted to prove, proved. I favoured the development because general hospital psychiatry, given the facilities, represents a turn away from the traditional County Asylum approach. At the same time, I am not sure that the day of the mental hospital is over.

But the DHSS research project contained a strong bias towards proving what they wanted to see proved. I said so, and went so far as to turn down some of the facilities offered. Instead, I said I would do some limited research, which is what happened.

They then set up a co-ordinating committee with me as Chairman, with Community Medical Officers, Directors of Social Work of the County and the town of Worcester, psychiatrists, general practitioners, and others concerned, including officials from the Department. We held quarterly meetings to examine what was going on.

Over a long period, what had been hoped for has largely come to pass. We have seen the rundown of Powick and the provision of new psychiatric facilities at Worcester and Kidderminster, which are the two main towns in Worcestershire, together with the development of community facilities, day hospitals, and things of this kind, all envisaged in the original project. The project has been not starved exactly, but pinched for money. At one time when things got critical, we had a very stormy meeting, because it looked as if the whole project was going to founder because of a financial squeeze.

I went to London and interviewed the CMO and Sir Patrick Nairne, who was the permanent secretary in the Department, saying, 'If you want this project to go on, you will have to find the money', and they did. The results, however, have not been an unqualified success.

The geriatric problem held us up. There are still geriatric patients at Powick and I don't know how they are going to be disposed of. There has been some talk of turning Powick into a geriatric hospital which, to a certain extent, nullifies the object of the exercise. The main thing we hoped to do was to close the wards and pull the hospital down. However, the two general hospitals and community services do seem to be containing Worcestershire's mentally ill.

BB   I see you have a Hong Kong Doctorate.

WT   In about 1975, I was asked to become Chairman of the Medical Academic Advisory Committee to set up an entirely new Medical School at the Chinese University of Hong Kong in the New Territories. I thought this a most interesting project and accepted. There was only one medical school in Hong Kong, at Hong Kong University which was not producing enough medical graduates. Our first medical undergraduates are now entering their clinical years and will graduate in 1985. It's been fun setting up a new medical school from scratch. The place has got plenty of money to do it, and lots of material; it makes a change from what goes on in this country.

BB   What will happen to it in 1997?

WT   I don't know; your guess is as good as mine. They gave me an Honorary Doctorate of Science for my services to the Chinese University.

BB   What do you think about distinction awards? Every year, the British Medical Journal publish an analysis of distinction awards, paying attention to the way in which psychiatrists of various kinds are discriminated against.

WT   Having seen the distinction award system from inside – as adviser in mental health both nationally and at a regional level – my view is it is probably about as fair as circumstances allow it to be. This is not to say that there is no discrimination against specialities. I would agree that probably psychiatry is not as well represented as it should be, but this is difficult to judge. People in the centre of things, in active hospitals, are advantaged by the fact that they are under the eye of their colleagues, and after all, it is their colleagues who put them up for distinction awards.

BB *What are distinction awards, what is their purpose? Are they to reward research ability, academic distinction, teaching ability, or are they for people who work hard for the benefit of the National Health Service?*

WT There has recently been a change. Originally, they were to reward academic distinction, research ability, and teaching ability, but there has recently been a change, at least in relation to C awards, towards rewarding long and arduous service, often in places in which people would not care to work – to my mind, quite rightly.

If a man writes lots of papers and is a well-known teacher, he is in the public eye and one knows first-hand what his abilities are and can form a judgement on whether he should be rewarded. But the man in some backward area, slogging away, doing a good job, his services isolated from his colleagues – the value of his work is more difficult to judge. This is the snag with distinction awards.

BB *There has been a problem in Birmingham with in-patient suicides?*

WT You would think so by the publicity. In fact, our statistics show that for 2654 admissions over a period of years, our suicide rate was 0.23 per cent (6 patients in all). I don't think anyone should complain at that.

BB *But the wards closed.*

WT This was because the coroner decided to hear three cases, which occurred in separate wards and over a period of time, all on one day, thereby exciting the national press, the local press, and the horror of the hospital administrators. There was a good deal of hysteria about it.

BB *Would you like to talk about that. I think the local press and their behaviour about local suicides can have a bad effect.*

WT Most psychiatrists agree that suicide is not completely preventable, so that one has to accept a minimum suicide rate, in the same way that one has to accept a small proportion of anaesthetic deaths and deaths from surgical operations. Short of chaining patients to the wall, I don't see how you can prevent them.

The dramatisation by the press is unreasonable. No good comes of it. It damages the image of psychiatry, gives pain to the relatives of the deceased, and hampers those of us working towards a more liberal approach to the care of the mentally ill.

4   Maxwell Jones

Interviewed by BRIAN BARRACLOUGH (1983)

Dr Maxwell Jones, CBE, MB (Edin) 1931, DPM (Lond) 1935, FRCP Edin 1935, MD (Edin) 1947, FRCPsych 1971. Dr Jones was born in South Africa in 1907, and died in 1990. He studied psychiatry at Edinburgh, in the United States, and at the pre-war Maudsley. He gained a gold medal for his MD thesis based on research into DAH (disordered action of the heart) which had established that this was a psychosomatic fear reaction. After the war he worked for the Ministry of Labour with emotionally disturbed unemployable people and developed the Belmont Unit. In 1959 he went to Stanford University, California as Visiting Professor and then for three years to the State Hospital at Salem, Oregon. He was Physician Superintendent of Dingleton Hospital, Melrose, Scotland from 1962–69.

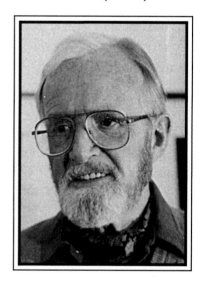

BB   *What is your family background?*

MJ   My parents' professional backgrounds were education and religion. I was born in Queenstown, South Africa, in 1907. My father went there at the end of the last century, when lots of young men were attracted to an adventurous way of life. We lived in Mafeking until I was five, when my father died.

BB   *So you came back to England in 1912, just before the war.*

MJ   Yes, it was a courageous thing for my mother to do because she had three children and, my father being a young man, we didn't have much money. Her father had emigrated to Indianapolis, when he became a millionaire. She knew no one in Edinburgh, but knew that a good, inexpensive education could be obtained there. This didn't please the rest of her relatives, but nevertheless, she did it.

BB   *Where did you go to school?*

MJ   Stewarts College, a typical Scottish day school – hard working, hard playing. I am a great respector of the Edinburgh schools. Plenty of competition among the numerous excellent schools.

BB   *Then what happened?*

MJ   I wanted to be a coffee planter in Kenya. I suppose I had some of my father's roving spirit. I needed £2,000, which the government required if you were to go to Kenya to develop a parcel of land. Unfortunately, no one seemed eager to lend it to me. So, I settled for my second love, which was psychiatry – the idea of knowing people. I had read many of the classics and thought the character studies were fascinating, and so I decided to study psychiatry. I slogged through medicine in order to become a psychiatrist. It wasn't a love of medicine at all, just an interest in people.

BB   *How old were you when you made that decision?*

MJ   I guess just school-leaving age, because I tried very hard to get the money to go to Kenya. I remember having to do some Latin at the last moment in order to get into university.

BB   *That was Edinburgh University – where you graduated in medicine?*

MJ   That's right. I suppose I was an average student. I wasn't thrilled with medicine. I was always inclined to look at the lot of the underdog. It may not be so bad now, but in those days, it seemed to me that patients were dehumanised; to see a young woman patient in a lecture theatre exposed physically to 200 students without being forewarned didn't thrill me – I thought it was insensitive, the lack of privacy, everything about it was so callous. And I never made friends with any of the lecturers. I resented their aloofness and lack of warmth, although I suppose this was inevitable given the size of the classes – 200 each year.

Still I count myself lucky to have been able to go to university and enjoy the athletics and so on. But my goal was quite clearly psychiatry, not medicine or surgery. That was unusual in those days, because it wasn't highly regarded as a profession.

BB   *Was there any psychiatry in the undergraduate curriculum in the 20s in Edinburgh?*

MJ   A little, because Edinburgh had the first Professor of Psychiatry in Britain, Rosy Robertson, and he was followed by Sir David Henderson, who really made a name and was the great high priest of psychiatry at that time. So I was able to make a good start in my training with Henderson.

BB   *Had he been with Meyer in Baltimore?*

MJ   That was *the* place to go at that time, and Henderson became his best known pupil. Meyer was a psychobiologist really, which is quite remarkable. He was ahead of his time.

BB   *What kind of teaching did you have as an undergraduate in psychiatry?*

MJ   Sir David gave lectures, we had the inevitable exposure to the 'loonies', and I was very unhappy at the rather cold 'objectivity' of it all. I liked good writing, and I liked rather romantic interludes, but it was all stark fact. I wasn't very happy until I began to see what I could do working with more exciting neurotic, psychopathic, and psychological disturbances. I worked for nothing for six months in order to get into the clinical field I wanted, and Sir David was apparently impressed by my motivation.

Then, to my amazement, in 1936, I was awarded a Commonwealth Fund Fellowship to the United States for two years. I was by now doing quite a lot of research in carbohydrate metabolism and enzyme chemistry, which no doubt helped me to get this Fellowship. In those days, it was considered to be prestigious, as they took only thirty people each year from the universities of the entire Empire.

I worked for a year at the University of Pennsylvania, where I continued to do non-clinical research and we had some exciting times – looking at cholinesterase and its effects on the transmission of nerve impulses, etc. I went for my second year, 1938, to Columbia University Medical Center in New York. By that time, I was determined to do animal work, which I had already begun before I left Edinburgh. I had a very good year studying hormones, using experimental animals, and then Aubrey Lewis invited me to come to the Maudsley. This was 1938.

I stayed with Sir Aubrey for five years at the Maudsley (evacuated to Mill Hill School). My psychosomatic interests and research resulted in my being asked to head a unit on cardiac neurosis or effort syndrome, a condition called neuro-circulatory asthenia in the USA.

I worked with Paul Wood, an outstanding London cardiologist from Australia, who stayed with us for 18 months. We did, I think, a pretty thorough bit of clinical research and demonstrated that this syndrome of left chest pain, breathlessness, giddiness, etc., had some real chemical indicators. We had a unit of 100 beds filled with army personnel for over five years.

The Harvard Fatigue Lab later confirmed our findings and agreed that the poor response to exercise pointed to a poorly integrated autonomic nervous system.

I wrote up all this work and got a gold medal MD from Edinburgh which was, I think, the first they had ever given in psychiatry.

BB   *Did you do that kind of work in America before you joined the Maudsley?*

MJ   No, this was all in wartime. The challenge resulted from the large number of Forces personnel with this condition.

BB   *It was a military problem?*

MJ   Absolutely. In fact, it was hardly noticeable in peace time, although sometimes affecting overstressed housewives, but in wartime, with increased physical output in army training, it showed up.

One other thing is relevant about the effort syndrome soldiers (100 men in all). As they all had the same clinical condition, commonsense dictated that we should begin to treat them as one group. So we had daily meetings with 100 men and all the staff on duty. We had nurses, etc., because in wartime, everyone was recruited. Some of these recruits were artists and they contributed audio-visual aids which we hung on the walls, showing the patients' symptomatology in a very dramatic way, including diagrams of the autonomic nervous system.

It was tremendously exciting, as patients and staff were working together in furthering treatment, with the patients themselves being a valuable resource for teaching. Moreover, it helped to undermine our unpopularity, as we were inevitably trying to get them back into army service. So they listened with open ears to their peers. We were there as resource people and didn't say too much, because there was always a nucleus of patients who understood their clinical state. They had learned that we had learned about the lack of homeostasis in relation to their exercise physiology.

This experience, over a period of five years, opened my eyes to the power of the patient peer group in treatment, and I began to wonder why much more is not done in a metabolic hospital ward with a diabetic group or whatever. You get an immense amount of material from the patients, much of it distorted or erroneous, which you can then modify and direct in healthy directions, but I don't think I have ever heard of anyone doing this. Anyway, that's how we started learning from patients.

BB *Where were these 100 beds?*

MJ   At Mill Hill. The public school was evacuated when we were moved there from the Maudsley. And the other half of the Maudsley, mainly organically orientated staff, went to the south of London to Sutton, Surrey, to the Emergency Medical Service (EMS) hospital there.

BB *And who was with you at Mill Hill?*

MJ   The more analytic crowd. Sir Aubrey, himself, Walter Maclay and Stokes, who later became the Professor of Psychiatry at Toronto, and those of the Maudsley staff who were psychodynamically oriented.

BB *Were you recruited to the Army?*

MJ   None of us were. The Army was in part associated with the Tavistock Clinic, and the Navy was with Desmond Curran and the St George's crowd. The Maudsley was the EMS.

When the war ended, the Maudsley were asked to take over a unit situated in a hospital near Dartford, Kent, for the rehabilitation of the most disturbed 100 000 prisoners of war returning from Europe and the Far East. I was asked to head this unit of 300 beds. It was a fairly natural transition from the physiology of the effort syndrome group to the sociology of the POW group. The army were doing much the same thing in their 17 civilian resettlement units – but what we had were supposedly the most mentally disturbed of the POWs.

BB *European prisoners of war?*

MJ   Yes. At Dartford, things were very well organised. The Government put all the Green Line buses we wanted at our disposal. These were needed for our plan to rehabilitate the men in real life situations. I went round the Dartford area on a push-bike and got 70 employers to agree to take our men, and help them to find their feet after being isolated in prison camps for up to five years during wartime. We had them in everything from ship-building yards, to market gardens, to shops, and the Green Line buses went round and dropped them off at their chosen places of work.

They worked for short periods, four hours or so, and were treated very understandingly by the regular employees, and then came back. We discussed their difficulties at work, their negative self-images, lack of confidence in social situations, fear of impotence after years of separation from the opposite sex, paranoid feelings about their wives and others.

The men were housed in six 'cottages', each with 50 beds. Each unit had a daily community meeting, along the lines we had developed at Mill Hill. We were still an annexe of the Maudsley and had retained most of our original staff. In a supportive environment where the trust level was high, the men discussed their fears about returning to society and to their wives and children born in their absence, their adequacy as husbands, and so on. We had a year at Dartford, with 1400 admissions in that year. We worked unbelievable hours, but the morale was high. A follow-up study of our rehabilitation results, done by the Ministry of Labour, showed that something like 86% were at work six months later.

BB *But, what were they cases of?*

MJ Of maladjustment, resulting from imprisonment and then release to their old world, but now feeling like strangers. Emotional reactions, depression, paranoia, and fear of impotence and inadequacy generally – so it was another syndrome like the effort one.

Now we had a 'POW syndrome', with a cluster of symptoms evidenced in a similar form in most of the cases, plus a few psychotic and other reactions.

BB *Were they men who had had a trial back in civilian life in England or had they come straight on release?*

MJ This was before release from the Army. They were screened, and if they were found not to be well enough to return home as civilians, the government said we must help to rehabilitate them first.

BB *Whose idea was it to have this rehabilitation emphasis at the Maudsley?*

MJ I think the Army must have said that the Maudsley should take some part in this process. We didn't have to collaborate with the Army. We did our own thing, but learned retrospectively that our methods and those employed at the Army units were very similar.

We were now asked by the Ministries of Labour and Health if we would tackle another social problem – the down and outs in London. Initially they were characterised as the 'hard core' unemployed. They were not just workshy, but also lacking in motivation to do anything approaching an organised existence.

And that was the start in 1947 of what I've spent the rest of my life on evolving – a therapeutic community. When we first saw these people, we soon realised that they were quite outside our previous clinical experience, and that our training to date wasn't much use. So we more or less taught ourselves as we went along.

The war was over and an atmosphere of change was in the air. We all wanted an end to wars and a better world for everyone, including the disadvantaged. The idea of accepting another challenge was appealing to us, especially as it was in a sort of 'no man's land' between medicine, social work, social psychology and economics.

We had a well balanced team of mental health professionals, including three psychiatrists, and were housed in a decrepit old building which was once a workhouse. The main hospital had been Sutton EMS Hospital during the war. It was now known as a neurosis centre, and the personnel there clearly disapproved of our proximity as well as our clinical outlook.

BB *What period are we speaking of?*

MJ   I'm talking about the 12 years I spent at Belmont, later called Henderson Hospital, from 1947 to 1959. We continued to evolve the community and group methods we had started during the war and relied increasingly on inputs from the 100 clients or 'patients' of both sexes for help. Most of them came from the very poor areas of London and had never known a stable or supportive home or social environment.

Psychiatry tends to label these people as sociopaths or psychopaths. I'd prefer to see them as anomalies of growth, probably environmentally determined. Unlike the mentally retarded with low IQs, these people were emotionally retarded.

Our aim was to create an environment conducive to social maturation. It had a 'family' atmosphere – no locked doors, no drugs, first names only (staff and patients), and an essentially democratic social structure.

BB *How did you set about that?*

MJ   We opened up communication of thoughts and feelings at our daily community meetings of all 100 patients and about a dozen staff. These were followed by small group meetings of around 10 patients with a staff leader.

What evolved has come to be called a therapeutic community. We aroused considerable interest in psychiatric circles, in this country, the USA and some countries in Europe – Scandinavia in particular. In fact, treatment facilities calling themselves 'therapeutic communities' are now commonplace, but often bear little resemblance to the original model.

Henderson Hospital has continued to evolve as a treatment centre for character disorders to this day, under the leadership of Dr Stuart Whiteley, and is spearheading a specific training programme in this field.

BB *What happened next?*

MJ   After 12 years at the Henderson, I needed a change and was glad to accept a teaching post in California, at Stanford University. There was much interest in therapeutic communities in the USA, and we had been given the Isaac Ray Award by the American Psychiatric Association in 1959 for our work in this field.

BB *Did you stay in America?*

MJ   I stayed for four years before returning to the UK. After the year at Stanford, I was offered a teaching post at Oregon State Hospital. I was eager to demonstrate that a therapeutic community was relevant to any psychiatric facility and not just in relation to character disorders. I went to Salem, the capital town, and stayed for three years, in which time a large traditional mental hospital was transformed to one which showed most of the characteristics of a democratic system. It would have been an impossible transition, but for the support of a very liberal Medical Director, Dr Dean Brooks.

BB *Why did you leave Oregon?*

MJ   What happened has become all too familiar an experience to me or anyone else attempting to be a change agent. Although the democratic system we were developing helped staff and patient morale, as well as treatment results, the new freedoms signalled dangerous signs of change to the conservative, hierarchical forces in psychiatry, in politics, public opinion, big business, and bureaucracy generally.

Disapproval emanated from the Governor's office, which unfortunately was situated near the hospital. Rumour, misinformation, and prejudice followed. I was made to feel that I was no longer welcome and it was hinted that I was a Communist!

A suggestion from Professor Morris Carstairs in Edinburgh that Dingleton Hospital in Melrose, Scotland, would soon become vacant proved to be an irresistible temptation. Nowhere could a social ecological approach to treatment and prevention be more likely to succeed than in this the first 'open' mental hospital in the English-speaking world, thanks to the pioneering work of Dr George Bell.

BB   And you went to Dingleton?

MJ   I was there from 1962 to 1969 and was able to satisfy myself that a traditional, autocratic mental hospital could become an open system, given time and sanctions from above. Clinically, this was the most creative period of my life and I have tried to describe the process of change over a period of seven years in a book of that name.

BB   Is The Process of Change published in this country?

MJ   Yes, by Routledge & Kegan Paul in 1982. I left Dingleton because I was nearing retirement age and, seeing no chance for further work in the UK, I returned to the US, having been offered a teaching post at Fort Logan Mental Health Center in Denver, Colorado and later a clinical Professorship at the University of Colorado.

BB   What do you feel about present-day psychiatry?

MJ   We seem to have regressed from the pioneering days of the post-war era and especially the 1950s and 1960s, when much of the excitement and change in social psychiatry stemmed from the mental hospitals, rather than the universities.

Men like T. P. Rees at Warlingham, Rudolph Freudenberg at Netherne, Denis Martin at Claybury, Duncan McMillan at Mapperly, David Clark at Fulbourn, Thomas Beaton of Portsmouth, B. M. Mandelbrote and B. Pomryn at Littlemore virtually created the field of social psychiatry.

It seems to me that both in the UK and the US, a rather dreary conformity predominates now and the abuse of power persists largely unchallenged. I know this will sound too extreme a view to many psychiatrists. But in an age when enormous changes are occurring in Western Society, whether technological or cultural, we in mental health are contributing far too little to the humanisation of our hospitals and social systems generally.

BB   Could you explain that statement further?

MJ   Take the authority structure in most mental health facilities. The doctor usually remains dominant and makes the final decisions. His skills are essentially organic and clinical, with little exposure to, or training in social systems, communication theory, learning theory, or the behavioural sciences generally. As a result, staff morale is often poor, with resulting high turnover and absentee rates.

It saddens me to see more interest in systems for change in at least some businesses where enterprising firms are re-examining their entire operation – their roles, role relationships, authority structure, values, attitudes, and beliefs. Everyone in their employ is being given a new importance and an opportunity to communicate and contribute to change and progress. If all this can happen in the name of profit, surely we have a similar responsibility to attempt to change hospital and medical systems generally in the cause of humanism.

BB *What exactly does that mean?*

MJ I find that nowadays, mental hospitals are unhappy places, with frustrated staff and relatively neglected patients. Compared with the 1950s and 1960s, these institutions seem not to be going forward or evolving. There are exceptions, of course, including therapeutic communities like Dingleton, Henderson, The Cassel Hospital, Fulbourn, etc. But cross-fertilisation with traditional facilities, including the universities, is rare.

On the positive side, Henderson Hospital and others have evolved a Therapeutic Community Association, which is developing training programmes in open systems theory and practice. These are organised by Graeme Farquharson, a social worker, and others. The *International Journal of Therapeutic Communities*, edited by Bob Hinshelwood, helps to integrate people who are interested in this approach on an international scale, and Dr Stuart Whiteley organises an annual conference at Windsor, which attracts many people from Europe and some from the US.

BB *Have you anything further you'd like to say?*

MJ I'd like to summarise how my work with open systems and therapeutic communities has shaped my own personal philosophy. I feel that the striving for freedom and peaceful conflict resolution which characterised much of our immediate post-war thinking became epitomised in the therapeutic community movement.

We played an important part in the evolution of social psychiatry, which helped us to see the importance of social ecology and the lessons we must learn from nature. These liberal qualities then became confluent with the social evolution in the Western countries, beginning in the 1960s, which is still gaining momentum. As Capra, a distinguished physicist, points out, we seem to have reached a 'turning point', where the familiar reductivist scientific approach to learning and growth is being implemented by an integration of Eastern and Western cultures and a new conceptual framework for economics, technology, physics, and medicine.

In a more specifically Western context, there are numerous cultural movements, including environmentalists, feminists, consumer advocates, peace movements, and many others. Part of this changing climate of public opinion is the growing disenchantment with the abuse of authority by the professions such as law and medicine and by government generally.

In this context, politicians seem to be more concerned with the retention of power than with societies' individual needs. If we consider a hospital to be a microcosm of society, then a therapeutic community is associated with all the foregoing problems of social structure, decentralisation, information-sharing, and shared decision-making at all levels of the social organisation from patients to governing bodies.

In the therapeutic community movement, we have come to have a deep distrust of reductivism in the form of scientific research, unless it is linked with a humanistic orientation and subject to constant discussion and recycling, with a view to achieving consensus with all the participants. We are not afraid of social values which highlight morality and the need to keep a constant check on the abuse of power. We evolved a democratic system which inevitably clashed with the more authoritarian and technocratic systems in other psychiatric facilities and in our surrounding environment, dominated by professional tradition, rationalism, and secularism.

At the same time, we became conscious of the effects resulting from our change from an individualistic society to one with a group identity. We began to experience new strength and a feeling of security, which was badly needed to combat the constant attempts to liquidate us which came from our own profession. This empathy among staff and patients was the start of a growing synergism, and we began to comment on our feeling of fulfilment, which at first as individuals we were at a loss to explain.

We even dared to recognise a growing spirituality, which helped us to explore new dimensions of consciousness such as intuition and the motivating driving force. Our group consciousness and open system organisation seemed to have something more than the aggregate wisdom of a number of people with their individual inputs and good will. In effect, it was synergistic and creative.

It is in this context that the therapeutic community has relevance. Its survival as a model for change, its positive healthy effect on the people involved, its answer to the abuse of power by delegation of responsibility and authority to the level in the system where it belongs, its conceptual framework of multiple leadership, social learning, growth, and creativity reflects one approach to the cultural dilemma of our time.

The general principles worked out in a microcosm of society, a hospital, can be applied to all levels of our cosmic society, if adapted to the culture and social environment as required.

It has taken me forty years to arrive at this point as one individual with, I hope, many peers who epitomise this spirit of change, which seems to grow daily everywhere. Can the gradual metamorphosis to holism be speeded up in time to prevent an atomic holocaust or famine on a world scale?

5 Edward Hare

Interviewed by BRIAN BARRACLOUGH (1984)

Dr Edward Hare, MA, MD (Cantab) 1943, FRCP 1961, FRCPsych (Foundation) 1971. Dr Hare was born in 1917 at Stoke-on-Trent, the third son of a Church of England clergyman. He studied at University College Hospital during the War, and qualified MB, BChir in 1943. Because of chronic middle ear disease, he was considered unfit for military service. Dr Hare began his psychiatric career at the Cardiff City Mental Hospital in 1945, and held junior posts at several county asylums. He won the Gaskell gold medal in 1953 (bronze medal 1952). He was appointed Physician at Bethlem Royal and the Maudsley Hospitals 1957. Dr Hare was editor of *The British Journal of Psychiatry* (1972–77) and Maudsley lecturer, 1982.

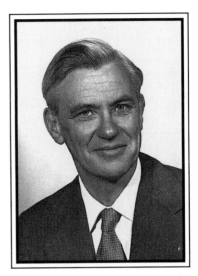

BB   *Did you come from a medical family?*

EH   No, I didn't. That's a disadvantage for a doctor, I believe. It means you lack the familiarity with medical ways of thinking which is inbred in children from doctors' families. But it may mean you come to medicine with less prejudice and are more ready to be objective about what it can do.

BB   *And your father?*

EH   He was a clergyman. In many ways, of course, a clergyman's work is not very different from a psychiatrist's. But he died when I was 13 and I greatly missed his guiding hand.

BB   *What determined your choice of medicine?*

EH   Probably my mother's wish that one of her children should be a doctor. My mother lived into her nineties and had a great influence on my life. I'd wanted to be a scientist, but at Cambridge, I failed to get the double first which was needed for a research job in the Biochemistry Department there. So I went to the counsellor on careers and accepted his advice to become a medical student.

BB   *What happened after that?*

EH   My clinical training was at University College Hospital, London, where I was fortunate in having eminent teachers – Sir Thomas Lewis, Sir Harold Himsworth, Sir Max Rosenheim, and the neurologist Sir Francis Walshe. Walshe was – and has remained – my image of the ideal physician. He was kind, suave, and witty, and had many caustic things to say about psychoanalysis – but that didn't stop me wanting to become a psychiatrist.

BB *It must have been unusual then, to decide on psychiatry before you graduated in medicine?*

EH   As an undergraduate, I'd read some Freud. But I'd also attended a course of lectures on abnormal psychology given at Cambridge by the Canadian, John MacCurdy. He wasn't a Freudian, but I think it was the excellence of his lectures and his sound common sense which really attracted me to psychiatry.

BB *What happened after you graduated?*

EH   It seemed proper to get a good background in general medicine, so I did a number of hospital jobs – medicine, surgery, obstetrics, ophthalmology – and some locums in general practice. I would have studied for the MRCP, but was advised this wasn't necessary for someone who only wanted to be a mental hospital doctor.

So I spent my spare time reading literature – *Don Quixote, Paradise Lost, Don Juan, The Decline & Fall.* Looking back, I think this was more help to me than the Membership would have been, as it taught me to write English and appreciate good prose. I loved Gibbon's irony, and have often felt his comment on the virtues of the clergy could be equally applied to doctors.

BB *What was your first experience of psychiatry?*

EH   As a houseman at the Cardiff City Mental Hospital (now Whitchurch Hospital): the hospital, where John Hennelly was superintendent, was well-known for the research done in its biochemistry department, but that department was closed at the time I came. When my six months was up, I had difficulty finding another job. I'd been unfit for war service (from deafness), and priority was understandably being given to doctors discharged from the armed forces.

But eventually, I found a job at Brentwood Mental Hospital, Essex, where I experienced the mild rule of Geoffrey Nightingale, the stimulating conversation of Thomas Power, and the bitter winter of 1946. My next junior post was at the Berkshire County Mental Hospital (now the Fairmile). I went there because married accommodation – in short supply then – was available in nearby Wallingford, from where I cycled to work each day. The hospital was set in lovely quiet country between the Thames and the Berkshire Downs.

I had no ambitions and would have been content to spend my working life in such a place. But the problem was housing. Our landlady fell ill and we had to move. Again, it was a matter of finding a hospital with married quarters. The search led me to Springfield Hospital, Tooting.

BB *What do you think about medical superintendents, having worked under so many?*

EH   They ranged from good to bad, as one might expect – from King Log to King Stork. I enjoyed my time with the good ones and was uncomfortable with the bad ones – though how far it was they who were bad or me who was awkward, I don't know.

BB   *In what respects were they bad?*

EH   It was the fault of the system really. The requirement was for an administrator, rather than a clinician. They had too much power and were authoritarian – some were benevolent despots, some were tyrants. Once appointed, often at an early age, a superintendent was there for life. He might do good work in his first years, but later would commonly be more concerned with avoiding trouble than with new ideas.

BB   *Was there training for medical superintendents other than learning on the job?*

EH   I don't think so, although they used to get together a good deal. The Medico-Psychological Association was founded as a society for medical superintendents.

BB   *Was there training for junior staff?*

EH   None at all. They picked it up as best they could. I came into that category. I never had any formal training in psychiatry.

BB   *How did you do it then?*

EH   I didn't do it. My concern was to get the Diploma in Psychological Medicine – you got £50 a year extra on your pay for that. I studied the textbooks, but the first time I sat the exam, I was failed in the clinical by Aubrey Lewis.

BB   *What was life like for a junior doctor in a mental hospital in the 1940s?*

EH   You were given some 'chronic' wards to look after, usually the male wards, as they were thought to be easier. Your job was to prescribe sedatives and make the periodic physical and mental examinations on patients, as required by the Board of Control. You did this, conscientiously or otherwise, and noted the findings in the case-record. The note was commonly limited to the words, 'no change'.

On visiting days, you saw those relatives who were content to see a junior doctor; and you replied to relatives' letters – though the replies were vetted and signed by the superintendent.

As I recall, there were no clinical meetings, no journal clubs, no medical libraries worth the name.

But there were perks, even for juniors. The food was good – free milk, cream, vegetables – and post-war rationing went unnoticed. It was a quiet, pleasant, dull life, still very much in the old asylum tradition.

BB   *What happened after Springfield?*

EH   I never wanted to work in London – too noisy and dirty – so I looked for another country hospital. My colleague Desmond Pond (we'd been students together at UCH) told me of the research going on at Barrow Hospital, Bristol. Barrow was then a country cousin of the old Bristol City Mental Hospital (Fishponds). It had been built in the countryside just before the war, with plenty of space, set among green fields and woods – and the lodge-keeper's cottage was vacant. So I applied for a post there.

BB   *As a senior registrar?*

EH   Yes, at first. Later, I was promoted to SHMO. The pay was meagre, the status not very grand, but it was a secure job. Security of tenure was important to me, as I didn't always get on with my superintendents.

BB *How long did you stay?*

EH   About three years. Barrow was a progressive hospital. There was a research department, a good medical library, and the occasional clinical conference.

BB *Was that the result of a progressive medical superintendent?*

EH   Yes. He was Robert Hemphill, later to become a professor in South Africa. A bit of a tartar in some ways, but he had an enterprising mind, was a good administrator, and encouraged research. I was able to do my MD thesis there.

BB *What was your thesis?*

EH   The subject I put forward to my Regius Professor was 'What do patients think about their stay in a mental hospital?' But he suggested a broader subject, 'The ecology of mental disease', choosing that title perhaps because a professor of ecology had just been appointed at Cambridge.

I think his use of the word 'ecology' was a bad one. It should have been 'epidemiology'. Ecology deals with the relation between an organism and its environment and can't properly be applied to diseases. All one had to do for a Cambridge MD was to review the literature and write up some case histories. But I found it a terrible struggle and almost despaired. My wife had to shut me up in the study and not let me out till I'd finished.

I was awarded an MD, and then it occurred to me to submit part of my thesis for one of the £10 prizes offered by the RMPA. Some months later, I was surprised to receive page proofs of this, as an article for the *Journal*. I'd never thought of submitting it for publication, but was very pleased. That started me off. As Byron says:

> 'Tis pleasant sure to see one's name in print;
> A book's a book although there's nothing in't.

BB *That was your first substantial study?*

EH   Yes. It led me to be interested in epidemiology and also in the writings of 19th-century psychiatrists such as D. H. Tuke.

BB *And after your MD?*

EH   My chief concern was to get a consultant post and be better paid. I tried for several, without success. Then, in the hope of improving my chances, I studied hard and sat for the Gaskell medal – in 1953. The number of entrants was small in those years and the papers not noticeably more difficult than the DPM, so the chances for anyone who'd worked hard were quite good. I was awarded the prize, jointly with the late Dick Pratt. Then, after one or two more attempts, I got a consultant post, at Warlingham Park Hospital.

The superintendent there, Percy Rees, had become renowned for his enlightened policies. He aimed to make his hospital a pleasant place for long-stay patients to live out their lives, and he used to tell them the fence round the ground wasn't to keep them in, but to keep other people out.

His first act as superintendent was to open the main gates, and they were kept open thereafter. He ordered – what was thought very risky – that the wards for 'suicidal' patients should be unlocked and the patients sent out on working parties in the grounds. He was a kind, benevolent Welshman, who encouraged his staff and made his consultants feel the importance of their rank.

BB   How long did you stay at Warlingham?

EH   Rees retired soon after I came and Stephen MacKeith took over. I was settling down to a quiet life when one day I was amazed to get a letter from Professor Lewis, asking me to see him at the Maudsley. When I got there, he said at once he wanted me to apply for a vacant consultant job. I protested that I felt quite unequipped, but he said he'd liked the papers I'd published and didn't think there was anyone he'd put up for a job at the Maudsley who had failed to get it. Encouraged by this, I duly applied and was appointed. I believe I was the first member of the staff not to have been trained there.

BB   And that was when?

EH   1957. Lewis certainly took a gamble.

BB   Would you like to say something about Aubrey Lewis?

EH   I admired him immensely. His scholarly and rigorous approach was what was needed then; his influence on British psychiatry – on world psychiatry – was profound. People said he was too sceptical, but I didn't think so. Because hard facts are so few in psychiatry, there's a constant flow of vague, hopeful hypotheses, and these need to be met with proper scepticism or they'd soon swamp the place. As he used to say, scepticism is only the wish to look more closely.

BB   So you feel he was an influence for the good?

EH   Oh, undoubtedly. Looking back, I think he may have been wrong in wanting to exclude undergraduate teaching and in stopping consultants having part-time appointments at other teaching hospitals. I used to wish we'd had medical students at the Maudsley. They're not committed to a speciality and often have fresh and original ideas. Postgraduates may be more knowledgeable but – as in much of medicine – their originality tends to be stifled by the need to pass higher exams.

BB   How did you find the change when Sir Aubrey retired and Sir Denis Hill became professor?

EH   I think Sir Denis felt that part of his task was to redress the balance from Lewis's sceptical and biological approach. No doubt that was a fair way of seeing it. But to my mind, the balance was swung too far. Hill championed the psychotherapists and wanted to create a school of psychotherapy at the Maudsley. He once said to me – I could hardly believe my ears – that he thought psychoanalysis the most important part of psychiatry. But he was sound on clinical matters and had quite outstanding gifts as a committee man.

BB   At the Maudsley, you were in the same post throughout?

EH   I was there 25 years, full-time NHS, and retired at 65.

BB *It's unusual for an NHS consultant to be as productive as you have been in writing.*

EH   The stimulus came from Aubrey Lewis, who told me, when I was appointed, that I should be able to devote half my time to research. I kept that in mind, and after a few years, started to take a research day each week. Some of my colleagues were a little surprised by this, I think; but in later years, when my clinical commitments were less, I used to take two days.

BB *Could we now turn from your career to your clinical experience? What, to your mind, have been the most notable changes in clinical phenomena, comparing today's cases with those you saw at first?*

EH   My strong impression is that patients are not as ill as they used to be. In the 1940s, there were many patients with advanced degrees of what was called 'dementia'. And there were patients with severe chronic catatonia – I remember one who slept with his head raised off the pillow and had done that for 20 years, the nurses said. I don't think such cases are common now. Schizophrenia and manic–depression seem to run a milder course.

BB *Milder? In what ways?*

EH   Both in symptoms and prognosis. I can remember cases of 'acute delirious mania'. I saw many patients admitted with acute schizophrenia who didn't improve and became so 'demented' within two or three months that their discharge was impossible. It may, of course, be just a matter of what cases you happen to see, but I don't think that sort of deterioration occurs much now. The change to milder cases is commonly put down to better treatment, but I think there's good evidence that this is not the only reason.

BB *What evidence?*

EH   Professor Ødegård[1], for instance, showed that the prognosis of schizophrenia improved steadily in Norway between 1920 and 1960 – so it was happening before insulin coma or ECT, or the phenothiazines came in. He also found that the incidence of schizophrenia, in terms of first admissions, was decreasing. Manfred Bleuler[2] says the prognosis of schizophrenia in Switzerland improved during the 1940s, and he didn't think it was due to drug treatment. Others have found much the same.

BB *What can be the explanation?*

EH   I think many diseases – perhaps all – vary a good deal in their signs and prognosis over the years, for reasons which aren't clear. There may be changes in the virulence of infectious agents or in host resistance. In medicine, treatments tend to change as much from fashion as from improvements in efficacy. And it shouldn't be forgotten that if a disease is getting milder from 'natural' causes, the efficacy of treatment will appear to increase.

---

1. ØDEGÅRD, O. (1967) Changes in the prognosis of functional psychosis since the days of Kraepelin. *British Journal of Psychiatry*, **113**, 818–22.
2. BLEULER, M. (1978) *The Schizophrenic Disorders*. (Translated from the German (1972) by S. M. Clemens.) Yale University Press.

BB *Do you think the symptoms and signs of illness which are taught in the books correspond to those that we see now? Some texts are based on observations made on patients a long time ago.*

EH   If the manifestations of a disease are changing, then any textbook description will become out of date. I think psychiatric illnesses are apt to change quicker than other kinds, because their manifestations are more dependent on social factors. I also suspect that the manifestations of any psychiatric illness vary from place to place. If these things are so, then it's hard to provide a description which is valid for long or valid for different countries.

The danger of textbooks, as I see it, is that they easily lead a student to see his cases in terms of what the books say he ought to see. If the description doesn't match what he sees, then he may Procrusteanise his judgement, or lose confidence in himself. But he should remember that it's his teachers who may be out of date.

BB *What do you think of the Present State Examination?*

EH   I never had much experience in the use of structured questionnaires. They are entirely proper for a particular research, of course, but I had reservations about their use in clinical work.

A structured questionnaire may introduce an inappropriate rigidity into a clinical interview, and it may contain leading questions which prompt a perhaps bemused patient towards certain answers. I could rarely bring myself, for example, to ask about the 'first rank symptoms' of schizophrenia: they seemed to me altogether too curious. Instead, I came to think a patient's answers to questions were of minor importance – he might not have understood the question in the way it was intended, or he might have chosen to answer in a way which suited him.

The best clinical guide is not the way a patient answers questions, but the way he behaves – as you observe him or as told to you by a fond relative.

BB *Let us turn to the British Journal of Psychiatry. When did you become editor?*

EH   In 1973, when Eliot Slater decided to retire after a ten-year stint.

BB *You were elected?*

EH   It was the first time an election for editor had been held under College rules.

BB *What do you think of electing an editor?*

EH   At the time, I thought it wrong. I thought an editor should be appointed by Council, because most members with a right to vote probably wouldn't know much about the candidates.

BB *But the editor is also an Officer of the College, so that might be one reason why election was decided on. And perhaps another reason was that some previous editors were thought to have stayed too long.*

EH   I think the ten-year period now laid down by the College is about right.

BB *How many years did you serve?*

EH   About four and a half, and then didn't seek re-election. I found myself over-worked. The editorship of a monthly journal is a hard job for a man with a full-time clinical commitment – and for a time, I was also chairman of the Medical Committee at the Maudsley.

BB   Do you think it right the NHS should subsidise the College in paying for the editor's time?

EH   There seemed no other way then. College finances would have made it impossible to appoint a paid editor.

BB   What kind of shape did you find the Journal in when you became editor?

EH   A ship sailing steadily along. Under Slater, the *Journal* had improved both in scientific quality and in prestige. It changed from six issues a year to a monthly production, at a time when I think Slater had retired from clinical work. But the honorary editor of a monthly, who still has clinical duties, will be under much pressure unless he can devolve the work-load. You yourself were kind enough to relieve me of some of the strain.

BB   You were the first editor who paid serious attention to the business side of the Journal.

EH   At the Council meeting I attended after my appointment, someone suggested the new editor should look into the *Journal* finances. As I've always liked dealing with figures I was quite ready to do that.

The accounts of our advertising manager were routinely sent to the editor, and I studied these. But it was only after some months that I found that our printers sent accounts to the Treasurer's department, which were not shown to the editor. I asked to see these, and immediately recognised that the cost of printing advertisements was greater than our receipts from the advertisers – in other words, that the *Journal* was paying to carry its advertisements. Looking back over the past records, I found the *Journal* had been losing some £2,000 a year on advertising over a ten-year period.

Our advertising manager knew nothing of our printing costs and had been increasing the advertising rates on a routine basis. We appointed a new agency, whose manager proved altogether more efficient.

BB   That wasn't the only financial aspect you looked at?

EH   No; it led me to look more generally at the *Journal* finances. I found that about half the recent losses were due to advertisements and the rest was partly because printing costs had risen steeply – faster than inflation – and partly because the increases in the *Journal* subscription rate hadn't kept pace with inflation. I saw, too, there were various ways of economising – for example, by reducing the weight of the *Journal* paper (lighter paper costs less to buy, less to print on, and less for postage). But all this was only half the battle.

Over many years – indeed, since the 1860s – the annual reports of our Association contain a debit sum under the heading 'the cost of the *Journal*'. When I first suggested to the Journal Committee that the *Journal* might make a profit for the College, the idea was not well received. Longstanding members thought it sounded too business-like for a learned society and feared a profit might attract the attention of the tax-man.

Just then, however, the College was in some financial straits, and it was agreed the *Journal* accounts might reasonably show a surplus rather than a deficit. In the event, and in the circumstances of the time, the *Journal* became a useful source of revenue. This seems entirely proper to me. The *Journal* acquired its prestige and readership as the result of generations of hard work by its honorary editorial teams. The College, which owns and administers the *Journal*, should profit from this historical asset.

BB Did you enjoy your time as editor?

EH   I wish I could say yes, but I was so busy all the time. Perhaps it was my fault for being over-conscientious.

BB Should the arrangement of an unpaid honorary editor be continued?

EH   Perhaps; but if so, the editor should have had previous experience of journal or book production. I came with no such experience, and though this perhaps meant I came with a fresh mind, I made some mistakes from ignorance. Dr Crammer, my successor, had had quite a lot of experience, and I expect this was a help to him. Our present editor has also had previous experience.

BB Another approach might be for the Journal to be produced by a publishing firm.

EH   When I was editor, we were approached by a well-known firm to take over publication. I looked into the finances of such a deal, and although life would have been easier for the editor, it clearly wouldn't have been to the financial advantage of the College – at least not at that time, when we'd begun making a profit. But there's always something to be said for handing over publication to people who have special experience.

BB How do you think the Journal compares with other journals in the field?

EH   I've often heard it said our *Journal* was one of the most respected of its kind – but that may be only self-praise or propaganda. Yet our *Journal* has certainly had a long and honourable history – age hasn't withered it – and I'd say we're preserving our honour satisfactorily.

BB Have you read the very early issues of the Journal?

EH   I'm familiar with them. In the 19th century, there were some extraordinarily able British psychiatrists, who wrote excellent articles and fine textbooks – and of a literary standard which I'm not sure we've been able to match.

BB And their subject matter?

EH   Not very different from today's, in essence. The early issues of a hundred years ago are full of sound stuff by the standards then. Nowadays, there's more statistics, control, and technical equipment, but I don't think there's been any real change in quality.

BB Let's turn from the Journal to your research. You did some drug trials?

EH   I was concerned to publish articles so as to improve my chances of a consultancy, and the scientific aspect of the controlled trial appealed to me. By modern standards, though, my studies would seem naive.

BB Did you discover anything of importance?

EH   Two things – at least they seemed important to me. First, controlled trials clearly showed that sedatives sedate and hypnotics help you sleep. Second, the other drugs I tested showed little or no advantage over a placebo. I concluded, for instance, that antidepressant drugs were effective only by virtue of their sedative effect.

BB *Do you still hold that?*

EH   Yes, but I continued to prescribe tricyclic antidepressants because they seemed to have one remarkably useful property. Unlike most sedatives, they didn't cause dependence.

BB *You were involved in a lithium trial?*

EH   With Alec Coppen, Ronnie Maggs, and others. I think it was the first test of lithium prophylaxis by a controlled, prospective trial. It was well organised and produced a clear result. But one should always be cautious of accepting positive results from drug trials, because that's the result everyone hopes for.

BB *You had reservations about the findings?*

EH   I was the more ready to accept them because they were the opposite of what I'd expected. I'd thought that in the absence of any sedative effect, the findings would be negative.

BB *Did you have doubts about the long-term value of lithium?*

EH   There were a number of reports of damage to the kidney and liver. But there was also the problem of the 'lithium clinic'. Patients attended year after year and often saw a different doctor each time. It became hard to tell if they continued to benefit. And there seemed to me a danger of the patients becoming dependent on the hospital – some patients like having a regular hospital appointment, but it's not necessarily to their benefit.

BB *You also looked at reserpine?*

EH   Reserpine is interesting because it may have been responsible for the myth (as I take it to be) that antidepressants take a week or two for their effects to begin. When reserpine was introduced for hypertension, its full effect took two or three days to develop. This, I think, led the people who did the first trials of reserpine in anxiety to wait a week or two before assessing the effect, so as to be on the safe side that the drug had had time to act. Now if, in conditions like anxiety or depression, you claim a drug takes some weeks to act, then any natural improvement which occurs during that time can be put down to the drug. The purely sedative action of antidepressants comes on within a few hours, of course.

BB *Did you see any reserpine depressions?*

EH   I was inclined to think that was another myth. People with hypertension may become depressed, with or without a drug, and I don't recall any controlled trial being done. Patients receiving a new drug are studied carefully and any untoward change may be put down to it.

BB *You have a reputation as a sceptical physician. Do you think that's the reason you looked into compliance?*

EH   On an occasion when the merits of a drug were being extolled, I said no one could be sure how far patients took the drugs prescribed for them. I was scoffed at, so I thought I'd try to see what really happened. Urine testing seemed a fairly reliable method, and our findings suggested that both for in-patients and out-patients, about 50% weren't taking their drugs as prescribed.

BB *Do you think concern with compliance is an outcome of having effective drugs?*

EH It represents an advance in medical objectivity and a concern with economics – but it also revealed a wise provision of nature: patients don't always take their pills. Doctors tend to over-prescribe, especially in an age of high-pressure salesmanship, and don't always consider the long-term risks.

BB *Shall we turn from drugs to epidemiology? You made a study in Croydon.*

EH Yes, encouraged by Aubrey Lewis, who thought epidemiology might yield valuable results for psychiatry. We set out to study what were called 'the new-town blues'. The sociologists believed that poor social facilities were the cause of much neurotic illness in new towns. We compared a population on a new estate in Croydon with one in an old part, using a variety of indices of neurosis. The two groups showed no difference.

BB *Were you pleased with the study?*

EH Many other people made similar studies, and on the whole, found the same thing. This suggested an alternative to the sociologists' explanation. It suggested that the incidence of neurotic complaints might be much the same in any comparable populations, but because new towns were then in the news, the complaints of people who lived there got publicity.

BB *How do you think that fits in with Professor George Brown's view of 'life events' causing mental illness?*

EH My own view is that life events don't cause psychiatric illness, though they may precipitate symptoms in those who Lord Taylor has called the weaker brethren. My guess is that most psychiatric illnesses are due to genetic or physical causes, and that much of neurosis and psychopathy is the consequence of constitutional damage in early life – from injury, toxins, infection, or poor diet.

BB *You published papers on birth order and birth month?*

EH I liked doing research and writing papers; though not being an academic, I never had any research training. And as I was unlucky – or inept – at getting grants, I had to choose subjects which could be done on a shoestring budget – or on no budget at all. But I was fortunate indeed in my collaborators, among whom were John Price, Eliot Slater, and Pat Moran.

In the early 1960s, there were three interesting problems about schizophrenia. Was there any association between schizophrenia and birth order, or birth month, or maternal age? Several studies had found schizophrenia commoner among later-born. We repeated these – it was easy to get the facts from the case notes – and found the same thing. But partly perhaps because of the large size of our samples, we were able to suggest that the findings could all be attributed to an artefact. The argument was a bit complex, but I think it is being accepted now.

For birth-month, we were able to get very large samples from the national Mental Health Survey, and confirmed other findings that schizophrenics tended to be born in the winter, and we were also able to show this wasn't so in neurosis and personality disorder. There's no convincing explanation yet, but an environmental cause remains a possibility. When our papers on birth-month first appeared, quite a number of people asked me if I was interested in astrology. Partly in self-defence, I made a study of the history of medical astrology and read a paper on it at the Royal Society of Medicine. I concluded there was a close parallel between astrology and psychoanalysis.

BB *You were the editor of the Statistical Reports of the Bethlem and Maudsley Hospitals.*

EH   These reports had been started by C. P. Blacker in 1946. They gave an analysis of in-patient and out-patient numbers by sex, age, diagnosis and so on. One of the conditions of my appointment to the Maudsley – though not a serious one – was that I should take over the production of these reports. I did so for 15 years, and then felt I'd done enough.

BB *Have they been continued?*

EH   No – at least not in the same way. The hospital changed so much that our old way of presenting them became out of date.

BB *Do you think they had some value?*

EH   There was a belief, after the war, that keeping such statistical registers would be useful both for administrators and researchers. Ours had some value for the hospital when it wasn't changing too fast, and I think they retain some value as historical records. But routine statistics are double-edged. They're easily misconstrued, and a clinician may fear an administrator will use them for his own ends.

BB *You've written papers on unusual subjects – masturbatory insanity, for example?*

EH   I once heard an old charge nurse say of a backward patient that he'd never recover because he masturbated. This struck me as odd and led me to study the literature. The belief that masturbation caused insanity was firmly held during most of the 19th century (it was held by Maudsley, for example) – a classic example of confusing the rules of health with the rules of morality. Immoral behaviour is sometimes a sign of impending illness, but rarely a cause.

BB *Did you have many requests for that paper?*

EH   Rather few, as I remember. I thought it had fallen on deaf ears – or on covered ears. And I'd had difficulty getting it published. Fleming rejected it and so did the editor of *Medical History*, but then Slater took it. As I'd had the same difficulty with a paper I wrote on the history of GPI, I turned back to more ordinary subjects.

BB *Talking of memory, I remember your lecture on Faraday's loss of memory.*

EH   He was my childhood hero, my ideal of what a scientist ought to be. I liked reading about him, and then came across a manuscript account by his doctor of the short illness he had at the age of 45. It was after that illness that he always complained of a bad memory. I studied the evidence and concluded he'd probably had an ischaemic cerebral attack. But it didn't quite add up – ischaemic attacks don't usually cause an amnesic syndrome – and I don't think I made a real contribution.

BB   Talking of mental problems of the famous, you've written about Virginia Woolf?

EH   Only a review of a book about her.

BB   Did you form an opinion about her mental health?

EH   It seemed clear to me, from Quentin Bell's[3] excellent biography and from other sources, that she was cyclothymic and suffered attacks of atypical mania and depression. One unusual feature was the physical symptoms she had during her illnesses – palpitations, tremor, pallor. As a child, she'd had a severe attack of whooping cough, said to have left her a changed person. That might have been why her psychosis was atypical. But the diagnosis of manic–depression is supported by her family history.

BB   May I turn to an aspect of your own health? You suffer from migraine?

EH   I get a well-developed fortification spectrum, but not much head-ache. It occurred to me to map the spectrum – the semi-circle of lights – on a piece of paper to see how fast it expanded and how long it lasted. I did this for a number of attacks, though I had to force myself each time. To my surprise, I found the expansion rate was logarithmic and the duration always the same (about 21 minutes). That wasn't what the textbooks said, so I enlisted the help of some 25 volunteers (through the newsletter of the Migraine Society), who agreed to time their own attacks. In those whose spectrum was 'typical' (most were), their observations confirmed my own.

BB   What about sociobiology, a fashionable subject? You reviewed Edward Wilson's book.

EH   A fine book, I thought. He set out to base the study of social behaviour in animals, including man, strictly in terms of biology. That seems to me the only scientific basis there is for sociology, which otherwise becomes a tool of politics or religion.

BB   That leads us on to your remarks about social anxiety, which I found attractive. What did you mean by social anxiety?

EH   It always seemed to me there were two sorts of anxiety – about one's physical health and about one's social standing. I was led to write a paper on this (as my contribution to the Festschrift for Eliot Slater) from reading that remarkable book by Keith Thomas, *Religion and the Decline of Magic.*[4]

It describes how in 17th-century England, people resorted to advice from priests and astrologers when they had personal problems or worries, and how in the past 100 years, such people have turned increasingly to doctors, especially psychiatrists. But there's no reason to think psychiatrists deal better with such problems than anyone else.

I took the view that the best way in which our society could meet this need for counselling would be through a profession of psychotherapy – along the lines of the Foster Report.[5]

---

3. BELL, Q. (1972) *Virginia Woolf: A Biography.* London: Hogarth Press.
4. THOMAS, K. (1971) *Religion and the Decline of Magic.* London: Weidenfeld and Nicholson.
5. FOSTER, J. G. (1971) *Enquiry into the Practice and Effects of Scientology.* London: HMSO.

BB   Would you include in this osteopaths, chiropractors, acupuncturists?

EH   Oh no. The aim would be discussion and advice. There are people who have a natural talent for these things. They should be, and would want to be the members of a psychotherapy profession – which would be quite independent of medicine, though no doubt some psychiatric knowledge would be relevant.

BB   Do you think there are any effective treatments in psychiatry?

EH   Treatment is a difficult word. It covers everything from a quick prescription to years of psychoanalysis. Treatments tend to come and go, and our concern should be to find out if a new treatment is better, quicker, or safer than the last one. There are many treatments which temporarily allay the severity of a psychiatric illness, thus helping the patient – or at least those who look after him.

I think the real dangers lie in long-term treatment, where unexpected toxic effects may occur. There is a too-ready presumption that if a drug helps in the short-run, it will help in the long-run too. In any case, the effect of drugs may be more on the mind than the brain.

I remember a medical officer at Springfield who secretly arranged that the nightly sedative should contain no more than a whiff of paraldehyde. All went on normally until the secret leaked out some months later.

If one believes, as I do, that psychiatric illnesses have become less severe during the past 40 years, then the advances in treatment during that time must seem distinctly modest.

But physical treatment forms only a small part of management. The most important part is nursing care. I always thought the patient's relatives were the next most important part. Relatives are a long-suffering lot, too often held to blame. They've put up with a difficult or distressed person before his admission, and may well have to do so again after his discharge. If a doctor shows them appropriate sympathy and comfort, this will rebound to the patient's benefit.

BB   Would you like to say anything about the future of psychiatry?

EH   For over 60 years, psychiatrists have been taught, and have largely believed the Freudian theory of neurosis. Most of us don't believe it now, but what will replace it? There's no clear line between neurosis and normality, and neurotic symptoms are much influenced by the theories about them.

Just after the war, a nationwide survey of symptoms was made (by Percy Stocks)[6], and one of the questions was about constipation. A respondent who admitted to constipation was considered to show evidence of neurosis: but we wouldn't say so now.

I think the causes of neurosis will be hard to pin down, and will be discovered not by psychodynamics or sociology, but by biological study of what determines a person's constitution.

BB   And the psychoses?

EH   Psychiatry still faces what it's had to face for the past 200 years – the fact that nothing useful is known about what causes the common serious illnesses we now call schizophrenia and affective psychosis. We don't know how to prevent them and treatment is still largely palliative. The discovery of their causes remains the principal goal of psychiatric research.

6. STOCKS, P. (1949) *Sickness in the Population of England and Wales, 1944–47.* London: HMSO.

6 David Clark

Interviewed by BRIAN BARRACLOUGH (1985)

Dr David Clark, MB ChB 1943, MA (Cantab) 1946, DPM 1949, MD 1967, FRCP Edin 1958, PhD (Cantab) 1972, FRCPsych (Foundation) 1971. Dr Clark, born in 1920, was brought up in Edinburgh. He served in the Royal Army Medical Corps from 1943–46 as a parachute medical officer in Northern Europe and the Far East. He trained in psychiatry at Edinburgh from 1947–50 under Sir David Henderson and the Maudsley from 1950–53. He had a personal analysis and trained in group analytic psychotherapy with S. H. Foulkes. In 1953 he went to Cambridge as Medical Superintendent at Fulbourn Hospital and Consultant Psychiatrist at Addenbrooke's Hospital. He retired in 1983 and is currently Chairman of the University of the Third Age in Cambridge.

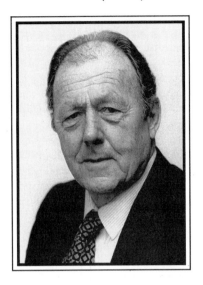

BB *Morris Carstairs says in the foreword to your book* Social Therapy in Psychiatry [1] *that you astonished your contemporaries by becoming, at 32, Medical Superintendent at Fulbourn from senior registrar at the Maudsley Hospital. Why did you do that?*

DC   There were two professional reasons – I wanted to improve the conditions of long-stay patients in the back wards of the mental hospitals, and I was fascinated by the social approaches being developed in British psychiatry then. I thought this was a chance to try them out. I knew there were the resources, in the staff of the mental hospitals, if they were given a chance to deploy them.

Of course, the prospect of consultant pay to a senior registrar with a growing family was attractive.

BB *Did you learn that at the Maudsley Hospital?*

DC   Most of it came before I got into psychiatry, in the Army, and from D. K. Henderson in Edinburgh.

BB *How did you come to learn it from the Army?*

DC   It goes back to my school days. I was at school during the thirties, and in Germany in 1935–36, and I was very frightened by Nazism. I came back from Germany saying there would be a war; the Germans were out to conquer

---

1. CLARK, D. H. (1974) *Social Therapy in Psychiatry*. Penguin. (Reissued in 1982 by Churchill Livingstone.)

the world and we would have to fight them. In 1939, the war came and I expected to become an Artillery Officer, but as I was a medical student, I was ordered to remain and complete my studies.

BB   How old were you in '39?

DC   Nineteen. By 1941, both of my best friends from school had been killed in the War – one in the Mediterranean and one in the Far East. I qualified in '43, and volunteered for the Parachutists. I got involved in the sharp end, because I wanted to do something effective quickly. They said at Crookham they wanted medical men in the Parachutists, so I went in.

I saw action in Northern Europe and in the Far East. Two things were particularly important in my service. One was the experience of the conquest of Germany. I was with the 6th Airborne Division that freed Belsen and other concentration camps.

The other was in the Far East. I was parachuted into Sumatra to a Japanese internment camp and was given instructions to take over and wait for the British Army to arrive. Three months later, there was no sign of the British Army, so I had to arrange the transport of five thousand people over the mountains to the British Army enclave on the coast.

BB   You had a command?

DC   I was sent in as a doctor, but I was the only British officer. I had to become commandant of the camp and chief liaison officer with the Japanese. It was a dangerous time. The camp was burnt to the ground two days after we left, and my colleague in the next valley was speared to death. But I got all my people out. It was these experiences that taught me of the extraordinary things that men did to one another and of the immense effect that the environment had on people. I developed a clear view of the power of social factors to help people to change, and this is what my professional life has been about.

BB   And Sir David Henderson's influence; he is not thought of as having been interested in social factors?

DC   His influence on me began when I was a medical student at Edinburgh. DK was the Professor of Psychiatry and one of the most impressive of the people that lectured to us. I found psychiatry, as he propounded it, deeply interesting because of his interest in people. He used to run an out-patient clinic in front of 150 students. Patients he had never seen before would be brought in, and he would take a case history from them, with the audience listening. You could say in a sense that it was a theatre, but it was more than that, because he and the patient became absorbed in the story that unfolded. I found this fascinating and thought that psychiatry was one of the subjects I might do. When I came back, I asked DK for a job, and did my first three years with him. The people with me were Ivor Batchelor, Kenneth McCrae, and Harry Stalker.

BB   So you did three years of postgraduate training in psychiatry with Henderson in Edinburgh and acquired the MRCP.

DC   I got the Edinburgh Membership.

BB *Was there an Edinburgh Membership in Psychiatry?*

DC   Yes, but I took it in neurology. Later, I took the University of London DPM.

BB *And then after Edinburgh?*

DC   I went to the Maudsley for three years as Registrar and Senior Registrar. I worked on the Professorial Unit under Aubrey Lewis and then in the Out-Patient Department with S. H. Foulkes. I had a personal analysis and learned a lot about psychotherapy and group psychotherapy.

The Maudsley in the early 1950s was full of the brightest and most ambitious young psychiatrists in Britain. They made an intensely competitive, but very stimulating environment. For a time, I even thought that I might stay there, and began to do some research and to write papers.

Then I was approached about the superintendent's job at the mental hospital at Cambridge. The job had been advertised and no appointment made. I didn't think it was a good job, but I wanted to get practice in facing appointment committees, so I thought, 'A trip to Cambridge, why not?' And so one March day, I came to see Fulbourn Hospital. It was an appalling asylum – locked (as they all were then) and grossly over-crowded; worse than most.

I thought, 'I can't possibly go there'; but then thought, 'they won't give me the job anyway, so why not try the interview just for the practice.' Half way through the afternoon, I realised there was a serious chance that I might be offered the job! I nearly bolted back to London, but then I thought, 'I'll give it a try and see.'

BB *What did you find when you got to Fulbourn?*

DC   A friend said he felt going out to Fulbourn was like cycling back into the nineteenth century. The same three medical gentlemen had run Fulbourn Hospital from 1925 to 1945, and one of them had remained on as superintendent until 1953. The NHS and the twentieth century made hardly an impression on the place.

BB *Whom did you succeed?*

DC   Treharne Thomas. He'd been a notable rugby player and won a Military Cross in World War I. He was a nice man, and kind, but unhappy with responsibility. He got the superintendency towards the end of his time and didn't enjoy it. The hospital was suffering from indecision at the top and poor management. It was overcrowded and demoralised. There were few student nurses and no women students at all. Of the five medical staff, three were under notice when I arrived.

BB *When was Fulbourn founded?*

DC   It was opened in October 1858 as the Cambridgeshire & Isle of Ely Pauper Lunatic Asylum. It was run by the County of Cambridgeshire, the Isle of Ely, and the Borough of Cambridge. Several active and lively men – Derek Russell Davis, Edward Beresford Davies – were working at Addenbrooke's and also at Fulbourn.

There was a lot going on in the admission wards, but the back wards had not been touched since 1939. The staff just kept things going, moderately clean and moderately humane. I applied myself to giving the nursing staff a chance to do for the patients the things they'd always wanted to do. There were quite a lot of male nurses that knew about active therapy and wanted to get the patients working, get the hospital cleaned up and opened up. They wanted to try opening the doors and seeing if it would work. What they needed was somebody who had the courage to stand by them when things went wrong, as of course, they inevitably did.

I had the most exciting and rewarding time of my life over the next nine years. In five years, we turned Fulbourn from a closed hospital to a completely open-door hospital. We got workshops going, halfway houses, we had Open Days, brought the public in, took patients out. We changed the place completely.

BB *How many mental hospitals in England had been reformed by 1953?*

DC Dingleton and Mapperley were open-door hospitals by 1953 and two or three others were a good way towards it. We joined them and moved briskly forward with them.

BB *Where did these reforming ideas come from?*

DC Various sources. It has always been known that you could open doors. Saxty-Goode did it at Littlemore in the 1930s, and it had been done in Scotland in the 1870s. The value of work for patients was known to Conolly and Pinel, and Hermann Simon had shown it again in Germany in the twenties. Much of what we did was a return to the principles of sound asylum management, known for a century. The principles had been lost in the development of 'scientific psychiatry' and in the overcrowding of the asylums during the latter part of the nineteenth century and early twentieth century.

Another source of ideas was the people who came back from the war determined to make things better. Bell at Dingleton for instance couldn't stand the squalid brutality of the old asylum. He said, 'Either I unlock the doors or I leave psychiatry'.

Then there were the sociologists – Goffman, Belknap, Dunham – who demonstrated the effects of prolonged incarceration on people, and suggested that a lot of what we called chronic schizophrenia might be due to twenty years in the environment of the back wards.

It was also partly the spirit of the times, of the Welfare State. We wanted to dismantle authoritarian, pre-War society and reform all institutions – schools, mental hospitals, hospitals, jails, and make them more humane.

BB *Do you understand what went wrong with the asylums? They started with good intentions.*

DC Fulbourn was much better in 1865 than in 1910. The history of Fulbourn, on which I am currently working, shows that clearly. The same happened in Germany, America, and France.

One element, undoubtedly, was increasing size. The asylums were made larger and larger. More and more patients were put in, but less and less money spent, so that they became impoverished, both in material standards and quality of life. Society's attitude towards unfortunates also changed. In the second half of the nineteenth century, with the influence of Social Darwinism, there was less concern for the unfortunate, and a feeling that the mad ought to be locked up.

The 1890 Act is very different from the 1845 Act, which was about running good hospitals; the 1890 Act is about locking people up. I believe doctors changed too. In the first half of the nineteenth century, a lot of gentlemen with medical degrees, such as Conolly, Kirkbride, Bucknill, and Hack Tuke wanted to improve society and were proud to work in the new asylums.

Then medicine became organised. Advances in knowledge came from strict attention to pathology and bacteriology. The doctors in the asylums, instead of going out and playing cricket with patients, sliced up the brains of deceased patients in the hope of finding the cause of schizophrenia.

BB *How did you come to be good at running things? Do you think it's inherited?*

DC   I think I learnt a lot of it in the Army. How many 26-year-olds have the chance to manage a camp containing 5000 people and then to take them out to safety?

BB *Was that your first experience of a large administrative task?*

DC   Yes.

BB *Well then, the Army couldn't have taught you how to do it.*

DC   I had small administrative tasks in the Army. The first was to take a heterogeneous group of reluctant men and turn them into a field ambulance section, to run a dressing station. Half of them were conscientious objectors and the other half were reluctant conscripts into the RAMC who found themselves together in this unit. It was my job to help them to see that our survival depended on our working together.

BB *I still don't find that a satisfactory explanation of how you come to enjoy and be confident at administering things. Perhaps you have always been well organised, and enjoyed making things work.*

DC   There may be something in my personality. I enjoy helping a group of people to find out what they want to do, and then helping them to get it done.

BB *What about your family background?*

DC   My father was a medical scientist, a pharmacologist, author of Clark's *Applied Pharmacology*.[2] He came from a Quaker family. My mother had been a teacher. We were brought up in a Quakerly way, with an emphasis on taking responsibility, thinking ahead, being orderly and planned and effective, so that certainly came from there.

BB *Did you go to a Quaker school?*

DC   No, I went to George Watson's, Edinburgh. When it became clear that I was interested in biology and fairly good at exams, my father determined that I should follow him. He got me into Watson's, which had good science teaching and arranged for me to go to Cambridge, to his old college, King's, so that I should get a medical degree.

---

2. CLARK, A. J. (1923) *Applied Pharmacology*. Churchill.

The war intervened and I had to go back to Edinburgh to do my clinical training. That was when things began to change for me; I realised that I was not going to make a medical scientist like my father.

BB *What did your father think of your choice of career?*

DC He died in 1941, before I had made my choice. He was only interested in pure scientific research. Whether I would have retained his respect as a psychiatrist, I don't know.

BB *What about others of your family?*

DC One sister, a doctor; one brother in the family firm; the other sister married a school teacher.

BB *Well, let us return to Fulbourn; had you worked in a mental hospital before?*

DC I had worked at Craig House in Edinburgh for three years. I knew all about 'bins', which was why I felt the Maudsley so unreal.

BB *What about the Social Psychiatry Research Unit?*

DC It had barely started in those days: it was much later that John Wing did such a magnificient job for those of us who are concerned about people in the back wards. But that wasn't the Maudsley in the early '50s.

BB *Can you describe what a back ward was like at Fulbourn in 1953?*

DC You were taken in by somebody with a key, who unlocked the door and then locked it behind you. The crashing of the keys in the locks was an essential part of asylum life then, just as it is today in jails. You'd be shown into a big bare room, overcrowded with people, with scrubbed floors, bare wooden tables, benches screwed to the floor, people milling around in shapeless clothing. There was a smell in the air of urine, paraldehyde, floor polish, boiled cabbage, and carbolic soap – the asylum smell.

Some wards were full of tousled, apathetic people just sitting; you'd see twenty people sitting in a row. Later, you learned that one of the reasons they were sitting in a row was that for twenty years, the nurses had been saying, 'Sit down, shut up'. Others were noisy.

The disturbed women's ward at Fulbourn was a phantasmagoric place. The women were in 'strong clothes', shapeless garments made of reinforced cotton that couldn't be torn. Many of them were in 'locked boots' which couldn't be taken off and thrown. There was nothing moveable, no knives; spoons were taken in and counted after every meal. The women all had their hair chopped off short, giving them identical wiry grey mops. As soon as you came in, they'd rush up and crowd round you. Hands would go into your pockets, grabbing at you, pulling at you, clamouring for release, for food, for anything, until they were pushed back by the sturdy nurses, who shouted at them to sit down and shut up. At the back of the ward were the padded cells, in which would be one or two naked women, smeared with faeces, shouting obscenities at anybody who came near.

If a ward was well under control, you didn't see many fights; the fights occurred after the medical staff had left. But if they were not managing very well, you'd see fights, hair pulling, screaming, with the nurses piling in on top and pulling them apart.

On some wards, there was an air of tremendous tension. You felt frightened the whole time, and watched your back. You knew there was a very real chance that somebody would try to hit you with something.

Then there were the airing courts. Grey, big courts, paved with tarmac, surrounded by a wall twelve feet high and a hundred men milling around. A few of them walking, some running, others standing on one leg, posturing, with the urine running out of their trouser leg, some sitting in a corner masturbating. A couple of bored young male nurses standing on 'point duty', looking at them, ready to hit anybody who got out of line, but otherwise not doing anything. A scene of human degradation.

BB   And what drugs were available?

DC   Paraldehyde. Barbiturates were used, but you had to be careful, because people died if you gave them too much. In an emergency, a compound injection of hyoscine and morphine was given to sedate. If it was believed a patient had been creating trouble deliberately, an intramuscular injection of paraldehyde combined sedation with punishment; it was very painful and often caused an abscess.

BB   And what did people do all day?

DC   Quieter patients often had jobs. The hospital was run by unpaid patient labour. They staffed the laundry, many workshops, the farm and garden, the kitchens, and scrubbed the corridors. At Fulbourn, there was a squad of women who scrubbed from one end of the hospital to another every week; then they scrubbed back again. Quite a lot of men worked out of the wards.

There were prestige jobs on the farm, in the gardens, in the stores, in the engineers' workshops. There were jobs enough so that the quieter, well adjusted, not too impaired patients led quite reasonable institutional lives. You didn't see them much on the wards.

The patients on the wards did nothing. The job of the staff was to see they came to no harm, and did no harm to each other.

BB   And night-time?

DC   That was unspeakable. There were 80 beds to a dormitory, with a chamber pot under each. The beds were so close together that the men could not get up between their beds, so they climbed over the ends to get out. It wasn't well ventilated, and on a summer's night, it stank of urine and of paraldehyde.

BB   How were the patients kept clean?

DC   Once a week was bathing day. They were all stripped and driven into the big communal bathroom where they were bathed, scrubbed, inspected for scabies and nits, and driven out the far end to get fresh clothes.

BB   How was time broken up?

DC   There was a pattern to the day. The patients were turned out to the airing court, counted out and counted in. Then they were sat at their tables for their meals; spoons and forks handed out and the food put on the table. The charge nurse said grace and they were allowed to eat. Then the spoons and forks were all taken in and washed by the staff and counted. Nobody left the table until all the cutlery was counted. As in the Army, everything took a terribly long time because there were too many people using inadequate facilities. People were put into the lavatories in batches and kept there until everyone's bowels had moved.

BB   *What about the week and the year?*

DC   There were the traditional festivities. The galas, such as the hospital Christmas and the annual fête and sports in the summer, were tremendous occasions. There were weekly film shows only for the better patients, of course, and there was the Chapel on Sunday. That was the one occasion that they had the chance of seeing the opposite sex. There was the hospital cricket team, which played regularly, composed mainly of staff, but when there were competent patients, they were taken into it. Parole patients were taken out to watch the cricket. And there were walks around the grounds. Twenty patients, one nurse at the front, one at the back, two at the sides, to make sure that nobody escaped; counted out and counted in of course.

BB   *And personal property?*

DC   On the privileged wards, patients were allowed a little property, but none on the disturbed or 'wet and dirty' wards. On many, the patients' clothes were rolled up at night, taken in, put in a cupboard, and issued again the following morning. No patient was allowed to have money; that was contraband, and they were punished if found with it.

BB   *And how was the institution run?*

DC   The job of the nurses was to watch the patients to see that they didn't escape or harm one another. The job of the doctors was to watch the nurses to see they didn't steal the patients' food and didn't abuse the patients.

One of your main jobs as a doctor was to examine bruised people, be told about how they acquired the bruises, and then decide whether it was so flagrant that you had to hold an enquiry.

In one hospital, I had a patient who was killed by the nurses; he attacked the nurses, they beat him up, and he died of a retroperitoneal haemorrhage. Deliberate violence by the staff to patients varied a great deal; there wasn't very much of it at Fulbourn, but there were always people among the staff who thought it was their duty to 'show them who is the boss'.

As a doctor, your job was to hold the balance; to see that it didn't get too far out of hand.

BB   *And the superintendent?*

DC   To watch the doctors, and also to watch other people and check thefts and abuses. For example, soon after I arrived at Fulbourn, the Group Secretary came to me and said, 'Sir, there is a leg of lamb missing from the kitchen. Would you hold the usual enquiry?' I spent a whole afternoon cross-questioning a set of shifty cooks to find out who had stolen the leg of lamb. I never did find out.

BB *What were the powers of the superintendent?*

DC   Absolute. He could fire anybody in the place, except for five named officers appointed by the Committee, but those he could suspend. Anybody else, he could fire on the spot if he saw fit. He would have to justify it later, of course. But Fulbourn Hospital had scarcely realised that the world had changed.

BB *When did medical superintendents begin?*

DC   The earliest asylums had various people in charge, but gradually the idea developed that medical gentlemen were the most suitable people to put in charge of asylums. It wasn't until the middle of the nineteenth century that the idea of a Hospital Committee appointing a doctor and making him all-powerful became established.

In the early days at Fulbourn, after an enquiry, the Committee put the clerk and steward under the order of the superintendent to prevent him stealing the patients' food, as the previous one had.

BB *What was the training of a superintendent?*

DC   Until the National Health Service began in 1948, the superintendent was paid more than the deputy superintendent and much more than the assistant medical officers. A doctor who went to work in the asylum and liked the life, and decided to stay, worked for promotion; in due course he became a deputy. Then, if he wanted to live well, he applied for superintendent vacancies. The doctors who became superintendents were mostly men in their mid-fifties, with many years of asylum experience behind them.

When the NHS came, all the senior asylum doctors became consultants and there was little money for being a superintendent, so nobody wanted a superintendent's job. That's why younger doctors like myself got them in the mid-fifties. Nobody with any sense took the job because you had to carry far more responsibility than any of the other consultants, but received little more than them.

The Committee, a group of city and county councillors, appointed the superintendents to run the place.

BB *Until retirement?*

DC   Yes. Ten years was the average. The superintendent was answerable to the Committee for everything that happened and also answerable in law.

If a certified patient escaped and broke into a house and stole, the only person the aggrieved householder could sue was the medical superintendent. So within the hospital, he had absolute power. In the thirties, when jobs were desperately short, the fear of instant dismissal was very real. Fulbourn was full of stories of people whom the superintendent sacked out of hand; for instance, when he saw a nurse hand a key to a patient, and fired him on the spot. So everyone was terrified of the superintendent.

There were signalling systems in the hospital, passing the message from ward to ward when the superintendent was coming round, by tapping with a key on the central heating pipes, one tap for the junior doctor, two for the chief male nurse, three for the superintendent. Another method was to have patients watch for the superintendent. In the 'disturbed' ward at Fulbourn, there was one patient who sat by the door and whenever I came in, he leapt to his feet and shouted 'Doctor' at the top of his voice.

At first, I thought he was saluting me, but then I realised his job was to warn the charge nurse to stop whatever he was doing, and come out in case the superintendent saw.

The place was run like a jail; authority was punitive and fault-finding. The hospital was riddled with curious covert devices. Part of the art of being a superintendent was knowing what was going on but not admitting that you knew. I learnt this from the Army. To be an effective commissioned or non-commissioned officer in the Army, you have to know the crooked things that people do, and you have to know how to stop them without openly declaring that you know. If you make it clear that you know, you then have to punish.

BB *What made you think you could be a successful superintendent?*

DC   I don't think I faced that question before I took the job. As I told you, I applied for the job lightheartedly, and only discovered the night before that they were taking my application seriously. I wanted to be a consultant and I believed that I could change things in the back wards of a mental hospital.

BB *You could see a job.*

DC   I had worked in hospitals that were in touch with the modern world, but I hadn't realised that Fulbourn hadn't moved out of the between-wars period.

The most powerful person in Cambridgeshire was the Lord Bishop of Ely. The Anglican Church still held vast power.

BB *How did that affect you?*

DC   I remember I was concerned about whether I dare affirm at inquest rather than swear on the Bible. It is a Quaker tradition and I was an agnostic. But I knew that it would cause a lot of offence and head shaking amongst the Committee, if they found out that they'd got a person who wasn't a member of the Established Church. It was the world of Trollope, of *Barchester Towers*.

BB *What about the superintendent and the other consultants?*

DC   The relationship of the medical superintendent with the other consultants bedevilled many hospitals right through the 1950s and 1960s, but it was not an important issue at Fulbourn.

The consultants working in Cambridge were far better clinicians than I was, so it never occurred to me to interfere with what they were doing. I respected what they were doing with their patients, and they came to respect what I was doing with the back wards, and we didn't interfere with one another.

BB *What did you feel you had to do when you got to Fulbourn. Did you make a diagnosis, as it were, and prescribe treatment?*

DC   My first job was to get the hospital running effectively; this involved listening to what people had to say. My predecessor used to see everybody separately but I thought this wasn't a very good idea. The doctors were coming to me to complain about the matron, the matron was coming to complain about the doctors; she also complained about the Group Secretary, who came to complain about the chief male nurse, who came to complain about the engineer.

I thought, 'This is silly!' So I arranged meetings of the medical and nursing staff, to decide about difficult patients. I started arranging meetings with the hospital officers to decide what jobs should be done next. This seemed to me obvious, but it was a revolution.

BB *Was there no regular meeting of the chief nurse, chief administrator, and so on?*

DC None, before I came. The introduction of democratic consensus methods was a wonderful change for everyone. They knew what was going on and they got on with things. Then, we began to consider improvements. I visited progressive hospitals, and came back with ideas. I said, 'Why don't we open some ward doors?' We talked about it and then we opened the doors of two or three wards, where all patients had parole.

Then over a period of five years, we opened other doors and found out what was possible. We did it by consultation and discussion. I had many meetings with the charge nurses – they were a wonderful powerhouse of change.

BB *You saw the group of charge nurses as the people who carried the hospital culture?*

DC This group of middle-aged men and women, who had worked in the place ten or twenty years and who had still got vigour and enthusiasm, were the carriers of the old culture, but they were also the creators of the new.

BB *Did you send them away to see Dingleton and Graylingwell?*

DC Those that wanted to. We promoted people who wanted to change things, rewarded people who changed things, and scoffed at those who didn't.

BB *How did you decide what to do?*

DC It was not a question of me deciding, but the nurses and myself deciding together. Many had worked in hospitals where there was activity.

BB *You have described how back-ward patients did nothing.*

DC There were hospitals in Britain where the patients were active, but the easier thing for the doctor in charge is to say, 'Don't let that patient out.' It's more difficult to say, 'Let him out rather more often'. When they say, 'What'll happen if he hits someone?' you have to say, 'I'll answer for that!'

I came to see in later years that my job had been to give people a feeling of security, of being backed, of being trusted – a belief that if they took risks, they wouldn't be abandoned to a Committee of Enquiry.

The therapeutic potential was there in those staff, but the tradition of medical management that had grown up in the twenties and thirties was an anxious checking of developments.

People like Duncan McMillan at Mapperley, T. P. Rees at Warlingham, and Joshua Carse at Graylingwell were doing all sorts of things, but many hospitals had old men in charge, who always said, 'No, no, don't do that; something dreadful might happen.'

That was the first phase, opening the doors. The next aim was to improve the life of the patients on the back wards. So I started picking up ideas, such as work for in-patients, getting the place cleaned up, and accommodation improved.

BB   *What does 'work' mean in that setting?*

DC   We put out gangs of men with hoes and dug up all the weeds; the hospital grounds were full of them. There was a great tangled overgrown shrubbery, that had got out of hand during the war; we took the men out and they dug it all out. One of our big projects was a new sports field. We built a complete sports field at the front of the hospital. I can remember times when we had fifty or sixty wheelbarrows going, with patients shovelling soil into wheelbarrows, wheeling it, dumping it.

BB   *For pay?*

DC   For reward, not pay. It was some years before we could give them money.

BB   *What were the rewards?*

DC   Tobacco, sweets, privileges. Later, I managed to get permission to pay. It wasn't very much money, but something they could spend as they wished.

BB   *That was to give purpose to the waking day?*

DC   Yes. Then we began to look at improving the quality of life. For instance, letting people have private property. We had to persuade the Management Committee to buy lockers for the patients – a new idea.

Then we began to review the penal restrictions. In 1953, out of 950 patients, there were fifteen who had town parole; each of the fifteen had a 'parole card' which had to be personally signed by the superintendent on Friday. I said, 'This is absurd. Let's scrap the whole system.' We extended the number of people allowed to go into town and the number of people allowed to go out of the ward into the grounds.

BB   *That's devolving responsibility downwards.*

DC   Yes, and dismantling the absurd and meaningless rules of the custodial structure. The rules had originally been quite sensible, but had been subsequently misapplied destructively.

I discovered for instance, that any patient who had ever had a fit, had to stay permanently on the 'disturbed' ward, and sleep in an observation dormitory with a hard pillow, because once, in the distant past, an epileptic had a fit in a non-observed place, and smothered in his pillow, and the coroner criticised the hospital. The result was that a number of well behaved, competent asylum patients, who had once had a fit, sometimes years before, were forced to live in a violent degrading place, and sleep in discomfort, in a grossly overcrowded dormitory.

I said, 'Let us review all these people; if there is somebody who has a fit every night, of course he must be under observation, but if somebody hasn't had one for over a year, let him take his chance.' I explained that we would point out to the coroner that all epileptics in general society accepted the risk of smothering, but that they did not let it cripple their lives. So this small group of elite workers were pathetically grateful for having been allowed out of the 'disturbed' ward.

Suicide caution cards were another. If a doctor considered someone suicidal, he made out a red card, with the name of the patient at the top. Every member of staff who came on the ward had to sign the card and a declaration that he knew the patient was a suicidal risk and must be kept under observation at all times. This procedure for setting up suicide caution cards was well established, but the procedure for cancelling them was not. So they were seldom cancelled. On the 'disturbed' ward, there were fifteen people on SCCs. Everybody solemnly signed the cards.

I said, 'Let's look at these people.' One had made a suicidal attempt three years before; it was completely irrelevant, yet he was still being watched, policed, harassed, and degraded. So we scrapped the system. We did give a lot of time and thought to people we thought were suicidal and arranged for them to be with someone, but we didn't routinise it. In any organisation, you have to revise the rules constantly to make sure that they remain sensible.

We had a slogan, 'Activity, Freedom, Responsibility', the three things we wanted to re-introduce into the lives of patients. Activity, we have talked about, freedom we've talked about.

We also wanted to give them more responsibility for their own lives. A simple device was self-governing arrangements on the ward, letting patients decide when they could have their meals, for example, which was first seen as revolutionary.

In the old asylum, anybody who was a patient was, by definition, irresponsible and unable to do anything. In fact, many patients were responsible and capable of dressing themselves, managing their money, and living their own lives, looking after themselves, and choosing when to have their meals. But because of the blanket rules, everybody had been treated the same way.

Beginning to challenge that and beginning to develop autonomy both for individuals and for groups within the hospital was the next thing we worked on in the sixties.

BB *Were the patients compulsorily detained?*

DC   In the middle-fifties, 90% of patients were certified. There were a few voluntary patients, who were on the admission wards, but on the back wards, everyone was certified.

BB *So that gave legal backing for total control.*

DC   In the decade before the 1959 Act, there was a ferment of discussion throughout British psychiatry, including experiments with relaxing legal restrictions. I started discharging people from their certificates. And when the appointed day came in 1959, we discharged the lot!

After a period of adjustment, we settled down to about 12% of our admissions and 8% of the resident hospital population as detained patients.

BB *You were talking about responsibility.*

DC   We tried to develop self-government. One of the first therapeutic communities at Fulbourn was run by Eddy Oram on Adrian Ward, a women's convalescent ward, in 1958–1960, and was published in *Human Relations*[3].

---

3. CLARK, D. H., HOOPER, D. & ORAM, E. G. (1962) Creating a therapeutic community in a psychiatric ward. *Human Relations*, **15**, 123–147.

In the early sixties, we began changing the disturbed wards, I ran a therapeutic community on the women's 'disturbed' wards. Then, we put the men's 'disturbed' wards and the women's 'disturbed' wards side by side, and ran them both as therapeutic communities. Then, we combined them, as 'Hereward House'[4,5].

That was the most exciting, the most interesting period of my work, and where I personally learnt a great deal. The patients and nurses challenged me about authority ploys that I'd taken for granted. Though I had been involved in bringing in humane and liberal reforms, I had maintained a considerable control over many areas. They forced me to see that some of these controls were no longer helpful. We looked at them, challenged them, and worked out our own rules – the patients and the staff together – within the therapeutic community.

BB   You came in as a benign tyrant. With the aim of introducing reform and giving people more responsibility over what they did, but you retained ultimate control.

DC   That's true of the first ten years.

BB   How far did you go in relinquishing control and how did you finally give it up completely, as I imagine you did?

DC   I came in '53 and found I'd got the paraphernalia of power of the superintendent of the previous generation. Not only that, but all kinds of bizarre tasks. I was told it was my duty to read the lesson in the Chapel at least once a month, and to examine the pigs at least once a week, and to do a post-mortem on every patient who died, so as to check whether the doctor had treated them adequately.

BB   You gave up the pigs?

DC   I continued looking at the pigs, because I enjoyed looking at them. But I made it clear that I could accept no responsibility for their welfare.

BB   And the lesson in the Chapel?

DC   Because I was an agnostic, that bothered me. First of all, I said I would only read the lesson at the great festivals, and then after a year, I refused to do even those. The post-mortems I did for about three or four months, and then said that I thought it was really absurd, and that if we had wanted to know what people died from, we'd better get a pathologist to do it. I started off by giving up a whole lot of the rather pointless aspects of the superintendency, but I was still responsible to the Management Committee for the way the hospital ran.

During the sixties, with ferment generally, a number of these things were challenged, and quite rightly; for instance, the old secretary retired and we got some modern administrators. They made it clear they were not going to

4. CLARK, D. H. & MYERS, K. (1970) Themes in a therapeutic community. *British Journal of Psychiatry*, **117**, 389–395.
5. MYERS, K. & CLARK, D. H. (1972) Results in a therapeutic community. *British Journal of Psychiatry*, **120**, 51–58.

be responsible to the superintendent. I thought they were entirely right, but I still retained a residual responsibility for the way the place ran.

Then in 1971, preparing for the cog-wheel reorganisation, we officially abandoned the title of medical superintendent. But really, for about five years before that, it had only been a title, and I hadn't used the authority inherent in it. The superintendency vanished in 1971, and I became the first Chairman of the Division of Psychiatry.

BB *Did you have your own Hospital Management Committee?*

DC   I was fortunate there. My first chairman was Lady Adrian; the next was Alderman Mallett, an ex-mayor of Cambridge, then Sir Henry Willink, an ex-Minister of Health and Master of Magdalen College, and the last, Mrs Pauline Burnet. All of them outstanding, able, charming people and all deeply committed to the welfare of the hospital.

In retrospect, it is clear that Fulbourn Hospital was fortunate. It had its own good Hospital Management Committee from 1951–1974. The members were interested in running the hospital for the benefit of the patients and saw to it that the patients' needs were predominant. They had their own budget; it was small but they managed it well. There was a great deal of building at Fulbourn during those 23 years, and the physical conditions were vastly improved.

The early seventies were unfortunate for Fulbourn Hospital because of the lack of money. But we were particularly affected because we were thrown in with Addenbrooke's at a time when Addenbrooke's was just moving into a new building that was inadequately funded. Any spare money in Cambridge was sucked into their vortex. The problem of getting a great big new district general hospital going absorbed everybody's energies.

There was a neglect of the needs of the mental hospital up the road. So there was a relative neglect of the long-term patients within Fulbourn. Because Fulbourn had a high morale, it has kept going far better than many other hospitals that I know, and it still is doing a good job. But compared with the '50s and '60s, when the hospital was getting public support and acclaim and really moving forward, they've had to battle on, looking after the long-term people without much help from either the financial side, the administrative side, or the newly appointed academics.

BB *So Fulbourn lost, you think, on balance?*

DC   Yes, compared with the way things were ten or fifteen years ago. It's all rather sad; but compared with the state that many mental hospitals are in, it's still good. I've been to places that I knew as good hospitals ten years ago, which have slid way downhill.

BB *What were you doing during these later years?*

DC   In the mid-seventies, I reviewed my work and took responsibility for the long-term patients. We developed the Cambridge Psychiatric Rehabilitation Service, which was described in an article in the *Lancet*[6].

---

6. CLARK, D. H. (1984) The development of a psychiatric rehabilitation service. *Lancet*, *ii*, 625–627.

D

In the last ten years, I built up a service which supports long-term patients out in the community. When I first met them, they were locked up, consigned to the back wards, where their only job was to live as long as they chose, and then to die and be buried in the asylum graveyard. There they were, herded into these warehouses, stultified by the way we handled them.

We showed that with freedom, activity, and responsibility, they could live a very much better life in the hospital. We then saw that many could move out of the hospital; and in the sixties, the people who moved out went off and we never saw them again. They managed perfectly well, having recovered first from the psychosis that took them to hospital, and then from the institutionalisation which kept them there.

BB   Do you think drugs played much of a part?

DC   They relieved tension, suppressed some symptoms, and made it easier to try things out.

By the seventies, we were working with people more impaired by their disorders and with residual deficits. How much they could do, we've slowly been exploring, and we've been forced to face the facts that despite all our modern drugs, and all our modern skills, there are still people who become long-term hospital in-patients. The number is probably not as great as it was, but there are a few every year, graduating to 'long-term status'. We showed it was 15 or 20 people every year in Cambridgeshire, from a catchment population of about half a million.

In the past ten years in Cambridge, we have been developing our psychiatric rehabilitation service. Most of the long-term patients are living out of hospital. Of 400 long-term patients, only 150 are on wards at Fulbourn, and only 70 in fully staffed wards; the others are in hostel wards, half-way houses, sheltered accommodation, and group homes. With a network of facilities, sheltered living daytime activities, and with skilled and devoted staff available to visit, support, and help through difficulties, most long-term patients do not need to be in a custodial institution.

BB   What is the future of the 70 on the wards?

DC   Difficult to tell. Some are youngish and disturbed, and there is a reasonable chance that by mid-life, they may be quiet and be able to move out. Others have multiple disabilities, for instance, a psychosis and a severe heart condition, or hemiplegic and simple minded, so that they require physical nursing and psychiatric nursing. How many people require residence in a fully staffed psychiatric institution is not yet clear. The number is uncertain, but small.

BB   Is a mental hospital necessary for them?

DC   No.

BB   You're looking forward to the demolition of Fulbourn?

DC   Not necessarily. The site so near the city may be useful, and some of the buildings are still good. But we must avoid another vast human warehouse, holding hundreds of people in impoverished and authoritarian conditions.

BB *Can a psychiatric rehabilitation service be run from a DGH base, without mental hospital back-up?*

DC I should think so, although I haven't seen it done. Doctors who are responsible for acute as well as long-term patients will inevitably neglect the long-term ones. They can't help it. Acute patients present acute problems which must be attended to at once; the others are forgotten, and then things go wrong. There will always have to be specialised institutions for patients needing security. In Fulbourn, we were able to contain and help people from secure hospitals, but that would be difficult in a DGH. It needs a lot more courage.

BB *Do you think it necessary to have one consultant whose sole job it is to run the service for the long-term patient?*

DC It is much preferable to have someone specialising, committing themselves. The problems of a long-term patient are very different from the issues that face a patient suffering from a short-term psychotic disorder. The problems of the long-term patient are often more social and educational than medical.

BB *Could we come back to your psychiatric training, that prepared you for this task.*

DC I can't say that my psychiatric training prepared me for the task of opening up the hospital, or for running therapeutic communities, or a rehabilitation service. It trained me to be a 1950s psychiatrist, not much else.

All we were taught, especially at the Maudsley, was individual – focused on the individual's mental state, the individual's physical state, the individual's psychopathology. It was only later, gradually, and mostly by myself that I learned something of the social factors in breakdown and in recovery.

BB *So whom did you learn your psychiatry from?*

DC At the Maudsley in 1950–53, Aubrey Lewis was the dominating figure. Then there was Dr Foulkes, from whom I learned a great deal.

D. K. Henderson was a man of warmth, charm, and ability. At the time I was with him in the late 1940s, he was holding prodigious, almost ludicrous power. He was the Professor of Psychiatry, superintendent of three hospitals, and ran the largest private practice in Scotland. So he didn't have enough time for any of them. He had an idiosyncratic way of teaching, but one learned a lot with him because he gave you a job to do and trusted you to get on with it. When one went to him in despair, his comment always was, 'Well, you'll just have to do the best you can'. If you went wrong, he told you. He brought out the best by challenging you and supporting you. One always knew that whatever happened, DK would be there and would back you.

I learned from DK how to help people grow, and from Aubrey Lewis, how *not* to help people to grow. Aubrey was a man of brilliance, of immense erudition, but the effect that he had on junior doctors was malignant. He terrified them. The only thing many of them learned at the Maudsley was to avoid being cut to pieces. Many of us learned how to avoid it – feed him a juicy fragment, and provided he thought he had scored off you, he would leave you alone. But if a junior doctor tried to defend himself, Aubrey would go on and on until he had reduced the registrar to a quivering heap. I remember him saying to a group of senior registrars, 'I can't understand why the registrars are so frightened of me; I'm only trying to help them to clarify their thinking. It is the Socratic method.' We came to understand why the Athenians put Socrates to death!

BB *You must have some good things to say about Lewis's achievements?*

DC He did much that was valuable and we are constantly being told about it! He ruled the post-war Maudsley, held it together, won the resources it needed, and fought for psychiatry amongst the physicians and surgeons and politicians. He lectured and wrote and summarised and reviewed endlessly, and was a powerful intellectual force for clear logical thinking and erudite writing. He ruled the Maudsley with a rod of iron, and his view of what a psychiatrist should be was enforced.

A lot of good people came from the Maudsley, but that was because they were good people before they went there, rather than because of what Lewis did for them. People came out of the Maudsley able to quote references and argue, but they were often incapable of taking responsibility for a difficult patient or facing a really nasty problem. And as for handling a disturbed ward or a group of angry staff, they just hadn't a notion.

To me, the Monday morning conference was one of the saddest things that happened there. I came down from Edinburgh and saw the eminent, pretty well all the great names in British psychiatry sitting like terrified rabbits while Aubrey seduced them into saying something, and cut what they said to ribbons with his logic. He had them all there and demonstrated their impotence.

BB *So you didn't like him?*

DC Personally, I liked him a lot. I found him charming, courteous, kind, and witty, once he had come to the conclusion you were all right. But I hated the way he ran the hospital.

BB *What did he have to say about your going to Fulbourn?*

DC He didn't try to dissuade me. I was told he wrote me a good reference. I think he felt I wasn't Maudsley material.

BB *Still, he had you for three years. Can we return to Foulkes. What was his career?*

DC Foulkes came from Frankfurt in 1933, a refugee from Nazism, like Stengel and so many others. After the war, he was at Barts part-time and he had a private practice in Wimpole Street. He came to the Maudsley, as many psychotherapists did in those days, to spend a few years there. It was a hard experience. They had contact with the bright young trainees, but they had to operate in an uncongenial and hostile environment.

I found in the Out-patient Department this nice, foreign gentleman who seemed puzzled about what was going on.

BB *He certainly gave that impression.*

DC I wanted to learn about group therapy, so I started doing groups with him. As I struggled, I found that a talk with Foulkes cleared my mind, and I came to value my sessions with him. To my surprise, I found that after a year or so, I was operating effectively as a group therapist. Clearly, I'd learned from him. Not until some years later did I realise just how much I learned from him and how good he was at allowing people to acquire insight. I kept in touch with him for the rest of his life through the Group Analytic Society.

BB *Foulkes is credited with discovering group psychotherapy, is that correct?*

DC   Yes.

BB *What did he discover?*

DC   He had started experiments with seeing psychotherapy patients in groups.

BB *For economy?*

DC   No, I think it was for theoretical reasons and research. He wondered where it would lead him.

BB *Where?*

DC   First in Exeter, but then at Northfield, the military hospital, where he and a bunch of bright young psychiatrists used groups a lot. Then they went back to London, to the Tavistock for example, to develop their ideas. He developed his own brand of group analytic psychotherapy, and then over the next 30 years he continued probing, refining, examining, and developing the technique.

BB *So how did you learn to be a superintendent?*

DC   Mostly by doing the job. But I was greatly helped by a course for superintendents run by the King Edward's Fund in 1957. I found myself for a month with Duncan McMillan, Rudolf Freudenberg, and a number of others from whom I learned a lot.

I learned most of all from Maxwell Jones. His Belmont Unit was at its most exciting and turbulent peak, and he expounded his ideas of the therapeutic community with brilliance, charm, and enthusiasm. I became a friend and have been learning from him ever since.

With Henderson, Lewis, and Foulkes, whenever I did anything and talked with any of them, I thought to myself afterwards, 'Well, he's a wise man and I'm a fool'. But what came next was the difference.

With Henderson I thought, 'Well, he's a wise man and I'm a fool, but strangely enough, he seems to trust me to do a decent job; I'll try and do better next time.'

After I had talked with Lewis, I thought, 'Well, he's a wise man and I'm a fool; he's made me realise what a fool I am, I'll not get caught that way again.'

And with Foulkes, I used to think, 'Well, he's a wise man and I'm a fool, but he seems to think that I may be able to grasp this, and I'm beginning to see something about what it's about.'

Those were three different ways of helping a student to learn and grow. Everybody has more capacity for growth than you think they have, and if you give them support and trust, challenge and opportunity, the most surprising people – the most psychotic patient, the most stubborn nurse, the most stupid registrar – will do far more than you ever thought they could.

DC   The therapeutic community has been the most important professional experience that I've had. My original concern was to make a better life for the pathetically imprisoned people. In doing so, I came to realise that the best ideas for changing things came from the grass-roots – to begin with, from the nurses.

Then I began to find ideas coming from the patients too. I realised that if you want to improve the life of people, one of the best things to do is to find out what they themselves actually want, rather than assuming that you know, and imposing it on them. So I started to listen to the patients, and realised that they had lots to say which was worth listening to.

About ten years after I came to Fulbourn, I began to apply directly the ideas I picked up from Maxwell Jones, who taught us to listen to the patients and then encourage them to tell one another about their problems.

I found that if somebody can't understand why he is being detained on a Section, other people who had been or were going to be detained could often explain it to them much better than I could. They would say, 'You're not fit to be running around loose just now, Dr Clark is quite right to put you on a Section.' There were occasions when the therapeutic community insisted I put someone on a Section, to protect them from themselves. I enjoyed this way of working, where the patients were doing so much of the work.

My job was to authenticate and support them with my authority and prestige. I found this exciting, challenging, immensely worthwhile, and I learned a lot. I have spent much time in the last twenty years, trying to understand the application of this to a psychiatric hospital and to other settings. I have helped to get therapeutic communities going in other settings, and have spent a lot of time working in the Association of Therapeutic Communities.

If you have a residential institution containing disturbed people, a socio-therapeutic approach is the only one that has any future. One of the challenges for psychiatrists is how to learn to do this, despite their medical training, with its authoritarian accent.

BB   *I believe you did quite a lot in the College at one time, and I believe you were the vice-chairman of the National Association for Mental Health.*

DC   That was an interesting phase of my life. For a decade, I moved amongst the mighty; I bowed to princesses, hobnobbed with peers and MPs, and with those who ruled and moved our land. And it was often exciting and exhilarating. I sat on committees and pondered great issues and passed resolutions; I would announce things in the press, appear on television, on the radio, and so on. I doubt how much value it had, although it was interesting to meet princesses, and very charming they were too.

After a time, however, I began to ask myself, 'Is this doing the patients any good?' It wasn't, so after a time I pulled out of it.

BB   *What about the NAMH?*

DC   In the late sixties, I was asked to help with it. It was a delightful organisation, which enabled psychiatrists, social workers, MPs, and peeresses, to work together with people of good will to encourage society as a whole to take a more enlightened and helpful view of the needs of the mentally ill and the mentally handicapped. A wonderful job was done from the time that they got it together in 1950 until about 1970.

Then, a new mood came. It wasn't only in the NAMH; it was general. There was emphasis on people's rights, rather than their welfare. There was a feeling against psychiatrists and psychiatry. Some was a just repayment for the arrogance that some of us had shown over the years, and some a reaction to disappointment that we'd failed to deliver the goods so exuberantly promised in the early '50s, when psychiatrists were saying that they would cure all mental disorder, abolish all suffering, and bring wisdom to a discovered world. But it was all rather sad.

NAMH became MIND, a civil rights, rather anti-psychiatric organisation, and I felt out of place. At that stage, I stopped being involved on a national scale, but continued to work in a local mental health organisation in Cambridge.

BB *How did that change in the NAMH occur?*

DC   I believe it corresponded with anti-psychiatric pressures in the country as a whole. If NAMH hadn't done it, some other organisation would have been set up to do it. They continued to do a great deal of positive work all through the '70s, but the civil rights work brought conflict. Instead of cooperation between them and the psychiatrists, there came hostility.

This was also at the time when psychiatrists were moving away from co-operation with other professions and a general concern with mental health, and turning inward and trying to become more and more professional, medical, scientific.

BB *You see the development of the College as part of the same process as the formation of MIND out of NAMH?*

DC   Yes. I was active in the Royal Medico-Psychological Association at the time the College was formed.

BB *You were for it?*

DC   Yes. I was sad that it turned into a body more and more obsessed with examining and failing people, setting up more and more complicated examinations. The paralysing effect that the membership has had on the learning of young doctors is unfortunate. In the '50s and '60s, the DPM was there and anybody who was any good got it. Now, they are paralysed by the exam for years. The College seems to me now to be a much more inward looking body than the RMPA was in the '60s.

BB *An academic department of psychiatry developed at Cambridge University in the 1970s. What effect did it have on Fulbourn Hospital?*

DC   Not very much. Its impact was not as damaging as the drying up of funds for development after 1974 and the paralysing effect of the progressive reorganisations. The Cambridge Health District has been in severe financial difficulties for the last 15 years because the New Addenbrooke's Hospital was never properly funded, so that what new money there was went to the exotic activities of Addenbrooke's, like kidney, heart, and liver transplants. Psychiatry, especially the care of the long-term patients, got very little funds or attention.

The same shortages affected the new medical school. When Cambridge University belatedly decided in the late '60s to have a medical school, they planned in the belief that the University would always have plenty of money, as would the NHS, so that a new medical school could be built from those two sources. They did not realise that both lots of money ultimately came from the public purse; when that ran dry in the mid-seventies, both of the funds ran dry too. So the medical school has been terribly hard work for everybody.

In the late 1960s, many of us had had great hopes of the new Clinical School and some, like Bernard Zeitlyn and I, spent years preparing for it. We had plans for an exciting curriculum using the ideas of Balint and Abercrombie, as at McMaster University.

BB *Would you like to say something about your experience at Palo Alto?*

DC In the United States, there is a postgraduate centre for social scientists called the Center for the Advanced Study of the Behavioral Sciences. They like to have a few foreigners, a few psychiatrists, a few lawyers, a few historians, and people like that along for flavour. It's a wonderful place, in a most beautiful part of California. They bring you and your family from wherever you live in the world, pay your salary for a year, provide a study and a secretary, and make no demands on you at all. It was a wonderful experience.

When I went there, I didn't believe I could write a book, but being amongst people who were all writing books, I got down to it and did get my first book done[7].

The year I was there, Eric Erikson and Carl Rogers were both Fellows, and I got to know them both and learned much from them.

BB *What did you think of Rogers?*

DC Delightful man, with the capacity to bring out the best in other people. One of the things that was most revealing to me about Carl was his opinion about book reviews. He said, 'I never do reviews. If you are required to do a review, you are required to think critically and spitefully about another person and I really didn't feel I wanted to spend my time doing that.' He is interested in helping other people discover what they can do, what their potentialities are, rather than pointing out to them their failings, weaknesses, and incompetences.

BB *And Erikson?*

DC Eric was a different figure. A big man with a bright red face, a great halo of white hair, charming, erudite, stimulating. He used to reminisce about summer holidays with the Freud family. He would bubble off in all directions about anything and anybody. His talk is slightly easier to follow than his writings!

BB *You have been a WHO adviser? I take it that your work at Fulbourn was the basis for your appointment.*

DC People came to visit Fulbourn in the early days, and some asked me to go to the States and lecture about what I had been doing. I saw unspeakable

---

7. CLARK D. H. (1964) *Administrative Therapy*. Tavistock.

places there, infinitely worse than anything in Britain. I realised that though clinical psychiatry was the same in most countries, the services provided are very different. It seems to depend on the primary health care services of the country and its attitudes to mental disorder. I did one or two things for WHO. They asked me in 1967 to go to Japan for four months.

BB *What was the point of going to Japan, from the Japanese point of view?*

DC The Japanese psychiatric scene was changing rapidly, and they weren't sure if they had got it right. Immediately after the war, after the destruction of Japan by the Allies, most of the long-stay patients had died and there were hardly any institutions for the long-term patient.

In the early 1950s, there were 80 000 mental hospital beds, for 100 million Japanese people. Their advisers told them they must build up the number of mental institutions. So they did, but with private hospitals. When I went there in 1967, there were 130 000 beds, and I found they were packed with patients, who were stuffed with chlorpromazine. The more patients a doctor got into the place, the more money he made. People were keen to get rid of their mad relatives, so they readily certified them; the patients were full of drugs, so they didn't complain. There was little concern for the life of the long-term patients.

I said to the Japanese, 'If you don't do something about it, then the numbers concerned will go up and up. In due course, you'll have a horrible problem.'

BB *To which Japanese people did you say this?*

DC I made a report to the Japanese Government. It was known as the Clark Report, and it was discussed in the Japanese parliament and caused a hullabaloo at the time. It was regarded as a widely radical document.

BB *What did you recommend?*

DC That they had to have rehabilitation services and an inspectorate for mental hospitals, and that they should concentrate on getting people out of hospital rather than in. They did not do these things. As a result, the numbers went up. At the time our numbers were going down, theirs were going up and by the mid-seventies, there were 300 000 mental hospital in-patients, or 32 per 10 000.

BB *Do you think, in retrospect, that your report was a bit too much for them to digest in one go?*

DC Giving advice to other countries is profoundly difficult. I had no beginning of an understanding of what it involved.

BB *Is the Clark Report now in use?*

DC It's widely quoted, and my books have been translated into Japanese, and they're read there. I've been back several times.

BB *And you've been to South America?*

DC I was asked to go to Peru. Peruvians are charming people. They took quite a lot of notice of what we said, but their economic problems since have made it practically impossible. They did set up therapeutic communities in the Larco Herera Hospital, but it came to nothing because of their economic troubles.

Then I was asked to go to Argentina in 1968. A shattering experience; we were nearly thrown out of the country for preaching democracy!

My wife said that she thought it would be a good idea if the nurses got themselves organised in the hospital. The medical superintendent banned her from entering the hospital again, saying, 'This is syndicalism and will not be allowed here!' I forced a formal apology (for the insult to my honour) from the Colonel in charge, but was left with a strong distaste for military government of mental hospitals! That was during the military regime. They are doing better now, I believe.

The WHO later sent me to Poland. The Poles sent me a letter saying, 'Your book is widely read and deeply appreciated, and we are all committed to social psychiatry'. This surprised me, but I found it to be true. The Poles had been taught their psychiatry by the Russians, whom they hated. But they had kept up their contact with the French, and the French have a strong social psychiatry movement.

The Poles discovered that if they called psychotherapy 'social psychiatry', they could practise it. So as far as Poland was concerned, 'social psychiatry' was a cover under which to smuggle in psychotherapy, psychoanalysis, Freud, Lacan, the lot!

BB *I see you have a PhD.*

DC   In Cambridge you can get a PhD for your published works. I was awarded it in 1972 for my writings on social psychiatry.

BB *What was the most rewarding period of your professional life?*

DC   There have been excitements and rewards in all periods. The first nine years at Fulbourn was an exciting period. The last decade was good too, creating a psychiatric rehabilitation service. There was a lot of fun and excitement then, and I think that by the end, we had demonstrated a solution to the problems which are bedevilling institutional psychiatry in developed countries all over the place. What the Americans call 'deinstitutionalisation'.

We showed that if you have a well-integrated, well-knit team of highly motivated staff (not many of them, but good), they can maintain people with long-term psychiatric disabilities in the community. There is then no need for hundreds of people to be locked up in dreary asylums, nor for lost, pathetic creatures to be wandering the streets of the big cities, raking in the rubbish bins.

However, I must say that the most exciting time was in the sixties, when we developed therapeutic communities at Fulbourn Hospital. In opening up the hospital, we had been doing what many people in Britain had already done, and we were following in others' footsteps, but with the therapeutic communities, we were striking out into completely new country. Nobody had ever taken all the patients from the segregated, locked, disturbed wards of a traditional mental hospital and put them together in one open-door, mixed-sex, therapeutic community. It was a challenging and at times terrifying period.

We successfully demonstrated that it could be done and that as a result, people who would otherwise be condemned to a perpetual back-ward life could make their way to a degree of independence and free living away from hospital.

But the reason I say it was exciting was because of what it did for me personally. In the community meetings, I was challenged and confronted by the patients and forced to rethink and modify many of the practices of unthinking authority which I had developed in a decade as a medical superintendent.

Exciting too was to meet the staff on equal terms and to hear from them something of their complex feelings about the doctors that they had been subjected to over the years. The hostility and the admiration, the envy and the comradeship, the resentment of the medical arrogance and tyranny, and the protection that that very arrogance gave them.

I learned an immense amount about myself and my profession during those years. It was a wonderful time.

BB *What do you see as the continuing theme of your professional work?*

DC   The exploration of the social factors in psychiatry. I learned medicine in the early forties, when the entire focus was on the individual patient and the things that were wrong inside his body and mind.

The psychiatry which I learned from D. K. Henderson and from Aubrey Lewis was much the same – continuous, assiduous, devoted examination of the pathology of the person and his mind. Even the psychotherapy of those days was entirely individual. We were not supposed to have any social contacts with our psychotherapy patients, nor even to talk to their relatives.

It is amazing how far we have moved since those days in learning to assess the social dimension and to use it to help the patient. My own personal interest has been social therapy within the institution: the development first of all of open doors and humane regime, then therapeutic communities and then rehabilitation.

There have, however, been many other social developments. There has been the whole development of family therapy, which arose directly from the awareness of the social dimension, and of course, the new growth therapies – encounter groups, psychodrama, etc, which are all rooted in the observation that for many people, their inner troubles are caused by their social relationships, so that the only hope of helping them is by exploring the problem in a social setting.

7 Kenneth Rawnsley

Interviewed by BRIAN BARRACLOUGH (1987)

Professor Kenneth Rawnsley, CBE, MB ChB Manchester 1948, FRCP 1967, FRCPsych 1971, FRCPsych (Hon) 1977. Professor Rawnsley was born in 1926 and died in 1992. He trained at the Maudsley, and was a member of the scientific staff at the MRC Social Psychiatry Unit at the Institute of Psychiatry. In 1964, he was appointed to the first Chair of Psychiatry in the Welsh National School of Medicine. He was a member of the Merrison Committee of Enquiry into the Regulation of the Medical Profession (1972–75), the Warnock Enquiry into Human Fertilisation (1982–84), and was a consultant to the World Health Organisation. He was Chairman of the Management Committee of the National Counselling Service for Sick Doctors. Professor Rawnsley was Dean of the Royal College of Psychiatrists 1972–77 and served as President 1981–84.

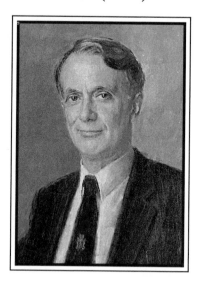

BB   How did you come to take up medicine?

KR   When I was about 14, I became interested in bacteriology; microscopes rather than bacteriology, I suppose because I had one through which I used to look at all sorts of things. Eventually, I focused on bacteria and decided that this was what I wanted to be, a bacteriologist. Not having any notion as to what was entailed and having no medical contacts in the family, I went to see the clinical pathologist at the Victoria Hospital in Burnley, Lancashire, which was where I was brought up, to ask his advice. He told me to take a medical degree first.

BB   That was standard form then, wasn't it, for a scientific career in biological sciences?

KR   I suppose so. His view was that a bacteriologist with a training in medicine had a more interesting career, with a wider choice later on. This was the main reason why I decided to do medicine, to do bacteriology. I applied for medicine in Manchester, and started there in 1943. During the first two years of anatomy, physiology, and chemistry, I was wedded to this idea.

But when I started clinical work, my view of the situation changed, and I became interested in clinical medicine as a career. At that stage, psychoanalysis, an earlier interest of mine, earlier than bacteriology, crept in. When I was a lad, my friends and I used to go and look round the Burnley public library, partly an intellectual thing and partly a social gathering point.

BB *Did Burnley have a good public library?*

KR   Very good. In those days, it had the highest rate for the issue of public lending library books in the country. I read Freud's *Introductory Lectures in Psycho-analysis*.

BB *Did you seek it out because of personal difficulties?*

KR   No, not at all; I read it by accident. It was on the psychology shelf, next to what looked like a book but was actually a block of wood. There was a label pasted on one side of the block with a list of book titles only available on application to the desk, the works of Havelock Ellis, for instance. Of course, I daren't ask at the desk, so I picked the next volume. I found it absorbing. It was written in a compelling style and the ideas were so new to me and so interesting that I read a great deal more in the field. Then, for a whole, I tended to look at everything in psychoanalytic terms and saw complexes everywhere.

BB *Did you have a psychologically-minded family?*

KR   Not a bit.

BB *Your mother had a shrewd understanding of human behaviour?*

KR   Yes, that is true. My parents were quite sensitively tuned in this way. But they would not have been interested in reading Freud. When I began clinical work as a medical student in Manchester, I found interest in the emotional, psychological aspects of the work in hospital wards. I suppose my interest in Freud when I was a teenager was a pointer to this. My passion for bacteriology became less intrusive and less persistent, and by the time I qualified, I had more or less decided on psychiatry.

BB *Do you see a link between psychoanalysis and bacteriology?*

KR   No. But there is between psychopathology and bacteriology – the detailed study of some aspects of life from a detached viewpoint. Anyway, I went on to do three house physician jobs during 1949 and 1950, the days before mandatory pre-registration years.

BB *How old were you then?*

KR   23.

BB *So you missed the war?*

KR   I even missed National Service later on because of eczema. I wasn't sorry about that. During my medical school years, 1943–45, the mind was concentrated by the fact that if you failed the exam, you got your ticket into the forces, promptly, so we all worked very hard.

BB *Did the Medical School stay in Manchester?*

KR   Yes.

BB *Not much bombing?*

KR   There was a lot of bombing in Manchester, but the School wasn't damaged, although the blitz destroyed part of the Royal Infirmary.

   I did not do all that well at medical school, very run of the mill. However, because I had come in without any biology and had to do it after joining the

Medical School, I took finals out of time, and that gave me the chance of a better house job than some of my colleagues.

My first job was with Robert Platt at the Royal Infirmary. He was the first full-time Professor in Manchester, and I developed a high regard for him. He was building up a new department, a galaxy of talent. His First Assistant was Douglas Black, later PRCP London, as was Robert Platt in his own day. Malcolm Milne was there, later Professor of Medicine at Westminster, and Bill Stanbury who was subsequently Professor of Medicine in Manchester. Acting as dogsbody for this lot was a daunting prospect.

Some of these able men were supernumerary medical officers, returned from the war. A number of medical students at that time and some of the senior people had been ex-servicemen and were funded in a special way that I never understood. Platt was a man of great intellectual power, but withal a good clinician and with a very keen eye for the psychological aspects of illness. Interestingly, his first wife, Muriel was a child psychiatrist.

BB *Judging from his autobiography, he had a cyclothymic personality.*

KR   He had black dog occasionally. His was my first important postgraduate influence, pushing me toward a clinical rather than a laboratory career.

After Platt, I did a neurology house job, tremendously demanding because Fergus Ferguson the chief, a first-class neurologist, worked you ruthlessly hard. If you could stand it, all was fine. After another house job in medicine, I had a year in clinical pathology, something often embarked on in Manchester by people preparing for the London MRCP.

I worked for a year in the Clinical Laboratory at the Royal Infirmary, under R. W. Fairbrother, whose textbook I won as a prize at school in my bacteriology phase. I chose this to the surprise and despondency of the headmaster. The bacteriology, haematology, biochemistry, and other things that you do in a clinical laboratory finished off any notions I had of becoming a clinical pathologist. When Fairbrother learned of my intentions to become a psychiatrist he was very upset, and went to a deal of trouble to dissuade me from a ruinous path. He said, 'You don't want to go into that subject; it's just a lot of mumbo-jumbo and guesswork. Stick to something scientific.'

BB *Did he want you to be a pathologist?*

KR   A pathologist or a physician.

BB *Do you think he was right, looking back?*

KR   No.

BB *What did you do next?*

KR   Manchester had a academic department of psychiatry, then in existence for three years, and I went as senior house officer for my first psychiatric job. I spent three years there, a happy time. The Professor was Edward Anderson and the Lecturer Bill Trethowan, who started work about the same time as me.

BB *It was Anderson, Trethowan, and you?*

KR   There were three others, Jack Kenna, lecturer in clinical psychology, May Irvine, lecturer in psychiatric social work, and Lawton Tonge, the Registrar.

BB *Situated in the Infirmary?*

KR Yes. We had eight beds in two medical wards. The level of disturbance we accommodated in these wards amazes me still. In fact, many of the very disturbed patients we saw were not ours, but surgical cases having post-operative psychoses or deliria, the demented elderly, and alcoholics with DTs. So it was a small in-patient experience but we did have out-patient work.

BB *Did you have mental hospital beds?*

KR No. Later, there were beds at The Cheadle Royal Hospital, a private psychiatric hospital near Manchester.

BB *Where did Anderson come from?*

KR He was a Scot who spent the greater part of his professional life in southern England, before coming to Manchester. Part of his early career was in Germany and he was particularly influenced by the work of Kurt Schneider and Karl Jaspers. When he was appointed to the Maudsley Hospital as a consultant, he carried the flag for the phenomenological school. He came to Manchester as the first Professor of Psychiatry in 1949.

BB *One of the first provincial chairs?*

KR It was an early one. There was nothing there apart from two psychiatrists who, pre-NHS, pre-1948, had been working in the Royal Infirmary. They were mainly concerned with private practice and came in, like the honorary physicians and surgeons, to do clinics in the hospital.

Anderson started from scratch, and found it hard adjusting from the Maudsley to what he regarded as a psychiatric wilderness. Nevertheless, he set about it. As an undergraduate teacher, he didn't come across well, but as a postgraduate teacher he was superb.

Up to then, I had thought of psychiatry as psychoanalysis. To discover that in Anderson's view, clinical psychopathology was essentially phenomenological psychopathology, and that dynamic psychopathology was something to talk about and discuss, but not a serious enterprise, was a shock. Of crucial importance to him was the ability to relate to patients in the traditional phenomenological way, the empathic 'living in the world of the other individual' and then to set down, in detail, the elements or morbid subjective life which emerged from the discourse, no theoretical position being taken.

Anderson's way of doing this was remarkable. He was, of all psychiatrists I have known, by far the most painstaking, the most penetrating, the most formidable in being willing to spend a long time discussing a problem with a patient, analysing the mental state and producing a phenomenological formulation. Having done that, he stopped. His interest was in the delineation of mental states and the making of an expanded diagnosis.

Treatment was not high on the agenda. He was a microscopist, if you like; perhaps this is why the approach appealed to me, a failed bacteriologist. He dissected problems into their elements and brought them into a sort of order. Although humane and sympathetic, he was a therapeutic nihilist.

In 1951, treatment in psychiatry was rudimentary. ECT, leucotomy, insulin coma, and modified insulin therapy were used, but there were no modern psychotropic drugs. If you believed in psychotherapy, this could be tried, but in Anderson's department, the psychotherapy in vogue was supportive, which he regarded as valuable in the management of chronic personality problems and for certain neuroses.

Anderson's prime contribution was in the approach he recommended, to take a good history and analyse the mental state fully, without theoretical bias. He gave me what he gave many other people – an orientation to psychiatry which is there as a basis whatever other aspects one pursues.

His second contribution was the time he was prepared to spend talking to his postgraduates. He didn't rush off to committees, and hardly ever went to London. He was there, and you could always take a patient in to see him; he would never refuse to discuss a problem. When I think about my own teaching of postgraduates in later years, I blush at how inadequate I have been, compared with Anderson.

He also taught me to be aware of the importance of personality in psychiatric diagnosis. Personality has a pathoplastic and pathogenic role in psychiatric disorder. Personality determines a range of conditions which pop up in the out-patient clinic and which one can easily be misled into thinking are related to something outside the character; but the character is the essential feature. I regard his training as absolutely bed-rock in this matter.

There was a University DPM, which existed before the Academic Department was established.

BB *The University of Manchester DPM?*

KR   Yes. A pre-War diploma.

BB *How did this come about?*

KR   There were a number of diplomas in various branches of medicine – public health, and so on. Psychiatry was one of them.

BB *Did he initiate research?*

KR   Yes. I worked with him on the psychopathology of the psychotomimetic drugs. We heard about lysergic acid diethylamide, which had been synthesised by Hoffman in Switzerland in 1943. We had no real idea of what it was or what it did. It became available in Britain and sounded interesting, so we decided to look into its effects. We first took it ourselves. I mean I and one or two other members of the staff took some.

BB *Did Bill Trethowan?*

KR   No.

BB *Too sensible?*

KR   Yes, absolutely right.

BB *And Anderson – did he take it?*

KR   No. There was myself and Bob Mowbray, a clinical psychologist, the late Dr Paul Scott, and the Departmental secretary, Miss Doris Bee.

BB *I have had it, so I know what you are talking about.*

KR   That was a very, very interesting experience indeed, but one I would never repeat. Later on, I took half a gram of mescaline and had a similar, but more muted experience.

BB *What happened with the LSD?*

KR   It was the first time in my life that I saw the world totally differently. Not just in terms of visual, spatial, and temporal distortion, but from the point of view of ego change – the sense of ego dissolution, a terrifying experience.

BB *What do you mean by ego dissolution?*

KR   I will try to describe it, but it's difficult. My percepts, the view of the door, the view of the table somehow became me. If somebody left the room, for example, they disappeared; they ceased to exist. Because I had perceived them, they were part of me and I was bereft if they left. This was threatening and worrying.

At the height of the experience, I decided it was too much to cope with, so I closed my eyes, a great mistake. Because all visual percepts disappeared, I felt I was breaking up, that the ego was somehow going up the chimney.

That was so frightening, I opened my eyes again and saw everything distorted and jumbled, but at least it was there, and I was there again.

I believe I realised for the first time what a patient with schizophrenia meant when he saw someone hammer a nail into the wall and said 'That nail is being hammered into my head.' My ego boundaries had dissolved. I was the wall, the table, everything around me, and the two things were indissoluble. If they were affected, I was affected.

The importance of that experience to me was very great for two reasons. I now had some personal understanding of the psychopathology of psychotic illness – organic states and schizophrenic states particularly. And secondly, I realised that one's everyday experience of the world is idiosyncratic and probably not shared by anybody else.

For purposes of communication, we assume we all see things in a similar way, but I don't believe this is true. LSD gave me a subjective view of personal psychology and a willingness to try and live into the world of the psychotic patient with a new sensitivity.

BB *Do you think the experience fitted a DSM–III classification?*

KR   Yes I do. An organic psychosis, fundamentally.

BB *Not schizophrenic?*

KR   No, organic. Not because of the fact that I had taken a drug, but phenomenologically. Whenever I have talked to patients with organic disorders, I have looked at their experience from this angle.

I'll give you an example of what I mean. I was given a problem by Trethowan to solve while I was under the influence of LSD. He said 'A train sets off from A at 60 miles an hour for B, and a train sets off from B at the same time at 40 miles an hour for A. A and B are 100 miles apart. How long is it before they pass each other?' Well that was absolutely impossible. If I thought about A, B didn't exist. I couldn't retain two ideas in my mind simultaneously; I couldn't blend them. The same thing happened with taste. I was given a plate of meat and veg for lunch, but I couldn't blend the tastes. I was either tasting the peas or potatoes or the meat, but there was no combination.

BB *And how did it end?*

KR   I had a good night's sleep. The next morning, everything was pristine, new, seen for the first time. Rather like Adam looking at the world.

BB *It's astonishing such a powerful drug has revealed so little.*

KR   We were excited about the drug. I went to talk to Elkes, who was working with LSD in Birmingham. It all seemed full of Eastern promise, but nothing much has come of it.

BB *Did you publish with Anderson?*

KR   Yes[1]. We also gave it to a number of patients. We did it not because we thought it would do them any good, but we wanted to see whether a schizophrenic patient could distinguish between the disturbances produced by LSD and the endogenous disturbance.

BB *And could they?*

KR   Yes. On reflection, it was not a good thing to do. Later on, I was against using LSD therapeutically. It is a powerful and dangerous drug and I have seen it produce persisting psychotic illness, both in patients and in 'normal volunteers'. I would never do it again.

BB *So you learnt about phenomenology, how to run a general hospital psychiatric in-patient service, out-patients, and you did some research on LSD. Anything else?*

KR   We did some research on induced psychosis. Anderson was interested in the Ganser syndrome.

BB *He kept up his German contacts?*

KR   We had visitors from Germany, who kept us abreast of the latest developments in phenomenology. Some of them were rather worrying, because they turned out to be psychoanalysts rather than proper phenomenologists.

BB *Anderson remained firmly on the continent?*

KR   He was in purer culture than any of the other British psychiatrists interested in phenomenology.

BB *Than even the émigrés?*

KR   Even the émigrés. Anderson was interested in pseudodementia and the Ganser syndrome. He set up an experiment.

Medical students were given a little brief to read. They had been arrested by the police on a murder charge and were to be examined by a psychiatrist. It was up to them how they presented themselves, but they were more likely to be leniently dealt with if they were found mentally ill. They were allowed to brood on this for half an hour and then put through a formal mental state examination by Anderson and Trethowan, to see what kind of stuff they produced. This was interesting and on one occasion funny. One student

---

1. ANDERSON, E. W. & RAWNSLEY, K. (1954) Clinical studies of lysergic acid diethylamide. *Monatsschrift für Psychiatrie und Neurologie*, **128**, 38–55.

produced a paranoid psychosis during interview and then at the end of the proceedings, Anderson relaxed and said 'Well Mr so-in-so, thank you very much you have been extremely helpful. We are grateful to you for helping with this research.' 'What research?' says the chap. 'Was this research?'

And he insisted on continuing this phase for some time afterwards, to the alarm of Anderson and Trethowan. They thought they had sent him over the edge. •

BB *Anderson wrote a successful short text didn't he?*

KR Later on, it was Anderson & Trethowan and now Trethowan & Sims.

BB *What were Anderson's achievements?*

KR His pupils were, in my view, Anderson's most important achievement. Perhaps too, the influence he exerted on other members of his staff who joined him after their training elsewhere. I left the Department in 1953 and Anderson retired in 1965, to be succeeded by Neil Kessel who was joined not long after by David Goldberg. Much occurred in those 12 years which I think of importance to understanding Anderson's achievements, some of which I would like to see recorded because I believe him to be underestimated.

BB *Who were his pupils?*

KR Trethowan came to him as lecturer from the Maudsley. He later had a distinguished career in Australia and in this country, where he became Professor and Dean at Birmingham – his interview with you does not give quite the same picture of Anderson as mine will. There was Lawton Tonge, who did some useful research at the Social Psychiatry Unit before settling in Sheffield with Stengel, and Clive Mellor, now Professor in Newfoundland.

BB *And Hoenig?*

KR He came fully trained to Anderson's Department, sometime after I left; he had a European training. Some time after Anderson's retirement, John Hoenig took the first Chair of Psychiatry in Newfoundland, preceding Mellor. He and Marian Hamilton together translated Jasper's *General Psychopathology*, which until then had only been available in the German. I count this a most important event. It must have had a great influence on the outlook of English-speaking psychiatrists who had no German.

BB *That is most of us, I expect.*

KR Anderson wrote the Introduction to the English edition of Jaspers, a tribute I think to his helpfulness and encouragement to Hoenig and Hamilton, who were in his Department at the time. Marian Hamilton, while still with Anderson, had earlier translated Kurt Schneider's *Clinical Psychopathology & Psychopathic Personalities*. Both books, through being accessible in English, have I think, had important influences on clinical practice and also on clinical research.

BB *What happened next to you?*

KR Anderson was keen I should go to the Maudsley. He was aware that the Manchester offering was rather narrow and that one should have the opportunity for wider experience. I went off there in 1954 having got my Manchester DPM after three years of experience, and not quite knowing what was going to happen.

BB   *Did you have your MRCP?*

KR   I had that before I joined the psychiatric department. I arrived at the Maudsley and was interviewed by the Dean, David Davies. He said 'You have been working with Anderson. What you need is some psychotherapy experience.'

So I was assigned to Denis Leigh, another Manchester graduate. We took to each other. He said 'I want you to go down to a mortuary in East London. One of my patients has died and you must get the brain because I am very interested in this case and I want that brain. Bring it back in this tin.' And he gave me a biscuit tin.

So I went down to a mortuary, somewhere in East London, and had a tussle with the pathologist, who wasn't keen to give up the brain. Anyway, I managed to get it off him and brought it back in the tin on the tram. I didn't have a car. That was my first day on the psychotherapy unit.

BB   *What was your aim there?*

KR   I had no aim. I knew my experience had been limited and that psychiatry was a big subject and there was more of it to be seen at the Maudsley.

BB   *It wasn't for an academic or research career?*

KR   I had no idea what I wanted to do up to that point. It was strange. I did learn quite a bit about psychotherapy with Denis Leigh; we were taught the Finesinger method. Ted Marley was on the firm with me and we had a good time.

I remember my first experience of the Special Problems Conference, held on Monday mornings. That was the first time I had ever seen Aubrey Lewis. I sat at the back of this large gathering of people in the out-patient room, Aubrey came in, and we had one of these remarkable conferences. I was intrigued by the widely disparate opinions expressed by the people present, in a way that later on, when you got to know them, became so predictable. At that time, I didn't know who they were.

And then I had contact with him at the journal meetings, which were on Saturday mornings. Unthinkable nowadays.

BB   *Isn't it; nobody would come.*

KR   I found his way of handling them interesting. Requiring people to defend their position, expecting reasonable background knowledge of what you were supposed to have read, and so on.

I quickly began to feel a little sorry for registrars and SHOs there, because most of them had come into the Maudsley to start their psychiatric careers. It was such a lottery to which firm they happened to be placed for their first experience.

The more I saw of it, the more I treasured my own experience of having the ABC of psychiatry, clinical phenomenology, to start with, rather than being put onto a specialised firm.

There was a feeling of uneasiness and uncertainty among many of the trainees. The level of feedback, the level of information coming out of the 'oracles' wasn't terribly high. People didn't know what their future was going to be, and they got worried about it.

After six months with Denis Leigh, I moved to the Professorial Unit to work with David Davies, a man for whom I developed a high regard. He had a balanced and broad-church approach to psychiatry, which appealed to me. The senior registrar was Michael Shepherd, who I found stimulating because he required me to think accurately and clearly and defend my statements.

After three months, Aubrey Lewis asked me to join his MRC unit, which was then called the Unit for Research in Occupational Adaptation and later became the Social Psychiatry Research Unit. He told me about the work of the Unit, although I knew something about it already. Lawton Tonge had preceded me to the Maudsley, and was working in the Unit. The Assistant Director, Morris Carstairs, later became Professor of Psychiatry in Edinburgh, and then Vice-Chancellor of York University. There were a number of interesting people working there: Jack Tizard and Neil O'Connor, both psychologists; Peter Venables, later Professor of Psychology in York, and Jacqueline Grad working with Jack Tizard on the mentally handicapped living with their families. George Brown was recruited after I joined. John Wing arrived later, about the time I moved to South Wales in 1957.

My first exercise was with Neil O'Connor to set up a workshop for chronic psychotic patients at Banstead Hospital.

BB Before you go on to that, what were the origins of the Unit?

KR   The Medical Research Council established it on Aubrey Lewis's request, in 1948. Aubrey had been interested in the social aspects of psychiatry and worked on the occupational patterns of the mentally ill.

BB A strange subject, don't you think, at least it seems so from this vantage point. There it is, the premier postgraduate institution in the English-speaking world and its first research unit set up by the MRC is concerned with work adaptation.

KR   Aubrey was a man of vision, and probably took the view that other aspects of psychiatry – genetics, neurobiology, psychology – would look after themselves.

BB Or were unapproachable at that time because of lack of techniques?

KR   They were running and, of course, he had given them all a good push within the Institute. I suspect Aubrey deliberately chose an important soft area, to test the boundaries and try to develop a scientific framework for the social aspects of psychiatry.

BB A soluble problem?

KR   Well, approachable, at any rate. The stuff I did with Neil O'Connor was looking at the effect on a defined measurable index of behaviour of a deliberate change in the social environment of chronic schizophrenic patients. We used the hourly production rates which these patients could develop under a certain stimulus in a hospital factory workshop. We compared them with control groups and groups under other kinds of work stimulation.

Although it was apparently a soft field, from the beginning we looked at it quantitatively.

I don't think I have answered your question about why he went for work adaptation – the prognosis of neurotic illness, and the importance of personality in adaptation to work. This had interested him since before World War II.

BB *Was it an important war-time problem?*

KR Indeed, but he also saw it as a general problem. Here are people with neurotic illness. Now what determines whether or not they do well? Is it the illness? Is it personality or character? How can we look at this? One index, which is more or less measurable, is adaptation to work, studied through a process of rehabilitation and assessment of output, related to psychological and social variables. That's certainly how it was being evolved as a research exercise, initially in the mentally handicapped.

BB *Did Lewis choose mental handicap because he was beginning something new and mental handicap appeared to be easy to define, easier than say schizophrenia or neurosis?*

KR He may have been interested in testing out the stereotyped view of the severely mentally handicapped being incapable of work. Now is that really true? You then discover that under certain conditions, the severely mentally handicapped can work, and show a learning curve not so very different from normal, except for taking longer to learn a skill.

BB *Was he trying to find out something about the handicapped or about techniques?*

KR I think both. But the methodology and the techniques which had to be developed he regarded as an important part of the exercise. He was happy for a lot of time to be spent on developing them.

BB *What part did he play in the Unit?*

KR We had regular meetings with him, mind-concentrating meetings. One of us would present a research proposal or give a progress report about ongoing research. He would take it apart, and one had to defend this as best one could.

BB *One of his least appreciated attributes, to some.*

KR When you say least appreciated, you mean they didn't like it?

BB *Hated it, were frightened by it.*

KR I don't agree with that at all. I don't think he was destructive in any malicious or negative sense. It was a constructive attempt to make one think clearly, cut away the sloppy thought, force you into the most economic mode of formulating an idea, testing an hypothesis if you like and producing the methodology and techniques to answer that question.

Provided you were willing to play the game, it was a bracing and stimulating way of tackling problems. You could sharpen your brain against his. You recognised he was cleverer than you were and knew more about the subject than you did. Provided you did not wilt or regard it as a personal attack, you learnt a tremendous amount about ways of thinking and ways of criticising, and you produced a much better project at the end of the day.

I accept that people were threatened by him. I think it a great pity. I came to know Aubrey Lewis well, as I worked with him for many years. He was a man of great sensitivity and humanity, of tremendous warmth, and he had the interests of his students at heart. It would have bothered him greatly to feel that people were being put off by his approach.

BB *He must have seen that some people were stirred up by it.*

KR I think perhaps he did. But at the same time, this is the way he felt one had to winnow the wheat from the chaff in ideas, thinking, procedures, and so on. I can only speak personally. People vary. There are some who need an entirely different, maybe a gentler approach, to bring out the best in them. I personally found it a stimulating and educational experience to have to present anything – a case, a research proposal, a set of ideas – to Aubrey, and let him have a go at it.

BB *What was his aim with the Social Psychiatry Unit?*

KR His aim, having started it off on rather occupational lines, was to let it grow, in whatever way seemed scientifically profitable.

I'll give you an example of that. When we agreed that I would join the Unit, he said 'I would like you to go abroad for a while. I want you to find somewhere to study social research methods.' He left it at that. So I went away very puzzled, wondering what to do. Various people came up with various suggestions. Anyway, we eventually agreed I would go to New York City, to the Columbia University Bureau of Applied Social Research, and spend some time picking up the latest American social research methods. So I went.

BB *Who was there?*

KR The Director was Charles Glock at that time, but his predecessor was Paul Lazarsfeld, who wrote an interesting book called *Mathematical Thinking in the Social Sciences*. He was an unusual, intelligent man, who tried to bring numerics into social research in a big way. Of course, this was in the early 1950s. I spent a few weeks there, but I found it a bit up in the air. I wasn't able to get into any particular research project. Eventually, I decided to look around. I fell in with Ernest Gruenberg of the Milbank Memorial Fund, who was kind to me. He gave me some advice and I worked out a deal with Professor Alexander Leighton and went from the humid heat of New York City in July to Nova Scotia.

BB *Was Leighton part of the Bureau?*

KR He was Professor of Psychiatry & Anthropology at Cornell University, which is in Ithaca, upstate New York. But he was working at his field station in Nova Scotia running a large-scale study with two teams, one of social scientists studying the communities, and the other of psychiatrists studying the same communities from the psychiatric point of view. They were supposed to be separate. Never the twain did meet, at least in terms of the data, to avoid bias.

Surrounding all this, he was building up a body of theory about the relationship between social structure and psychiatric illness. Broadly speaking, he predicted social disorganisation was positively related to mental disorder;

he defined social disorganisation operationally. The aim of the exercise was to see how the map of social organisation and disorganisation related to the map of psychiatric morbidity.

BB   *One hardly thinks of Nova Scotia as being a place of social disorganisation.*

KR   It's a complicated set-up. This was rural Nova Scotia, not Halifax; it was on the other side of the peninsula, with small fishing villages, farms, communities of mixed French and British origin. There were some areas which were pretty disorganised and some were affluent. Anyway, this gave me an opportunity. Leighton was helpful and kind to me; he gave me the chance to work with the psychiatric survey teams in Nova Scotia. For the first time, I was into epidemiology at a practical research level and learnt a lot about field work, both the social and the psychiatric sides.

BB   *What did Leighton find out?*

KR   About his hypothesis? Well, it was supported, broadly speaking[2]. I learnt a lot from him and much about the use of indices, both medical and social. For example, Leighton used lifetime prevalence as a major index of morbidity, but that is a difficult index to interpret. The work I did later on in South Wales used period prevalence and incidence.

Leighton later took over the mid-town Manhattan study, following the death of T. A. C. Rennie in New York City. They found the lifetime prevalence of mental disorder in mid-town Manhattan was 81%, which is meaningless really[3].

BB   *So you learnt from the way he did things and from the way you might have done them if you had been him?*

KR   I also learnt from Leighton the difficulty of working with an all-embracing theoretical framework, rather than less complicated, more tightly defined theories and hypotheses, which one could test in a more limited exercise than the huge surveys going on in mid-town Manhattan and in Stirling County, which was the pseudonym for the study area.

BB   *Is it a secret where Stirling County was?*

KR   The main place was Digby, a small fishing port on the Bay of Fundy looking over from Nova Scotia towards New Brunswick.

When I came back to the Unit, I reported all this and then went onto something quite different, the work with Neil O'Connor on chronic schizophrenics and their response to social change.

I had been doing that for about two years when we had a visit from Archie Cochrane, an epidemiologist working for the MRC in South Wales. He was studying the prevalence of illness, starting with pneumoconiosis, and spreading into coronary heart disease and diabetes. He had some well studied and documented communities in South Wales, in the Rhondda Valleys and in the Vale of Glamorgan, a rural area near Cardiff.

---

2. LEIGHTON, A. H. (1959) *My Name is Legion*. New York: Basic Books.
3. SROLE, L., LANGNER, T. S., MICHAEL, S. T., OPLER, M. K. & RENNIE, T. A. C. (1962) *Mental Health in the Metropolis*. New York: McGraw-Hill.

Archie Cochrane has a number of Aubrey's attributes; he is an iconoclast, a man who requires proof and demands hard evidence for statements made. Clinicians regarded him with apprehension. He came to the Social Psychiatry Unit and offered access to his communities in South Wales for a psychiatric study.

Morris Carstairs and George Brown did a reconnaissance. I told Aubrey I was interested. He said straight away, 'This is where you can begin to use your North American experience'.

BB   Had Leighton found something which Lewis thought could be pursued in South Wales?

KR   Only in methodology.

BB   You were explaining this as an example of the way Aubrey Lewis would take something and allow you to develop it.

KR   Yes. He accepted Cochrane's offer.

BB   What was Cochrane's background?

KR   He was a doctor who saw service with the Republicans in the Spanish Civil War. He was captured in Crete during World War II and spent three years in German prisoner of war camps working as a doctor, part of the time using X-rays. He was only a General Medical Officer, but did quite a bit of X-ray work in the camps with crude equipment. After the war, he became interested in the public health aspects of tuberculosis and other chest diseases and joined the newly set up Medical Research Council Unit just outside Cardiff, the Pneumoconiosis Research Unit, to look at the epidemiological side of pneumoconiosis.

BB   Was he interested in the social and psychological side?

KR   Yes, and in psychiatry. At one point, he said he had considered becoming a psychiatrist. When Aubrey accepted his offer, this meant a new chapter in the work of the MRC Social Psychiatry Unit, because the work in Wales was an epidemiological venture.

BB   There had been no epidemiology until then?

KR   There had in mental handicap; Jack Tizard did some at an earlier stage.

BB   A survey of the prevalence of it in London.

KR   A repetition of E. O. Lewis's study, but none in mental illness. My brief was to develop methods for the study of mental illness in South Wales.

The first thing was a social investigation to see how we could best get going epidemiologically. I was joined by Joe Loudon, a medically qualified social anthropologist, and Lewis Miles, a psychiatric social worker, who later went to Australia and is now retired.

We worked as a team in the context of the Pneumoconiosis Unit. Loudon concentrated on the Vale of Glamorgan for the anthropological study, but we worked together studying the process of the recognition of mental illness at different stages of declaration. For example, we studied how general practitioners recognised mental illness and referred it to psychiatrists. We looked at the way samples of the population recognised mental illness or aberrations of behaviour, defined it, and dealt with it. We were later joined by two psychologists, Jack Ingham and Jim Robinson, who produced instruments for measuring morbidity.

BB   *Did you develop new instruments?*

KR   Yes, we used modifications of the Cornell Medical Index. Ingham also developed sophisticated symptom rating scales which we applied to random samples of the population.

BB   *Not in a city, but the valley villages.*

KR   In two areas, the Little Rhondda Valley or the Rhondda Fach, a mining community with small villages and townships, and the Vale of Glamorgan, a rural area with a market town in the middle. We had private censuses for both areas and were able to draw straight random samples or stratified random samples.

BB   *Why did you choose such contrasting communities?*

KR   Because we wanted to study communities where we thought that attitudes, values, perceptions of mental illness, and the way in which people dealt with it differed. We knew from hospital records that prevalence rates were much higher in the mining valley than in the rural population. Was the difference due to a difference in grass-roots prevalence or a difference in recognition?

When it all came out in the wash, the answer was complicated. We found that however measured – as hospital cases, GP recognition, or morbidity by population survey – the mining valley prevalences were higher than those of the Vale of Glamorgan. The explanation we thought lay in the attitudes of the populations. The Rhondda Valleys are interesting demographically. The population had been sharply reduced since the 1930s; many people had left mining.

BB   *You were studying a survivor population?*

KR   Also with people who were aware of the dangerous nature of their work in coal mining. There was what might be called a rather low threshold for the self-awareness of pathology, by comparison with the rural area. People were much more ready to declare themselves ill or be affected by something or other, whatever it might be – backache, headache, depression – than in the rural population. I think the measures of morbidity reflected attitudes which prevailed in those areas.

That's about as far as we got. From that point on, you get into difficult waters methodologically, discussing the relationship between social factors and the pathogenesis of neurosis. The two things almost come together[4].

In the middle of all this, we had an interesting interlude in 1961 with the people from Tristan da Cunha. A volcanic eruption on this isolated South Atlantic island prompted evacuation of the whole population by the British Government to Calshot, near Southampton.

---

4. INGHAM, J. G., RAWNSLEY, K. & HUGHES, D. (1972) Psychiatric disorder and its declaration in contrasting areas of South Wales. *Psychological Medicine*, **2**, 281–292.

BB *How many were there?*

KR   About 260. They were studied from all angles by the Medical Research Council, particularly genetically and for chest diseases. Joe Loudon and I went to look at their psychiatric status and the structure of their society.

BB *Why the interest?*

KR   Tristan was a closed community. Nobody had left or joined it for 50 years, though people visited. There was a British administrator, a doctor, a padre, and one or two others – birds of passage. The Tristanians had retinitis pigmentosa, at least some of them did, and asthma. They were racially mixed, from America, Europe, and Africa, and in colour ranged from rather black to rather white.

They did not regard us as medical investigators, just hangers on – Joe Loudon particularly because of the way he worked. They complained to us about the other doctors who were messing them about: one chap insisted on photographing them naked against a scale for their physical anthropometry. A terrible thing to do, they said. We were harmless.

Joe did an interesting social examination of this group. Together, we did a psychiatric study, pure gold actually, because when we had finished, we found a publication from a Norwegian group 25 years previously. They had landed on the island, unannounced, and studied the medical and social aspects of Tristan. At the moment of landing, they found themselves in the middle of an epidemic of major hysteria. People were having fits, fainting bouts, and screaming attacks. The Norwegians were meticulous and tracked the spread of the epidemic, using personal initials for identification. Twenty-five years later, using the initials, we traced forwards and found these people. Most were women, but a small proportion were men. The hysteria had probably been triggered off by a Montagu and Capulet situation – two groups of people worrying about a prospective marriage.

We found the main symptom among the islanders, at the time of our study to be headache, described in a stereotyped way, both verbally and non-verbally using similar gestures. About 40% of them had regular headaches, and they recognised that emotion could bring on a headache. We correlated the prevalence of headache in 1962 with that of *grande hysterie* 25 years earlier. There was a close association between the two: a marvellous example of how predisposed people can take on board neurotic symptoms as a spreading epidemic, or as an endemic condition with stereotyped symptomatology. The same gestures, the same language, in a population on top of each other all the time, sharing values, sharing ideas, sharing symptoms. A simplified and crystal-clear example of neurotic epidemiology of two different forms – the spreading variety and the endemic variety.

Although this was in a special population, it is the sort of thing that I believe operates in more complex societies by example, contagion, imitation, sympathy, but is far more difficult to study in Western society, where everybody is moving around and rubbing shoulders with lots of other people, than it was on Tristan, where everybody was together all the time.

From the point of view of psychiatric epidemiology, it tied up in an interesting way with the social structure of the population, particularly the leadership patterns. It was the wives of the leaders who had a hypersensitivity to neurosis, which raised the question of assortative mating of leaders with neurotic women, or whether being married to a leader is pathogenic.

BB   *What happened to the Tristanians?*

KR   They were fed up with Britain, and didn't like it at Calshot. They all went back except about three, who married British people. The longer they were away, the greener the island became.

BB   *You were asked by the MRC to do this survey?*

KR   We dropped everything and spent a lot of time with the Tristanians.

BB   *Worth it?*

KR   A powerful example of the pathogenic and pathoplastic nature of social factors in neurosis.

BB   *It is in the literature.*

KR   It has been mentioned[5]. But it loses its impact in the telling. I was more impressed by the Tristan neurosis than any other bit of epidemiology that I have ever come across, because it just shouted at you.

I will tell you something interesting. Joe Loudon went with them as ship's doctor on the voyage back. This *grande hysterie* had not happened for 25 years, but when the ship came in sight of Tristan, three or four people went off into fits and swooning attacks.

BB   *After studying the Tristanians, you went back to Wales. What was the relationship with Sir Aubrey Lewis and the Social Psychiatry Unit?*

KR   He was the Honorary Director. We were a detachment, if you like, of the Unit.

BB   *He was responsible, ultimately, for what you were doing?*

KR   I saw him regularly; he was helpful and supportive. Aubrey retired in 1966 and there was concern about the future of the Unit.

BB   *Your branch of it?*

KR   The whole thing. In the event, John Wing became Director and the Unit carried on.

The Welsh National School of Medicine created a Chair in Psychological Medicine in 1964. I applied, partly in order to secure a base for the continuation of the MRC work when Aubrey retired. My part of the Unit carried on for five more years before dissolving.

BB   *What were the achievements of the Unit in Wales?*

KR   We showed it was possible for people from different backgrounds to work together to produce a methodology which transcended the boundaries of social anthropology, psychiatry, and sociology. That it was possible to examine random samples of disparate populations, using reliable instruments on both the social side and the psychiatric side which were independent of whether or not people had chosen to seek medical advice. Then to address the question of

---

5. RAWNSLEY, K. & LOUDON, J. B. (1964) Epidemiology of mental disorder in a closed community. *British Journal of Psychiatry*, **110**, 830–839.

whether the apparent differences in prevalence of mental disorder between a mining valley and a rural area were due to differences in patterns of seeking advice or to frequency of mental illness.

We showed there was a fundamental difference between the two areas in South Wales, but that this conclusion begged a lot of questions about thresholds of awareness, of response sets to questions, about illness, and symptoms springing from local culture. We finished up answering some questions but posing many more, which I think touch on the fundamental issues of what is neurotic morbidity. Can it be defined independently of attitudes, values, and culture? How can one try to measure these things in different sub-cultures or societies?

I see the work of the Unit more in breaking new methodological ground than producing answers of value in aetiology or for the provision of services. It is a subject which still has not been fully explored.

BB *Your involvement in this sort of work then came to an end. But it didn't come to an end for some of the other members of the Unit; Ingham continued it.*

KR Yes, in Edinburgh with Kreitman. He has done some good work in general practice in Edinburgh and extended the methodology developed in Wales to answer rather more practical questions about prevalence.

BB *Who else from your unit carried on with research?*

KR Joe Loudon went to the Department of Sociology & Anthropology in Swansea. He continued to have an interest in this field, though he became involved in teaching and did little more fieldwork. Lewis Miles did a prevalence study on the Isle of Anglesey which had practical importance for service development. Jim Robinson carried on looking at the relationship between hypertension and personality in the local populations. So there were strains of the work which continued, but I got absorbed into developing the new Department in Cardiff.

BB *You were the first professor?*

KR Yes. There was a lot of goodwill and a certain academic tradition at Whitchurch Hospital, but I had to build the foundations of a teaching programme for both undergraduates and postgraduates, so it was a long time before I could start to recruit people for research. Most of the researchers who did come into the Department were not doing epidemiological work, but biological psychiatry and evaluation of services for the mentally ill and mentally handicapped. Epidemiology was not a main feature of the Department.

BB *What do you do when you are a new professor?*

KR That's a very good question. One of the problems is the expectations which are very high, that you will produce a first-class undergraduate and postgraduate teaching programme, develop a lot of interesting research, and produce a rapid improvement in the psychiatric services over a large area, in this case the Principality of Wales. Also, that you will relate to the Health Authorities and the Welsh Office and make a case for psychiatry in various contexts. Challenging.

BB *Including clinical opinions on the distinguished citizens of Cardiff and their wives and relations?*

KR I certainly saw a great many special patients. I thought this one of the privileges of the job. It is time consuming, but I thought it important to try in all ways to foster good relations and to develop contacts with colleagues throughout the Principality.

I felt greatly supported at all times by the psychiatric community in Wales. I have found that there has been a readiness to go along with proposals that I made to support the improvement of postgraduate training; a very heart-warming situation. It does lead to dilemmas of how to husband resources and how to spend one's time, more particularly later on, when I became involved with bodies outside Wales.

BB *In the first few years, how did you divide your time?*

KR Much time was spent building relationships with the other Departments in the University College, the Medical School, and Cardiff Royal Infirmary, which was the main teaching hospital before the building of the University Hospital; time spent consulting physicians, surgeons, and other medical colleagues both in Cardiff and outside. I was appointed by the Welsh Hospital Board as Adviser in Psychiatry for Wales, which meant spending a fair amount of time talking to people in the Welsh Hospital Board about planning of services for Wales.

BB *What qualifications did you have for that?*

KR None whatsoever, except I suppose some sort of knowledge of the range of clinical problems which were to be found in a population and my scientific outlook as an epidemiologist was of value.

BB *Who taught you administration?*

KR I picked it up by osmosis, by watching a few people operate.

BB *Do you think the undergraduate professorship, as you have described it, which is pretty standard around the country, is reasonable?*

KR In one sense, no. It is a bit of a nonsense because it's a Leonardo-type expectation. The professor has a lot of influence. Rightly or wrongly people look to him for help and advice. Someone purely concerned with research or teaching could not have this kind of potency. It is a paradox in a sense; if you have a broad range of interests and roles, then you are regarded as an oracle. What you say carries weight.

BB *Is it the same for the other chair-holders in the Medical School?*

KR The other disciplines are not so aware of the need to develop services. Psychiatry is a complex profession when it comes to building services and there are many variables to be taken into account. Psychiatrists are more aware of the need to develop the infrastructure of services, the teams required to produce a good service, and are willing to devote more time to this, than surgeons or physicians. That is because of our preoccupation with the social aspects of medicine in psychiatry.

For good or ill, your average professor in the provinces has to be willing to take this broad and extended position, wearing a lot of hats and being willing to forego the luxury of spending vast amounts of time doing any one thing to perfection.

BB *I suppose he can be more effective if there are subordinates to whom he can delegate. What does the President of General Motors do all day, one wonders?*

KR He has a clear desk. But it's not like that in professional psychiatry. You cannot organise your life as you would want to because you are always looking after patients. Whatever else I was doing, I would always have beds, and out-patient clinics, and domiciliary visits. That seemed to me absolutely essential, otherwise you took off into the clouds, lost all touch with the realities. But people ring you up and ask 'What you are going to do about Mrs Bloggs?'

BB *What were your achievements, in Cardiff, since you have been the professor. You were appointed in 1964 and retired in 1985. Twenty-one years is a long stint.*

KR The Department started with a professor and a secretary in 1964. In 1985, we had four senior lecturers, three lecturers, and a number of research people. Psychiatry was well represented in the undergraduate curriculum. We had developed a good rotational training scheme for registrars and also for senior registrars. There were two main research units, one of which was concerned with the biochemistry of mental illness based in Whitchurch with David Shaw and the other with the evaluation of mental handicap services in Wales, run by Roger Blunden. We had a senior lecturer in mental handicap, Valerie Cowie, who since has been given a personal chair in mental handicap in Wales.

I used to feel depressed towards the end of my stay. The University recession, I thought, had touched a low point, and I believed things were never going to be so good again as they had been. However, the Department became well established, gave a good account of itself on the teaching front at undergraduate and postgraduate levels, and at least in the latter half of its life, was beginning to turn out some research. For a new department to build up a research head of steam takes at least ten years, I would say.

BB *Perhaps we can turn now to the Royal College. Were you involved with its foundation?*

KR I was a member of the Royal Medico-Psychological Association Council, but I wasn't in the inner circles, if I can put it that way. I didn't see the inside machinations, but I was aware of some fierce infighting going on between different factions.

Some people were much opposed to any change in the RMPA, or if there was a change, they thought it should be to a Faculty of the Royal College of Physicians of London. Others were sure there should be a Royal College of Psychiatrists. There was acrimonious debate. Many people felt the RMPA 'establishment' had been for long an inward-looking and self-perpetuating oligarchy. The Council and the Officers were people selecting themselves, or were being selected by a small coterie. The President was, in effect, elected by the Council, as were the Officers. There was much dissatisfaction; I remember one or two quarterly meetings of the RMPA when things were pretty rough.

Eventually, a referendum of the Membership gave the clear result in favour of a Royal College. After that, there was a long series of discussions with the Privy Council for the Supplementary Charter.

BB *Do you understand why, constitutionally, it should be the Privy Council, as opposed to Parliament? It seems to be a thoroughly unrepresentative alternative system of government.*

KR   The Privy Council represents the Queen. The Queen promulgates the Charter on the advice of her Privy Council. Somebody once said negotiating with the Privy Council was like trying to argue with a black man in a coal cellar at midnight, to find the right questions to ask in the first instance. That's the system; that's the way it operates.

BB *I can see you are a man who believes in working with systems.*

KR   I do.

BB *Not to change them.*

KR   It would be a waste of time to try and change this particular system. I believe there were one or two bodies in the medical establishment very much against a College of Psychiatrists, who put in a number of oars to prevent it.

BB *You're not going to name them?*

KR   The London Royal College of Physicians was one of them. They were keen on a Faculty of Psychiatrists within their College.

BB *And the other Royal Colleges?*

KR   The surgeons would see it as an irrelevance. The Royal College of General Practitioners were supportive and welcoming, when our College was established.

BB *Were you involved in the negotiations?*

KR   I was not privy, except to reports from those negotiating, like Ben Monro, secretary of the RMPA, a key figure. When we became a College, and got our Supplementary Charter, it was agreed we would go straight ahead preparing for the Membership examination.

BB *Before the election of the Officers of the new College?*

KR   There was a transitional period, and then the Officers were elected. I was elected Dean.

BB *How did that happen? There had been no Dean in the RMPA.*

KR   The RMPA equivalent was the Registrar. William Sargant had been Registrar for years and years. Then there was a President who served for a year.

BB *So he had no power.*

KR   By the time he had decided what was to be done, he was off.

BB *Martin Cuthbert was the last President.*

KR   Martin was both last President of the RMPA and transitional President. Then Martin Roth was elected as the first President of the College, by general election. This was one of the key changes in the Constitution. The Officers, with the exception of the vice-Presidents, were to be elected by the membership.

BB *Roth would not have been the first President otherwise.*

KR   I'm sure that's right. But he was clearly elected.

BB *With the publication of the votes – a practice which has ceased. I regard this as a retrograde step don't you? It is a political office and you stand in public to be elected.*

KR You think it should be published for all the Officers?

BB *Why not?*

KR It can be embarrassing if someone has attracted say three votes.

BB *They will think twice before standing again. How did you come to be nominated as Dean?*

KR I was a member of Council and was a Council nominee. Some people are nominated by Council and others by members.

BB *Martin Roth was not nominated by Council.*

KR He was nominated by a group of members. Not that it matters one way or the other, because that doesn't appear on the ballot paper. Perhaps people thought I was interested in education. Anyway, I was elected and immediately found myself in the middle of all kinds of strong currents of emotion and pressures.

BB *What was the Dean's job?*

KR The Dean is the chief academic officer of the College; his job is to oversee the examinations of the College. I know there is a Chief Examiner, but the Dean's job is ultimately to ensure the exam operates. It's the Dean's job to ensure the educational and training functions of the College are in good order. One of the first things I had to do was to get cracking on a system for approving the training programmes throughout the UK and Ireland.

BB *Was that your idea?*

KR The idea had come out of the RMPA Committees. I had to implement it.

BB *There must have been something existing before that. There was for the Conjoint DPM.*

KR That wasn't anything to do with our College.

BB *I realise that, but there was a pre-existing system whereby certain hospitals were approved for training.*

KR That's right, but there was no inspection; it was a bit of a nonsense really. I had to get on with the business of constructing what became the Approval Exercise, from scratch.

BB *Nothing had ever been attempted on this scale by any College?*

KR There were inspections of a kind at registrar and SHO levels by some Colleges, but nothing on the scale we attempted. We devised a scheme and did four pilot visits. I took part in them. On that experience, we drew up a plan for the United Kingdom and for the Republic of Ireland, because the College writ extends throughout the British Isles.

BB *Isn't that extraordinary?*

KR Yes. I had to decide how to work it and which Divisions of the College would visit other Divisions. I tried to do it in such a way that if, let's say, Scotland was approving Ireland, then at no time would Ireland approve Scotland. There had to be a cunning Latin Square design; it was a bit hairy to begin with. First of all on the question of who was going to pay for it, travelling and so on. We got the money through the Health Service, eventually.

BB *Because the DHSS was in favour?*

KR   To raise standards. We were approving hospitals as suitable for preparation for the Membership exam. Without a Membership exam, we would have had no reason to go around the country looking at these places. So the Membership exam was a good excuse for the Approval Exercise.

BB *Were there criteria?*

KR   A list of criteria refined over the years.

BB *Applied uniformly?*

KR   Yes, because of the way the thing was designed. We had a Convenor from each of the College Regional Divisions, who took the main initiative in carrying out the visit. They recruited people from a panel to go on visits. Reports were prepared. Then the Convenors, ten of them altogether, one for each Division, met in a body called the Central Approval Panel, of which I as Dean was chairman. This set the standards. The Court of Electors ratified the decisions of the Central Approval Panel.

The whole thing went far more smoothly than I ever dared to hope and nowhere more so than in Eire, interestingly enough, where people were quite uncertain how it was going to work. There were good centres in the Republic, but some difficult areas too; we never had any problems there and were always welcome.

The Approval Exercise involved a great many people looking at other people's training programmes. In this way, good ideas were communicated in both directions, for the people going around doing the visits and the recipients of visits.

My policy was a gradual elevation of standards. We started off at a low level, but have slowly screwed the standard up. On the whole, I think the exercise has gone well and has improved standards of clinical practice as well as educational standards. The two go hand in hand. That is the most important thing I did as Dean, far more important than getting the exam going, which was done mainly by the Chief Examiner, Bill Trethowan.

The Deanship I found an entirely new experience: my introduction to psychiatric politics, with a small 'p'. It involved chairing committees, relating to other colleges, and relating to other bodies in medicine to do with education and training. I began to learn the rather labyrinthine set-up which operates in Britain in postgraduate education and how to work it.

There was a lot of hassle, understandably, from people who at the inception of the College had been members of the RMPA but were not entitled to be Foundation Members of the Royal College. I had to deal with this as Dean.

BB *What was the criterion?*

KR   If you were a consultant in the National Health Service or equivalent at the inception of the College then you were entitled to Foundation Membership. There was a lot of ill-feeling about this, from people who thought they were being disadvantaged. It took a lot of sorting out.

BB *These were holders of non-consultant posts, at a senior level.*

KR   There were SHMOs and senior registrars who had to take part of the new membership exam. There were people abroad in equivocal posts, difficult to equate with the British job structure. All this caused a lot of resentment, which still grumbles on.

BB *It must happen at the foundation of any institution. Did you get through one round of the Approval Exercise while you were Dean?*

KR   One and a half really, because it was a three year cycle, and I was Dean for five years, re-elected each year. Five is the limit.

BB *What's going to happen now, do you think? Will the new DHSS venture into making the number of training posts equivalent to the number of anticipated vacant consultant posts result in hospitals that have been through the turmoil of being approved losing their trainees?*

KR   I have always seen this possibility, before the DHSS got into this act. I have taken the view that the College must be prepared to face the situation in which some psychiatric hospitals and units no longer train registrars and senior registrars. They may nevertheless deliver a good service and train other personnel. On the other hand, it's a mistake merely to have a few mini-Maudsleys up and down the country, for training registrars. You need a compromise situation in which you have a moderate number of centres.

BB *Each one based on an undergraduate professorship?*

KR   Mostly.

BB *You can foresee some medical schools not having professors of psychiatry.*

KR   I think they will all have professors of psychiatry, even the London schools in time. I was envisaging a training programme operating without necessarily too much involvement of the local university. Broadly speaking, I think the training programme of the future will have a rotational element. It will have a university link and most important, a 'critical mass' of postgraduate students to relate to one another, rather than at present, where three or four people can be in an isolated setting.

There is a problem which can be dealt with at senior registrar level. This can be seen at the Maudsley, where people are trained in a hothouse atmosphere which does not, in a sense, prepare them for the hurly-burly of life in the sticks. These senior registrars, as well as having time in the 'teaching centres', should be alternated to where they are less part of an academic community, where they are more likely to find themselves in three or four years' time as consultants, practising the art in relative isolation. This could be catered for in the higher training level.

BB *How much of your time did the Deanship take up?*

KR   About two days a week in London, plus a lot of homework and preoccupation away from the office.

BB *Good fun.*

KR   Tremendous.

BB   Shall we talk about distinction awards? What's the justification for them?

KR   The justification is the goal, a stimulus, an incentive to work, to become involved in a range of things in the service. And to live in hope.

BB   You have been an Adviser?

KR   I was an Adviser for Wales. Now, I'm the College representative on the Central Distinction Awards Committee, I hope for not much longer.

BB   Do you think the system is fair?

KR   A tremendous amount of trouble is taken to ensure that all people, using multiple criteria, are given a fair whack. Evidence is collected from a range of sources by the central body. There are a lot of fail-safe arrangements for people who might be missed out. I believe that it's as fair as you can make it.

Having said that, I think it is difficult to run a system like this in a rational way. To start with, if you serve on an awards committee in a region or a district, you are required to compare, let us say, radiologists with physicians. People's names are put forward and it is impossible to assess merit across specialities, and for any one person to do this. It has become even more difficult because it is no longer just distinction, but distinction and meritorious service. Meritorious service has become more important.

BB   Can you explain the difference?

KR   Meritorious service means what the late Sir Hector McClennan, who was a Chairman of the Central Distinction Awards Committee, termed 'the heat and burden of the day'. He meant the consultant who has served conscientiously and in a way which is regarded as worthy and satisfactory for a long period. They may never have hit any high spot, published any papers, achieved fame or notoriety, but nevertheless have done a very good job.

BB   Labouring away in the hope of an award.

KR   Or even in the hope of helping people.

BB   It was you who introduced hope of an award.

KR   I think that's true, but I am not saying that everybody who gets a distinction award gets it because that's been their main aim in life.

BB   We were discussing whether it's fair. You discovered it is difficult to find and apply objective criteria, to apply a uniform standard across specialities. The solution to that is quotas of awards to each major speciality.

KR   That presupposes the cohort of people coming into each speciality is of equal merit, which is unlikely to be true. In practice, however, there is a tendency for this thinking to operate, for the apparatus to say – the anaesthetists are falling behind; we must see they are given better consideration. Or geographically, that the north-west of England is falling behind the south-east. Let us keep an eye on that. This quota thinking, when it comes to fundamentals, is wrong. But it does operate, though the figures show there are discrepancies between specialities and between regions, so it is not the sole factor.

BB *Published figures are attacked along the line you have just described, of lack of equilibrium. And people accept that as a valid argument they are not fair.*

KR I don't think that's right.

BB *Do you think it has a corrective influence, of making them more equal, irrespective of merit, when Bourne & Bruggen publish their comments.*

KR I think it has an effect. However, I don't think that vitiates the main function of the award system. God knows how you could have a perfectly 'fair' system. It is difficult within a speciality and worse across specialities. But the fact that it is difficult to implement to everybody's approval, even if they approved of the idea in general, does not mean you should throw the whole thing out.

BB *How did distinction awards start?*

KR When the National Health Service was established in 1948, Aneurin Bevan agreed to this extraordinary way of making it possible, for what was then regarded as the elite of the consultants, to 'have their mouths stuffed with gold'.

BB *Is it unique?*

KR I think so. I don't know of anywhere else that has it.

BB *After you finished being Dean, I think you stood for President.*

KR I wasn't elected. Desmond Pond was.

BB *How did you feel about not being elected?*

KR I had mixed feelings really. I was disappointed on the one hand, but on the other relieved. I thought I could have another go in three years' time. It gave me a breather anyway, to catch up in Cardiff, where my presence had been somewhat diluted while I was the Dean. I quickly got over the disappointment and got on with what I was doing.

Three years later, I put my hat in the ring again. I was uncertain about how it would go, because I've learnt to be chary of taking bets on College elections. I think they are unpredictable, especially those involving the general membership.

BB *You became President for three years. That's the limit of the office. Re-elected each year. Why was that put in the Constitution?*

KR To make it possible to get rid of somebody incompetent. If it was obvious after six months that they were useless, then the machinery of putting another candidate forward could be started. So far, it has not been used.

BB *How did you see the office of President?*

KR Quite different from being Dean. The President is the Head of the College, and has to relate to other bodies, to the other Royal Colleges, the DHSS, the postgraduate education bodies such as the Council for Postgraduate Medical Education in England & Wales.

I found this to be an interesting side to the work, seeing how other organisations function, how they run their affairs and also viewing the medical scene from a general platform. The Joint Consultants Committee for example. The President is a member, and therefore comes into contact with the British

Medical Association hierarchy. You see the political battles that go on between the organisations such as the BMA, the Colleges, and the DHSS; you take part in them. Very interesting. You get something of the flavour of the balances that operate to keep the whole thing rolling along.

The President has to take a lead in matters of major importance. Thinking through the range of things I had to do, there were three matters to which I had to devote a lot of energy. The Mental Health Amendment Bill, which eventually became the new Mental Health Act, was put forward during that time. Secondly, the arraignment of the Russian Psychiatric Society came up when the World Psychiatric Association had its meeting in Vienna in 1983. The third matter was organising my thoughts and taking soundings in the College about the future role of the consultant in psychiatry.

BB *Did you also play a part in the day-to-day running of the College?*

KR   The President is concerned with everything, in one sense. The Dean looks after the educational side of the College. The Registrar is the chief administrator of the College. But the President copes with a range of things from basic housekeeping to enquiries from the DHSS which need an urgent response, or from the media. It's quite a busy job, busier than the Dean's. I spent half the week at the College on average, as well as being involved when I was at home. It's a major commitment.

BB *What effect does it have on your Department? This is a general question about all Royal College Presidents and their Officers, I should think.*

KR   It's one of the interesting things about the British medical scene. You don't find them on the continent of Europe – these important organisations like Royal Colleges which rely on voluntary labour of a large number of people to run them. If you are appointed to a College office, the expectations are that this takes priority; the first thing you must do, even though it's not your paid work.

Inevitably, what you are supposed to be doing at home suffers. As far as I was concerned, I had colleagues in Cardiff who were generous and willing to take over a lot of the work of the Department. I suspect the whole thing got along very much better in my absence than it would have done if I had been there, in many ways. But there is a dilemma, a sense of guilt that wherever you are, you should be somewhere else.

BB *What did the University think about it?*

KR   The Medical College and the Health Authority were happy to allow me to do the work. They saw it as bringing kudos to Cardiff and to Wales.

BB *Can we talk about your experience with the Mental Health Act while you were President?*

KR   I had not before been involved in detailed parliamentary work and it was an eye-opener. The Bill started life in the House of Lords.

BB *Is that normal practice?*

KR   Bills sometimes start in the Lords, but usually in the Commons. We were heavily involved during the Bill's passage through the Lords, lobbying peers and trying to steer the thing the way we thought it ought to go. When it went to the Commons, the Government took the unusual step of setting up a Special Committee to examine the Bill in detail.

BB *Who was the Minister?*

KR Kenneth Clarke had the main responsibility, although Norman Fowler was Secretary of State. Clarke attended meetings of the Special Standing Committee of the House. We gave evidence to that Committee both written and oral; I, together with some colleagues, appeared before the Committee and was grilled. I believe we modified a number of clauses in the Bill, some of which were initially a bit outrageous. Then, unfortunately, some things slipped past us which caused a great deal of concern. I don't think we could have done much about some of them.

For example, at a very late stage in the progress of the Bill in the Commons, a Member moved an Amendment that certain treatments, such as psychosurgery, should be subject to a mandatory second opinion from the Mental Health Act Commission, even if the patient was 'not liable to be detained'. That was put forward from the floor of the House and to my horror, was accepted straight away by Kenneth Clarke for the Government – to the amazement, I believe, of his advisers who were in the House.

That was a major setback. It meant that the consultant and the patient together no longer had the right to work out between themselves what was the best treatment, even though the patient was informal. The overriding feature was that under that part of the Act, the Minister had the power to include other treatments if he wished.

It seemed to me that we were in danger of a situation where many of our treatments could be subject to mandatory second opinions, in out-patients or even in general practice, because the Act applies to all mentally disordered persons. We tried hard to get this overturned when the Bill went back to the Lords. With their traditional good sense, the passage of the Bill in Scotland did not include that clause; in Scotland, there are no such restrictions on the use of psychosurgery. I wondered whether we would have clinics in Gretna Green.

We had asked for the Mental Health Act Commission, created by the Act. I am not sure it has worked quite as we would have wanted. The Commission is an unwieldy body containing some people who I think have very little appreciation of the realities of psychiatric work. They take an impractical, ideologically based view of what should happen. It is still too early to say how that Act is going to work out in practice.

There is a powerful anti-psychiatric feeling among many Members of Parliament. I think it might have been part of a general anti-medical feeling, but it was clear and it is worrying. It alerted me to our standing and our image in the public mind. I've been preoccupied with it ever since, and I voiced my concern in my Presidential Address to the College[6]. We are at risk of being reduced because of misconceptions about our role and our function by the uninformed.

---

6. RAWNSLEY, K. (1984) Psychiatry in jeopardy. *British Journal of Psychiatry*, **145**, 573–578.

BB   Do you understand what led up to the new legislation?

KR   There were anxieties fuelled by the enquiries and scandals which occurred in mental and mental deficiency hospitals. The feeling had grown that detained patients were not adequately protected by the 1959 Act. A major factor was to improve the safeguards before detaining patients. The other element, which the College was sympathetic to, was to have an inspectorate to keep an eye on what was happening in psychiatric hospital practice. Since the dissolution of the Board of Control under the 1959 Act, that had not been happening, except through the Health Advisory Service, which does not have strong teeth.

BB   The mood of Parliament and of influential people in the period leading up to this Act seems different to their mood leading up to the 1959 Act.

KR   The 1959 Act was in keeping with the spirit of that time. There had been an extraordinary revolution in psychiatric practice, particularly in hospitals in the 1950s – the unlocking of doors, the discharge of large numbers of patients, and the great increase in the numbers of voluntary patients.

There was a feeling of optimism, of a revolution if you like, in psychiatric practice, reflected in the 1959 Act. A good example is the de-designation of mental hospitals. Before 1959, mental hospitals were designated by Act of Parliament as places which could receive detained patients; it was not possible to have detained patients in others. The 1959 Act removed the distinction, and it was then possible to have detained patients in any hospital willing to take them.

BB   What went wrong, do you think, if anything did go wrong, to produce this feeling? Did psychiatrists overplay their hand? Or was it a direct outcome of the scandals, for which scapegoats had to be found for the underfunding which lay behind?

KR   It's a complex question and I don't know the answer. There is, I believe, a general anti-professional, anti-medical movement, and anti-scientific also: don't trust professionals. That view was fuelled by emotion coming from the civil liberties lobbies.

So the whole thing became transformed into an issue of building in safeguards. It's not good enough to let the doctors get on with it. We must have clearly defined safeguards under an Act, and bring in other people who are not psychiatrists, to keep an eye on them and take part in the process of detention, approval of certain treatments, and so on.

It's a downgrading of the professional role. I believe this is potentially bad for clinical practice, and for patients. I also think it has been seized upon by organisations which involve other professionals in the health field, for their own aggrandisement.

BB   What are you thinking of?

KR   I'm speaking generally, because the majority of people in these professional groups would not work in this way. But there are elements in, let us say, social work or in clinical psychology which have chosen to harness this energy for their professional advancement; the upgrading, if you like, of their activities in the mental health field. Sometimes, this has been done rather unscrupulously.

BB Do you not think that ultimately, the problem lies in the comparative lack of technical skill in psychiatrists?

KR   I don't agree with that view. I had the scales pulled from my eyes when I got into epidemiology and saw physicians in action. For example, we regard X-rays as a precise tool. I was involved as a spectator in some systematic evaluation of X-ray reading, on a big scale. I was amazed by the amount of observer variation and bias in these readings.

When I worked in clinical pathology, I had always thought of the laboratory side of pathology as an exact science. There was a test used for estimating globulin in cerebrospinal fluid, the Pandy Test. You put something into a sample of CSF and it went milky. The globulin was determined by comparing this milkiness with a standard set of scales or tubes with variable milkiness. This was about the most imprecise thing you could imagine, and absurdly vague in practice. Some of this technical precision is actually pseudo.

Robert Platt, that master clinician, taught that the most important element in making a diagnosis was the history, and that is notoriously imprecise.

The high-technology side of medicine, though I applaud it in many ways, must not blind us to the fact that precision can be practised by psychiatrists just as well as it can be by physicians and surgeons. The ability of psychiatrists to alter the course of illness is actually good – high in many cases. If you look at some of the terrible problems of general medicine, which really can't be cured even by high-powered technology, we are not so badly off.

BB Did you find MPs aggressively against psychiatry?

KR   Yes. Many of them. Some were sympathetic.

BB As energetically as the others were against?

KR   Yes, especially in the House of Lords. A number of peers took a great deal of trouble to find out and present a point of view which was balanced and reasonable. I was impressed by the standard of debate in the House of Lords – much better than the Commons. You might say they had more time.

BB You mentioned the Russians.

KR   I had been a member of the College Special Committee on the Political Abuse of Psychiatry for some years. When I first joined that committee, I was a sceptic. I didn't believe it was an important problem. I thought a lot of the stuff being put about was propaganda and disinformation. However, when I looked at the data, I decided it was a real problem and a very worrying one.

When I became President, I regarded it as a major issue for the College and myself too. The Russians, by incarcerating dissidents in mental hospitals for no better reason than their speaking out against the Soviet state, prostituted our discipline – something which had to be opposed in the strongest possible way. To try and perhaps secure the release of these unfortunate people would right a wrong and remove a major blot on our professional image.

I spent much time on this matter and became involved in the movement through the World Psychiatric Association to find out what was going on in the USSR. The World Congress of the Association, which happens every six years, took place in Vienna in the penultimate year of my presidency. The College mounted a strong campaign to arraign the Russian Psychiatric Society.

BB   *Were the other WPA member countries allied with you?*

KR   Not all; some were much opposed. The American Psychiatric Association was our principal ally, and some of the European psychiatric societies. When the Motion was put in the pipeline to be debated in Vienna, which would have led to the expulsion of the Russian Psychiatric Society from the WPA, the Russians pre-empted us and resigned from it a few months before the meeting.

We went ahead nevertheless and had a debate at the Congress, a very acrimonious debate. There were a number of Russian supporters, even though the Soviets weren't there themselves. Attempts were made to have the whole thing set aside. But our resolution, re-worded at the meeting, was passed by a substantial majority. In effect, it criticised the USSR for what was happening, at the same time saying that the WPA would welcome the Russian Society back into the fold when evidence was clear that the offending practices had stopped. We made our point.

Since then, things have happened in the USSR with the 'glasnost' policy of Mr Gorbachev, including the release of some prominent dissidents which we had campaigned for, including Anatoly Koryagin. There is evidence that incarcerating dissidents has eased up, although still going on. We have to keep pushing.

BB   *It is largely a political, rather than a clinical matter. Could Russian psychiatrists stop it?*

KR   I don't think they could. The number of psychiatrists involved is small and most are well up in the hierarchy of Soviet psychiatry. I don't think they would desist without a clear directive from above.

BB   *You see this issue as important for the reputation of psychiatry outside Russia? Even more important than what was happening to the dissidents.*

KR   As far as the College was concerned, we were not trying to tell the Russians how to deal with dissidents, but we were saying you must not regard them as mentally ill when they are not. You must not give them injections of psychoactive drugs and lock them up in mental hospitals for years for saying things which the Soviet Government does not like.

BB   *Do you think the involved people in the Soviet Union knew what they were doing, or that they believed that dissidents were mentally ill because of a different view of what is mental illness?*

KR   I believe some knew the truth, but continued to operate the system. Others I'm not sure about. They may have persuaded themselves that anyone who has the temerity to speak out in public against Soviet policy was *ipso facto* insane. Even if that were true, it would not justify committing a person to a mental hospital for years or to use these powerful treatments. Under the Soviet constitution, in theory, there is the right of free speech. The dissidents were not a danger to themselves or to anyone else in any ordinary sense of the word.

BB   *The third matter that you felt was important while you were President was the role of the consultant.*

KR   The business of the Mental Health Act and anti-psychiatric feeling seemed to be knocking the image of the consultant psychiatrist, which led me to think hard about this question. Especially the authority of the consultant in modern psychiatric practice, particularly in the multi-disciplinary team. The feeling that the doctor should be one member, with no special authority, and accept corporate decisions for managing patients.

I tackled this by writing a paper on the future of the consultant[7]; I circulated it through the College to Divisions and Sections for comments. I then reformulated the paper as recommendations to Council. Council debated these issues and, broadly speaking, supported what I recommended.

Essentially, they endorsed a policy statement made some years earlier by the College on the role of the consultant – that the consultant should be primarily responsible for the care of patients, should have the major responsibility for making decisions, certainly with advice and help from other professional groups, but that there should be no question about where the prime responsibility lay.

There were other aspects to the paper. For example, the relationship between consultants and general practitioners, and the question, for instance, as to whether it was desirable to have direct access to consultants, walk-in clinics, this type of thing. On the whole, Council was against them. It took the view that the general practitioner should be the central figure in medical practice and the consultant, broadly speaking, should operate through the general practitioner wherever possible.

BB *Why do you think the consultant's position was threatened?*

KR   To some extent because of indecision and uncertainty on the part of consultants themselves. Some became unsure as to whether they did have special skills, whether they did have a particular expertise in psychiatry in comparison with, let's say, psychologists and social workers.

This is in part a result of the erosion of confidence which has been one of the products of the anti-psychiatric feeling; they have become unsure of themselves, listening to critics. Many of these consultants, perhaps working in isolation, were persuaded there was nothing very special about being a doctor in psychiatry. One should just be a member of the investigation and treatment committee.

That is a recipe for disaster.

BB *From the patient's point of view?*

KR   Yes. Language is one of the problems we have to cope with. For example, people say 'Well, you know, you shouldn't rely on the medical model; it's very narrow, and a very partial way of looking at problems'. If you accept those words, then you are accepting a false statement, because medicine in general, and psychiatry as a branch of medicine, is actually a broad subject.

The medical man or woman, by virtue of the training they have received is able to draw on a biological standpoint, a psychological standpoint, and a social standpoint, all of which should come together in the assessment of the clinical problem. The imputation of the term 'medical model' is that it has to do only with organic factors, drugs, and a mechanistic way of looking at patients. This is quite wrong.

The medical model, as I define it, brings in all angles from the biological to the social. A good doctor uses a complex, elaborate point of view, in assessing a clinical problem. It's a unique perspective, the product of a long training.

---

7. RAWNSLEY, K. (1984) The future of the consultant in psychiatry. *Bulletin of the Royal College of Psychiatrists,* **8**, 122–126.

BB *By unique, you mean it is not held by any other profession involved in treating patients?*

KR   Yes. It is a broader perspective than that of any other professional group in the health field. By virtue of that, the doctor, the psychiatrist, should hold pride of place in decision-making about patients. It's not a popular view.

BB *Why doesn't everybody believe it?*

KR   I think if they believe that, they would feel their own professional development was being imperilled. Bear in mind that clinical psychology and social work are young professions by comparison with that of medicine. They have to make their way in the world, build up their image and their standing. To do that, they must make territorial claims which, inevitably, will be at the expense of existing professions.

When developing something new, you tend to push hard and perhaps overplay it. Their contributions are great, but they have to be fitted into a scheme of management for patients where the doctor, the psychiatrist, must be the key figure in making decisions.

BB *How is the confidence of the doctor to be improved?*

KR   It is a major function of the College. The College has a duty to promote this point of view through its educational programmes, through meetings and through conferences; to infuse a sense of confidence and a proper appreciation of the doctor's ability and skill to take a leading part in the management of the patient.

The College must maintain a sense of integration, of family if you like, in our profession. Because of the complexity of psychiatric medicine, and the many specialities within psychiatry, so many orientations, there is a factious tendency which could be dangerous.

The College is the only organisation in Britain which has the power, the resources and, I hope, the will to keep the family together. There have been times when I thought we were going to lose a chunk of our brethren, that certain sections might hive off. I won't go into detail, but it was averted. It's something to be watched and pre-empted, if it looks like happening.

BB *So you had three years as President and you seemed to have enjoyed them.*

KR   I did, except that during my penultimate year, I wasn't well. I developed an illness which, because I chose to have the treatment in London, meant paradoxically that I spent rather more time in the College than I otherwise would have. Even so, it was quite a nuisance during that last year.

I had been having symptoms of prostatism for some years and put off doing anything about it; I couldn't really be bothered. Eventually, I had it investigated because it became difficult. I went in for what I thought would be a routine prostatectomy, and it turned out to be malignant. Quite unexpected. I then had to have radiotherapy, which wasn't too bad in itself, but it meant going every day or so to hospital, so I had to cut down my activities. But because I was staying in London, I was able to carry on at the College.

The illness itself caused me to see life in different terms. It's amazing how when you develop a potentially fatal illness, you take stock of the situation and paradoxically savour certain aspects of life more keenly than before.

That certainly happened with me. In other ways, it was a major nuisance. I haven't often been ill, but whenever I have been, particularly if I have had to have treatment, I have regarded the experience as one to be treasured from the professional point of view.

The experience of illness in oneself as a doctor is beneficial, or can be, in enhancing one's empathy and sensitivity to illness in patients, making one more aware of the anxieties, the immense dependence which patients develop. And of the importance of a sensitive, careful response on the part of the clinician. And not only the clinician, but all the staff who are concerned with you. From that point of view, it had its positive side.

Eventually, some two years after, when I got secondaries, I decided to retire from the Chair of Psychiatry at Cardiff. I took the view that with the form of malignancy I had, the pace of life was going to be important in influencing prognosis, and I wanted to cut down my activities to a large degree. As it has worked out, with further treatment, and perhaps because of a different way of life, I'm not feeling at all bad at the present time.

BB   Do you think the prognosis would have been affected adversely if you had remained at work?

KR   I think so. The endocrine-sensitive cancers, particularly, are, I believe, likely to be influenced by the general state of vitality, as well as by outlook. There is some evidence on breast cancer outcome to support the idea that mental attitude affects survival. This could well be true of prostatic disease. It is no doubt mediated by hormonal influences.

BB   Did you have a sense of anger, having been given this disease?

KR   More of frustration. Perhaps that's linked to anger. I did feel frustrated by having to undergo all the treatment and waste a lot of time going to hospitals and seeing doctors. I also felt irritated.

When I went to Vienna to represent the College's view on the Russian affair, I was partly incapacitated by symptoms. My experience of Vienna was largely as a map of the public lavatories in the city to which I could have urgent recourse. I remember sitting through the meetings and occasionally having to nip out, being careful not to do so when a crucial vote was about to be taken. I wondered how much of the British Empire had been lost through a prostatic absence at a crucial time.

BB   Perhaps this is an appropriate time to move on to a different kind of sick doctor.

KR   You're thinking of my interest in sick doctors and the development of the National Counselling Service. That was prompted by my work on the first Merrison Committee, established to look at the regulation of the medical profession.

This Committee, which reported in 1975, looked at the function of the General Medical Council in respect of sick doctors. At the time, the GMC could only deal with alcoholic doctors, and other doctors failing professionally through illness, by its disciplinary procedures. One of the outcomes of Merrison was the new Medical Act, which made it possible for the GMC to set up a Health Committee, a more humane, rational way to deal with doctors who failed through illness.

I was impressed by the evidence we received in that committee about the extent of the problem of sick doctors, and it led me to try to think of ways and means in which we could develop machinery to help doctors before they had to be picked up by the GMC. An opportunity arose when the Association of Anaesthetists wanted to set up a scheme for their own members and our College helped them with that.

BB *It's mainly a problem of addiction.*

KR   With the anaesthetists, yes – drugs and alcohol. But later on, it seemed appropriate to broaden the service. Initiatives were taken by Sir John Walton for the General Medical Council and by Mr Tony Grabham for the British Medical Association.

I was asked to set up a national service with a small management committee, to be autonomous and independent. This service opened in October of 1985 and covers the United Kingdom. It has a network of advisers and counsellors willing to help doctors.

A number of things struck me forcibly about this service. The first is the way in which the profession has been willing to help. Of some 300 people that I have approached to help, not one has refused – a remarkable tribute to the profession's willingness to look after its own.

BB *Are you talking of 300 psychiatrists?*

KR   Doctors of all kinds. The second is that so far, the scheme has worked smoothly. We're running a referral rate of about 10 new cases a month. It's confidential and private, so one doesn't know what's happening to the patients. So far, there have been no major hiccups. I hope it is doing some good, but I don't know for sure.

BB *You act as a central referring agency?*

KR   We have a hotline telephone in London, which is manned by doctors. I act as a co-ordinator, with a small management committee. The DHSS pays, although it doesn't cost much.

BB *The Service finds a doctor to care for the referred doctor?*

KR   Yes.

BB *The Service doesn't know who the referred doctor is?*

KR   The central body doesn't know who the referred doctor is. The purpose is for a worried colleague of a sick doctor to get in touch with the scheme. They can then be linked with an adviser who will try to approach the sick doctor and persuade him/her to accept help. A fifth to a quarter of the referrals are sick doctors themselves ringing up saying they would like help, but they don't want to consult local colleagues. It's easy for us to put them in touch with someone outside their own region.

BB *Do you mean a worried colleague who obtained the name of an adviser would then go to the adviser, share his worry, and the adviser would then, as it were, unilaterally approach the object of worry?*

KR   A delicate undertaking.

BB It would be interesting to know the outcome, wouldn't it? Is there a way of finding out?

KR   I had a meeting of national advisers recently in London. It was to some extent impressionistic data which came out; certainly, there are cases taken on board as a result of this approach, but one doesn't know the ultimate outcome. It is going to be difficult to evaluate.

BB Would you like to say something about your views on the future of psychiatry?

KR   I have an optimistic view, in one sense. I believe psychiatry as a profession will continue to exist and tackle the problems of mental illness for a long time to come.

I am more sceptical about major breakthroughs in the diagnosis and treatment of mental disorders. There will be developments, particularly in dementia. But the crystal ball is dark in predicting the changing limits of psychiatric involvement in human affairs over the next decade or two.

This is an important issue, in which there could be useful research jointly between psychiatrists and general practitioners. General practitioners do the bulk of psychiatric work in this country and are often unsure about the proper limits of their involvement in human misery, unhappiness, and discontent.

The limits of psychiatry are constantly refined in terms of values and expectations of the profession and of the general population.

BB Is distress a medical matter?

KR   For the most part, no.

But distress may be the cause or consequence of some disturbance of psychological or physical function where a doctor may be able to help. There is a risk, as happened in the United States in the 1950s, that psychiatry becomes too extended, proclaiming its interest in territory which is well beyond its proper scope. It's a matter of fine judgement as to where these limits should be set. And they do keep on shifting. We should be more aware of limit-setting, if you like, and look at it from an operational point of view.

BB What do you mean by that?

KR   Look at it from the point of view of the validity of our power to intervene effectively in situations and in ways which other professions or lay people cannot.

8 Peter Sainsbury

Interviewed by HUGH FREEMAN (1987)

*Dr Peter Sainsbury, BA (Cantab) 1938, MB
BChir 1941, DPM (conjoint) 1947, MD 1950,
FRCP (London) 1975, FRCPsych (Foundation)
1971, FRCPsych (Hon) 1983.* Dr Sainsbury was
born in Horsham in 1916. He served in the RAMC
in West Africa and Germany from 1942 to 1946.
An interest in suicide led to appointment as
Professor Aubrey Lewis's research assistant at the
Maudsley Hospital. In 1957 he was appointed
Director of the MRC's Clinical Psychiatry Unit and
Honorary Consultant at Graylingwell Hospital. The
team's research work at Graylingwell led to many
publications on evaluation of psychiatric care in the
community, on suicide, on psychophysiological
studies and on research methodology. Dr Sainsbury
was Chairman of the Special Committee on the
Political Abuse of Psychiatry 1978–86.

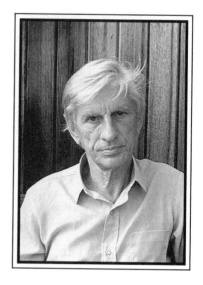

*HF   As psychiatrists, we are supposed to be interested in people's early life and background,
so I wonder if you would tell me something about yours and if you think it had any relationship
to your later career?*

PS   I was born to a middle-class family in 1916. My mother and father were
'bright young things' in the 1920s, and part of that set. I was sent as a boarder to
a prep school just up the road in the street where I lived, when I was five-years-
old. I think that might have had some influence on my future development!

But I suppose things started becoming interesting in relation to my career when
I was at Stowe school. I was placed in the bottom form and got stuck there.
Nevertheless, I was very interested in science and used to read a good deal. In fact,
I knew a lot of biochemistry at that age and also read a bit of psychology and
physics; but at the bottom of the school, one did not study the sciences.

The headmaster, Roxburgh, was one of England's great headmasters: an
admirable figure whom we all tried to emulate, particularly his language. He
would complain 'what a lamentable performance, Sainsbury'; or 'egregious
student'! We delighted in his love of words, and this remained with me. He
worried about me being stuck there and started quizzing me about why this
was. Then, I was able to tell him that the only thing that really interested me
and that I felt I was any good at was science. So he broke the rules and let
me study chemistry and physics.

From then onwards, my academic career took off and the interesting thing
is how one's performance at other subjects improves as well, as soon as one
gets going. I was told I got the highest marks in England in my school certificate

134

in chemistry, 99%! Next, my interests turned to biology, and so I started on the path to studying medicine.

HF   I would like to ask you two things next. Firstly, what was your home atmosphere like – you say your parents were 'bright young things'. And secondly, what was your experience of boarding schools?

PS   Home was really quite exciting; my parents were always going to cocktail parties, treasure hunts in motor cars, and such like. My brother, sister, and I were left to the care of our nurse, whom I adored and visited often, until she died last year. But they attracted into the home a lot of interesting people, who had quite an effect on me.

My father started an amateur theatrical company, the Horsham Players, which became quite well known, and people like Miles Malleson used to produce the shows; but these theatricals instilled an enduring fear in me of public performances. And when I was a bit older, I became very attached to Allen Lane, and helped to choose books for the first series of Penguins.

I did not like boarding school, but Stowe was about the best option one could have at the time. It was fairly progressive and the buildings and grounds were very beautiful – the headmaster taught us to share his love of 18th-century architecture. So Stowe not only helped me to become a scientist, but also excited an enduring pleasure in buildings, gardens, and music too.

HF   I would like to ask you now about the point when you left school and how you then started on your course towards medicine.

PS   I left school when I was taking my Higher Certificate. This was early, as I did not really enjoy being a boarder, so I went up to Bart's for a year prior to going to Cambridge. I did very little studying at Bart's; it was really a year off in London, the sort of thing young people do nowadays between school and university.

Then I went to Trinity, when I was 17. Cambridge was a fascinating place in 1935. There is a lot of fuss these days about the left-wing traitors in Cambridge, but it was part and parcel of the ethos of the young men and women there. We sought a brave new world; a lot of my friends joined the Communist Party, and some of them went to Spain. A friend of mine, John Cornford, who was at Stowe with me, was killed there on his 21st birthday. That was how people thought in the 1930s. You either hated and demonstrated against Mussolini, Hitler, and Chamberlain, joined the Left Book Club, and were part of that set, or missed out on the great issues of that age. We undergraduates were among the first to take up the cudgels against Nazism, and were re-labelled 'patriots' as the war approached.

At Cambridge, I enjoyed the opportunity to get down to studying physiology and biochemistry. The biochemistry department was very exciting, inhabited by people like Needham, Bernal, and Hopkins. It was at this time that I first developed an interest which was going to be important to me for the rest of my working life. I was fascinated by Cannon and the physiology of fear and emotion, and had a fantasy that this was what I was going to study. In fact, some of my first research at the Maudsley was in the psychophysiological area; but it was unrealistic in 1935 to think that I might have opportunities to study disorders of that kind.

HF   Are there any of your fellow undergraduates that you particularly remember from that time?

PS   The ones who are most relevant to what we are talking about now were the radical young scientists, one of whom had been Head Boy at Eton and became a communist. Four of this group became directors of MRC Units.

HF   Who were the other three?

PS   Waterlow, Humphreys, and Gell.

HF   Let's talk now about the point when you left Cambridge and went on to hospital work.

PS   After Cambridge, I went to the Middlesex Hospital, where my father had been a dental student. But teaching was disrupted by the war, and after a year there, we were evacuated to Aylesbury.

There, I made my first contact with psychiatry, with Skottowe who was just introducing ECT at St John's Hospital. Then we came back to London, but were again evacuated, this time to Wolverhampton; but for some reason, I went via Cambridge, where I got a job as a houseman because they were so short of junior doctors at Addenbrooke's.

So I studied for my surgery and got paid for it at the same time, while living in a fantastic house – the Granary on Silver Street Bridge, part of Darwin's home. It belonged to the Director of Education, who revived my interest in architecture. He had people like Gropius come to stay and the young modern architects of the time, who were designing his 'village colleges' and schools. These were pioneering endeavours, which provided the pattern for many of the post-war schools.

So that was a happy year, but it did not go down well with the Middlesex Hospital, as I should really have been at Wolverhampton. But still, I and a friend from Stowe struggled through our exams and passed them.

As a student, I was interested in psychosomatics, and found it natural to see stress as a factor in illness. I remember being shocked when a senior cardiologist went into paroxysm of rage with a patient who complained of tachycardia and extrasystoles of a nervous kind. He seemed to feel that this unhappy man was there just to tease and provoke him!

HF   You qualified in medicine then and started out on your first medical job. What were your experiences then?

PS   My emotional ties were with Cambridge (where I married a German refugee), so I applied for a job as a house physician in Bury St Edmunds, at the Royal West Suffolk Hospital.

But one knew then one was just marking time until joining the RAMC. There, I met up again with many old friends from Cambridge and the Middlesex. I particularly remember my entrance into Crookham, saluting smartly at the gate, and knocking my cap off. I was that sort of a soldier!

Eventually, I was sent on a tropical medicine course and boarded a ship to India, which I was really looking forward to. I had lots of books on the subject. However, we stopped off at Freetown for training in Grafton Valley, which the Malaria Unit told me had the highest infection rate for mosquitoes in the world; this was where the Army sited the hospital! Consequently, I got malaria there and was in a sort of semi-coma when the Unit moved on to India and Burma, and this I always regretted.

However, I did then have a fascinating job in Sierra Leone: they made me Recruiting Medical Officer for the colony. We went up country on a tiny railway and then walked through the bush for a couple of weeks, going from village to village picking up recruits for the army. I think each headman was told to produce so many volunteers. This was pristine, untouched tribal life such as it would now be difficult to find anywhere.

It was a really unique experience and my sorrow is that I did not have an anthropological training to take more advantage of it. There were Leopard and Baboon societies, through which a chief of a village imposed his influence and exercised power; tribal dancing and drumming, and primitive rites for pubertal men and women were still practised, as was voodoo: natives who violated tribal laws died, yet we found nothing at post-mortem.

HF   I believe that after leaving Africa, you had a short spell in Germany at the end of the war, and then came to your demob.

PS   When that happened, I still had this crazy idea about wanting to study the pathophysiology of emotions, so I decided to try and get my Membership and then go to a mental hospital and get a grounding in psychiatry.

My rather vague notion was that I would become a physician who specialised in those disorders in which there is a large emotional component, rather than becoming a psychiatrist, of which I think I was a little bit nervous. In the event, there were more of us demobbed than there were jobs and I became tired of going on refresher courses.

I decided instead to reverse the order and do my stint in the mental hospital first, and then go and improve my general medicine afterwards. So I went to Bexley Hospital, which was then go-ahead with Leslie Cook in charge; he was a nice man to learn from and work with. While I was there, I took my DPM.

HF   What were your impressions of your first experience of a mental hospital?

PS   I was really rather alarmed and horrified when I first went in. It was so unlike the tidy, orderly, clean atmosphere of a general hospital.

An early impression was how skilled and devoted to their patients the male nurses were at that time. A lot of them were men who had come down from the north during the Depression. The male wards needed so little paraldehyde, compared with the female ones, and I found this remarkable.

Very quickly, I got extremely interested in the work and attached to the patients. Also, of course, we were very spoilt then. We had a farm, and wonderful food, much better than they were having at the Ritz: strawberries and cream and marvellous great joints used to come up to the wards – for the patients as well.

Another aspect of the place was the sense of community in the hospital; nurses and doctors were still rather alienated people, so we tended to cling together.

Also some of the patients were much more treatable than at first appeared – and how a success could bolster one's confidence! I recall, for example, a lady who had been in the hospital for some years. I established that she was suffering from bromide poisoning. On stopping her bromides, another condition emerged; she was suffering from an agitated depression and when we gave her ECT, she got better and went out. This made me feel that there was a lot more one could do than I had first imagined.

HF   What was the next stop after Bexley?

PS   I got my DPM and apparently, but I did not know this, there was a job advertised for a registrar, or the equivalent to it, at the observation ward at St Francis in Dulwich.

Dr Cook was away and Dr Comerford, his deputy, was in charge; a warm, kind, and rather eccentric man. He wrote to St Francis in my name, applying for the job. He thought I ought to get a move on! I certainly was rather stuck at Bexley in a way; my wife was very ill in a sanatorium nearby and it never occurred to me to leave and apply for the job.

But he had me up, and said, 'You've got a job at St Francis observation ward', and – this is rather typical of me – I said 'Well, this is the way it is,' so off I went. Dr Comerford was quite right.

The observation ward provided a wonderful experience in acute psychiatry and I enjoyed it, especially Professor Lewis' fortnightly visits to advise us on the more difficult cases. I got on very well with him. I used to tease him about coming down on the tram and wondered why he made the social workers cry when he quizzed them about the patients. He liked this and it was only later on that he made me nervous too!

One day, I told him I was perplexed by the suicide attempters and indeed why people killed themselves. This set him off saying 'Oh Sainsbury, haven't you read Faris & Dunham?', 'No sir', 'Do you know Durkheim's work on suicide?', 'No', 'Do you know Booth's survey of London?', 'No', 'Oh well, you might find something interesting there'. It took me a year to see what he was getting at, to read these books, and to gather that he was suggesting that I did some kind of social epidemiological survey of suicide.

HF   Was this how you got interested in suicide in the first place?

PS   I often think of this encounter with Aubrey and wonder why was I interested in suicide. Prior to joining the observation ward, I had never had to talk and cope with people who had seriously wanted to kill themselves. I think I was genuinely concerned and amazed; it seemed so unbiological and somehow tragic.

HF   What was your next move then, from St Francis?

PS   Aubrey Lewis asked wouldn't I like to come up to the Maudsley and, he hinted, do research? But he added that I needed to fill in the gaps in my psychiatric experience, and proposed I go to child psychiatry first. So I did six months with Kenneth Cameron and that was a very interesting period.

Then it really baffled me when Professor Lewis said he wanted me to go full-time into research, and suggested that I devoted myself to this study of the ecology of suicide for my MD and a Maudsley monograph. Within a month of starting it, I realised I was on a good wicket, that there was not only an immense reservoir of statistics on suicide but also of social data on the London boroughs, and that they could be related to one another in all kinds of ways. It quickly became evident that this was very economical research. Here was a wealth of data which could easily be exploited, and so I was soon able to tell Aubrey Lewis that I was making good progress, and this seemed to please him.

He then arranged what, I suppose, was the next step in my career. He appointed Sidney Crown and me to be full-time research workers at the Maudsley, with rooms in the basement of a house on Denmark Hill. His suggestion was that tics and other spontaneous movements merited study, and with this end in view, he had already begun negotiations with an electronic expert at St Thomas's, Peter Styles, who had developed a device able to record and count the activity in muscles – something that was quite novel at the time. So he presented me with this wonderful apparatus and told me to get on with it, which I did with relish, using this apparatus and frame analysis of ciné-photography to count tics and relate their occurrence to a variety of circumstances.

I became particularly interested in 'muscle tension' and the kind of symptoms psychiatric patients complain of: backache, writer's cramp, headaches, and so on. So together with John Gibson, I began some studies on anxiety and these muscular symptoms.

My next step was to use the same device to measure gestural activity in psychiatric patients. To do this, we gave the patients interviews in which we first discussed bland topics and then stepped on their psychiatric corns, while counting the changes in gestural activity which occurred when the emotionally disturbing topics were introduced. Gesture was an aspect of behaviour in which I remained interested for the rest of my working life.

HF   There came a point then when you had to decide whether you were going to devote yourself to a life of research or go into more direct clinical work.

PS   I rather panicked at this point and as there was a clinical job going at the Westminster Hospital, I applied for that. I felt anxious about devoting myself solely to research, I was not confident of my ability for it, and I was very contented doing clinical work. So I started with Garmany at the Westminster.

During this time I had to give a lecture about my work at the Maudsley on movement and muscle tension, and Aubrey Lewis was in the Chair. *While* I was giving the lecture and in the gap between slides, Aubrey said 'would you like to join the MRC?'

I was never a good lecturer and this made me even more incoherent than usual. So a few days later, I formally applied for the post of Director of the Research Unit at Graylingwell.

HF   Was that the job which had been vacated by Martin Roth?

PS   The reason it was vacant was because Martin had just been appointed to the Chair at Newcastle, but his outstanding work at Graylingwell had prompted the MRC to take over the clinical research there, though this had not yet been implemented.

In 1956, the MRC was assessing research being conducted in all NHS hospitals with a view to supporting those departments they approved of. As Martin was no longer available, they needed to grab someone.

My interview at the MRC was amusing and quite typical of Professor Lewis. While I waited my turn, other applicants came away from their encounter with remarks such as 'My God, it's rough in there', so I entered with some trepidation, but it so happened that as each question was put to me, Aubrey Lewis was ready with my answer! There was going to be no doubt about who was to have the job, and he was not going to let me mumble and fumble and put them off.

HF   How did you feel about your life being directed in this way?

PS   It's most satisfying – making choices is very unsettling. But this is a question I often ask myself. Perhaps I'm a bit of a fatalist. In this instance, however, this opportunity was so manifestly attractive that I would have been a fool and a coward not to have had a go at it. As on other occasions, some generous patron had formed a more optimistic opinion of me than I had.

Looking back on my life, I can see that fortune and kindly people have indulged me. Aubrey happened to like me, he was my sponsor, and urged me along in a way I could not have done by myself. Given my sort of diffidence, I can only feel grateful to those who took on the task.

HF   So at that point, you left London and moved to Chichester.

PS   Then there was the problem of what the research programme of the Unit was going to be. I have always preferred dry facts to juicy theories, and clinical research tends to be the applied kind anyway.

Through my own inclinations and the staff that were available, there was a premium on work on the psychophysiology of symptoms, and on the epidemiology and statistics of suicide and other disorders. The Unit's early endeavours involved a study on personality and psychosomatic disorders in all patients attending the general hospitals in Chichester, as well as a survey of mental illness in a New Town, Crawley, which was in our catchment area. Indeed, my choice of projects was often determined by the particular opportunities our district presented to us. In West Sussex, for instance, we had a quite unique opening for research into the psychiatric services, and this was something that tallied nicely with my interests.

Dr Carse, the Superintendent of Graylingwell had, in 1957, just introduced the Worthing experiment – a real innovation in community care. This was a psychiatric service in which every patient referred was first seen in the community, either at home or at a day hospital. Moreover, the patients were then treated as far as possible in one of these settings, rather than by admission. It was a 24-hour service, efficiently organised, and operated in close conjunction with the GPs. But it also provided the research unit with a novel opportunity. So we started an evaluative study, comparing this community service with a hospital-based service in Salisbury, a district which is demographically similar to the Chichester one.

A lot of our findings and comments on community care nearly 30 years ago now have an all-too familiar ring about them; that it can only succeed clinically and avoid burden and distress in the family if the service ensures that adequate social and psychiatric support is provided in the community. Without that, everyone is in dire trouble, but given the facilities and skilled personnel, community care does work because, on the whole, patients' families and GPs prefer this alternative.

HF   Do you happen to know how it was that Carse got on this track in the first place?

PS   I don't know how he got in touch with Querido, who had set up a service of this kind in Amsterdam. But Carse went over to Holland, saw what they were doing there, got sold on their ideas, came back, and introduced and adapted them to meet the needs and circumstances of West Sussex.

HF One criticism made at the time of the Worthing experiment was that it was done rather in isolation from the local authority community services.

PS   This was absolutely the case. It was remarkable to see how the social workers in the hospital reacted too. They were so used to taking clinical histories for the psychiatrists that they were quite at a loss as to their new role. They could not get away from the habitual way of working. But oddly enough, the social workers in the hospital-based service in Salisbury clearly recognised their function as one of supporting the patient's family and coming to grips with the problems of out-patients.

HF You did find, though, that a greater degree of hospital care reduced the burdens on the families, at least for some categories of patients.

PS   The burdens were relieved on families when the patient was admitted. Nevertheless, families in the community service were very tolerant of the extra burden which they had.

Although the burden on the family was increased for those in the community support was given to the family, but in Chichester it was usually given by the psychiatrists. They visited the patient at home and collaborated with the GP. Where this kind of support was provided, the burden was reduced as much in the community service as in the hospital one, and it was found to be more acceptable to the family. The family were prepared to take on a lot of extra commitments, providing they were assured of some regular backing, whether by the day hospital, the psychiatrist, the GP, or the social worker.

HF Was it true to say, as I think some people said at the time, that Graylingwell at the beginning of the experiment had an unusually high admission rate, compared with the rest of the country?

PS   I am not too sure of that. All I can say is that in our controlled comparison of the two, 80% of the referrals to the psychiatrists in Salisbury were admitted, whereas only 14% were admitted in Chichester. So even if Chichester had a high admission rate, this would not explain this enormous decrease.

HF Are there any other implications of this comparative work of yours for the situation that we are in today with the mental health services?

PS   I think that a lot of what we said at that time about the problems that are entailed in establishing an effective community psychiatric service are now recognised as evident. You cannot do community care on the cheap.

The Department of Health was very interested in our study to begin with, because I believe they saw it as an economical way of providing care. Our original intention was to include a cost-effectiveness study in our evaluation, but we were unable to recruit an economist. Community care is costly on personnel. Indeed, it's almost irresponsible to introduce such a service unless this fact is honestly faced, as well as recognising the importance of ensuring an effective organisation not only for maintaining contact with patients being treated extramurally but also for providing skilled support.

Another aspect of the study, though of a different kind, that made a great impression on me is the enthusiasm with which all levels of staff in a mental hospital welcome, assist, and do their best to promote a research project. Providing its purpose and their contribution is made clear to them, they enjoy collaborating and sharing in the endeavour. This was true of the GPs too. So one ends up with a really fine research team of nurses, doctors, social workers, and others.

HF   What about the practical difficulties of carrying out a large research programme and getting all the data into a published form?

PS   We had two problems. We did not publish nearly as much of this study as we ought to have done, partly because we were always in a hurry to get on with the next thing, but also because this was the first large-scale survey of any kind to go on a computer.

The Atlas in Manchester was the most advanced computer in the world then and a program was developed to analyse our data, but the whole thing just would not quite work, so we have never fully exploited it. Nor did I really get down to the huge task of taking it all off Atlas and reprogramming the data for a later generation of computer.

This has always been a terrible regret of mine. I should have put other things on one side and got a new member of staff to recode and make the data available in another form.

HF   Could you talk about some of the other things that you were interested in at your unit?

PS   One of the projects that I and other members of the Unit got very interested in were case registers. Here was an immense pool of information waiting to be exploited, and we tried to use it in various ways.

John Birtchnell did some valuable epidemiological studies using the North-East Scotland case register, and Jackie De Alarcon set up one in Southampton which was specifically tailored to evaluating services. This case register accumulated details of the type of care patients received over the years, as well as recording social and clinical items.

Unhappily, funds were withdrawn when the NHS policies were revised, and the plan agreed with the Region to evaluate the mental health services in Southampton by comparing the half of the city based on a District General Hospital with the other half based on Knowle Mental Hospital had to be abandoned.

What an absurd waste of money, opportunity, and work: administrators and doctors are still asking the questions we hoped to try to answer 15 years ago. Now, even the register is closed. It makes my back ache!

However, Birtchnell's epidemiological studies on birth order and early bereavement in relation to psychiatric disorder are nice examples of the uses to which registers can be put. Richard De Alarcon set up a register and undertook an interesting and pioneering survey of drug dependence in our district, but very sadly, Richard became ill, and much of his work was never published.

I found uncompleted work to be a major difficulty in directing a research unit. A psychiatric project often takes two or three years to plan, implement, analyse, and then write up. The real problem arises at this last stage of publishing. What happens is that as the researcher's appointment comes to an end, he applies for and obtains a consultant post. He really believes he will finish writing up the work after leaving, but in fact never finds the time. This happened to three or four good projects. I should have been tougher and made sure the work was finished.

Other projects which especially interested me and which we did publish were Kreitman and Nelson's work on mental disorder in married couples, a study on the psychophysiology of hypertension, and an ultrasonic device to measure gestural and psychomotor behaviour, developed with Mr Haines. (As a psychiatrist, I was always very proud that this apparatus was exhibited at the physicists' annual exhibition at Alexandra Palace.) Dr Shaw was with the Unit from day one, and made some very original contributions to methods of analysing the EEG, which had important clinical implications for dyslexics and schizophrenics. I must mention Dr Levey's interesting studies on classical conditioning and Dr Knowles' on the placebo response, while Mr Jenkins and I enjoyed working on a commission from WHO to investigate the social and other factors affecting suicide trends in Europe, and in particular its decline in England. But the best of the work on suicide and that which brought me most pleasure was that of Brian Barraclough. I had not intended to reply to your question at such length!

HF   Have you any ideas on how research could be better organised in the future, so that it would be more productive and make better use of its resources?

PS   That question is more important than ever in this miserly and illiberal age. The MRC, of course, really had the right idea and one which used to make it the envy of research workers the world over; namely, its policy of giving a good proportion of its scientific staff tenured appointments. This not only attracted people to a career in research, but enabled them to undertake more ambitious, long-term investigations.

But such support is currently not very popular, so short-term grants, which often allow one to touch the edges of a problem, now tend to prevail and they are not now as amply provided as they should be in this country with its research ethos (which will wither if it's not nourished).

I think we need to ensure more opportunities both for young psychiatrists to be exposed to research and for more formal training in research design and methods. We might provide some regional organisation whereby panels of experienced research workers would be available to advise, assist, and direct psychiatrists who are seriously intent on investigating a problem.

I tried to promote a scheme of this kind when I was Chairman of the RMPA's research committee, but it never really caught on. I very much like the idea of the College setting up a research department. It could provide some of the facilities I have just mentioned.

Attracting funds for psychiatric research is another matter. In the RMPA committee, I made quite good progress in liaising with the pharmaceutical industry's institute on research. They were keen to collaborate, but for some reason which I never understood, the rest of the committee did not like it. I think it might be worth trying again.

As an aside, I would like to mention that I strongly favour placing research departments in the mental hospital (and its district services), rather than confining them to the universities. The day-to-day problems of clinical psychiatry and of providing psychiatric services are most conspicuous there, and opportunities for getting pertinent ideas present themselves daily.

HF   Since your retirement from the Unit, have you continued to work on your research data to publish new findings?

PS   I have done a bit of publishing, but I think I had intended to do more than I have done. I mentioned that we did a quite interesting study on Suicide Trends in Europe for WHO. One of the things I had resolved to do was to write this up for publication, and this is still on my list of tasks; otherwise, I have written some papers for conferences, chapters in books, but very little new work.

HF   Could we talk about your College activities?

PS   The College (and RMPA) and my various assignments with the two institutes have been of the utmost importance to me in both my professional and personal life. I think I have been, at one time or another, a member of every committee they have managed to devise, despite my ineptitude in that role.

When I became Director of the MRC Unit at Graylingwell, I instantly inherited Professor Roth's position as Chairman of the RMPA's Research Committee. This, and other commitments to the College, kept me in touch with other psychiatrists and many friends, and this was a continuous source of pleasure. The College was a kind of club that spared me becoming a recluse in the Sussex steppes.

I cannot remember how I became a Vice-President, when Linford Rees was the President, though I know I felt very proud to be one.

In that office, it fell to me to interview Plyusch, the first Russian 'psychiatric' dissident to come to the College. This was one of the events which led Council to set up a Special Committee on the Political Abuse of Psychiatry, of which I became Chairman. Its deliberations were always engrossing, often led to interesting decisions, sometimes to real successes in helping dissidents or in influencing attitudes, and once, with Sidney Levine, to a remarkable encounter at the Soviet Embassy.

HF   Have you any summarising thoughts on your career in psychiatric research, particularly which might be of interest to those who are starting out today on a similar road?

PS   I do feel if one is sufficiently motivated and there is a problem which you really know you want to pursue, this is probably the essential preliminary to research. It is amazing the extent to which things become possible when you know what you want to investigate.

I know I have had a lot of luck. Nevertheless, I do believe that if there is an idea, an area of inquiry which truly enthrals and preoccupies you, then the motivation to read about it, worry about it, and then to formulate a viable research project will follow. The funds, or even recruitment to a research team, despite the current squalid neglect of support for psychiatric research, will also materialise.

9   Sir George Godber

Interviewed by HUGH FREEMAN (1988)

**Sir George (Edward) Godber, GCB, BA
1930, BM 1933, DM 1939, Oxon, FRCP 1947.**
Sir George Godber was born in 1908 and was
educated at New College, Oxford and at the
London Hospital and London School of Hygiene.
He became Medical Officer, Ministry of Health
in 1939 and from 1950–60 was Deputy Chief
Medical Officer. From 1960–73 he was Chief
Medical Officer, Department of Health and Social
Security, Department of Education and Science,
and Home Office. He was Chairman of the Health
Education Council from 1977–78. In 1973 he was
made an Honorary Fellow of the Royal College
of Psychiatrists. His publications include *The Health
Service: past, present and future* (Heath Clark
Lectures) (1974) and *British National Health Service:
conversations* (1977).

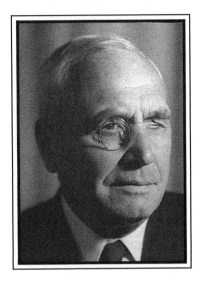

*HF   Could I ask you about your first exposure to psychiatry in your medical training and how
it struck you at that time.*

GG   My first exposure came during my fourth year at Oxford, when I was
doing pathology and pharmacology, in the six months of clinical work that we
used to be able to do then.

One of the regular things was that we went once a week to Littlemore Mental
Hospital, out on the edge of Oxford, where we were taught, after a fashion,
by the medical superintendent.

HF   Was that Dr Good?

GG   It was indeed Dr Good, and he just talked, and talked without really
carrying a great deal of meaning to the people to whom he was talking. So
I couldn't say that I got a very good impression of mental health there. I didn't
have any more, of course, until I did my main clinical training at The London
Hospital, and I wouldn't say that the training in pyschiatry was very good
there either.

The psychiatrist who did the lectures and was the main teacher did take us
to one or two mental illness and mental deficiency hospitals, but it was regarded
by most of my fellow students, I think, as a not very onerous half day out.
I don't think we got any real sympathy for psychiatry or for mental illness,
and it didn't seem to figure very largely in what other teachers at the hospital
were trying to give us.

HF   After qualification, did you have any contact with psychiatric illness?

GG   I didn't do any work in psychiatry – didn't do a job in a psychiatric hospital, for instance. I next came into contact with psychiatric patients when I was doing some work for the Ministry of Health in 1939, helping to prepare for the Emergency Medical Service hospital programme. This included visiting a number of mental illness and mental handicap hospitals to propose ways in which some of their buildings could be used for casualties, if indeed we had to use that number of beds for them.

I encountered a number of senior psychiatrists then, but it was hardly an introduction to effective psychiatric work, because those hospitals were mainly of the custodial type. There are one or two people one remembers, like Macmillan at Mapperley, who was a very impressive personality, but I can't say that I got much else out of it.

HF   Any particular aspects of the wartime experience which are of interest in this connection?

GG   Not insofar as the management of mental illness is concerned because, as you know, a fair number of patients were crowded up or moved out of mental hospitals then, if any of their buildings were being used for the physically ill or military patients.

But I did have some contact with this problem, because I was one of the team of hospital surveyors who looked at all the hospitals in the country. As Regional Medical Officer for the Ministry, I did the survey of the North Midlands with Sir Leonard Parsons of Birmingham and Clayton Frye of Leeds.

I was always puzzled by the way in which the mental hospitals were excluded from that particular survey. It was largely, I believe, because the Board of Control treated this as their separate empire, and if anything was to be done about provision for psychiatric illness, they thought that was within their compass; they didn't want the advice of these people from outside. And they could have been right about that, because I don't think any one of the three of us knew a great deal about mental illness.

HF   Before the War, was there really any thought that things would change, so far as the treatment of mental illness was concerned?

GG   I don't think I am in a position to answer that, because I only went into the Health Department in the early part of 1939, and was almost straight in to the preparation of the emergency services.

There had been a certain amount of change in the general hospitals by then, in the introduction of more out-patient services, and I don't think we should forget that between the Wars, there was quite a lot of new building for the handling of early cases. Many mental hospitals had good modern admission units, though some of the patients they were admitting would probably eventually graduate to one of the long-stay pavilions. There was some good accommodation in mental hospitals; it was the old and very inhospitable dumps that needed to be cut down.

HF   In the discussions about a future health service that went on in the latter part of the War, what was the feeling initially about the place of mental and mental deficiency hospitals?

GG   Nothing very positive. The management of services for mental illness was really passed by in much of the thinking. Yet it didn't seem practicable to devise a hospital service, certainly of the kind that was required by the 1946 Act, under which all the hospitals were going to be taken over, to organise a comprehensive health service without taking the mental hospitals into the same organisation. An argument went on about mental handicap, but there was really no-one else with whom that particular problem could have been left, with any degree of fairness to the mentally handicapped.

HF   I think it's true, isn't it, that the first actual plan for the NHS excluded the mental hospitals from the general services?

GG   I think that is true. I wasn't really involved in the detailed exchanges centrally, in the early 1940s. One saw, of course, the published reports of the Medical Planning Commission and Medical Planning Research – that group of younger doctors – and I think that the general view of most doctors directly concerned with psychiatry was that the arrangements for the mentally ill would conform to the same pattern as the rest. In 1943, I was engaged in doing this hospital survey. One only became aware of the problems of linking up the mental hospitals with what was being done for the physically sick because of odd exchanges with the staff at the Board of Control, who were then responsible.

HF   When the NHS was set up, all the mental hospitals and all the mental deficiency hospitals were given separate management committees. Do you know why that was?

GG   I think it was largely at the insistence of the Board of Control. They believed that only they had the requisite background, and that there should be people locally who had this special, isolated interest in mental illness or mental handicap to supervise those hospitals.

There were attempts by some regional hospital boards to get the large mental hospitals incorporated in mixed groups, and some of those were referred back and altered at the insistence of the Ministry, because the Minister had to approve all grouping schemes. There was no reluctance locally to having mixed management groups – it was the Board of Control's influence.

HF   Coming to the time after the establishment of the NHS, I suppose that what must have become clear to the Ministry was that there were very serious problems in the mental hospitals.

GG   Yes, that's true. The line generally taken by the people on the Board of Control side, which now doubled with being the Mental Health Division in the Ministry, was that we needed more hospital beds than we had.

The emphasis really was still on care within institutions, much more than on out-patient care, and it was only in odd places like the Marlborough Day Hospital that there existed real facilities outside for looking after people who were mentally ill. There were, of course, out-patient sessions, some of them at general hospitals and some not, but in the very early days there wasn't really forward looking promotion of out-patient care, short respite stay, and support in the community.

There were a few people doing this, like T. P. Rees at Warlingham Park and Macmillan at Mapperley, who were trying to get across the idea that you shouldn't approach mental illness first with the idea of incarcerating the person suffering from it and trying to put him straight, away from the whole of his ordinary background.

I think it was the Manchester Region, where you work, that really began to see the opportunity of providing short-stay units, day hospital, and out-patient care – chaps like Arthur Poole, who was established in Oldham before you went to Salford. I remember Poole well and Chalmers Keddie, the MOH with whom he worked, and being very impressed on visiting them with the way they were trying to do so much more for the mentally ill, without taking them out of circulation. And there were people like Joshua Carse at Graylingwell, whose 'Worthing Experiment' was widely publicised.

It seems to me that too little credit is given as pioneers in this field to T. P. Rees and the MOH of Croydon, Dr Wright, who was very constructive, and was one of the youngest of the County Borough MOHs. The thing that always impressed me was that you got this progress going where you had support from community services. It wasn't something that just the psychiatrists were going to do, from the base of their mental hospital.

HF   I think what you are saying is that these ideas started in the periphery, and then the Ministry became aware of them and perhaps began to change its thinking. Would that be true?

GG   Yes, partly. It was a subject that exercised the Standing Mental Health Advisory Committee right at the beginning.

There were reports of a day hospital (an experimental one) in Montreal, and it happened that when I went on a WHO travelling fellowship to the United States and Canada in 1951, I was asked by Sir Alan Daley, the then County Medical Officer for London, who was Chairman of that Committee, if I would visit the place and report back. Along with John Pater, my administrative colleague, I went there and was very impressed by Ewan Cameron and by the work that he was doing; when I came back, I reported favourably on it to the Committee.

They used that, I think, not as an original idea reported from North America, but as confirmation of the advantages that could be gained by this kind of approach. And they came out strongly in favour of development of day hospitals and short-stay care.

HF   Apart from the day hospital in Montreal, did you see anything that impressed you particularly in North America?

GG   We were there for a specific purpose – to examine their programmes for training in administration in hospitals, and this was an incidental which I was asked to look at.

I did see an enormous mental hospital outside Chicago from which I got one of the funniest comments I have ever heard from a medical superintendent. I was talking to him about his staff and what they did, and he said 'Well, of course, I don't have much to do with the patients. I deal with the political end'. I had got his figures about hospital administration and said 'How on earth do you manage to admit 200 patients a month?' And he said 'Oh, it's quite easy. We have so many escapes'.

HF   Did the Standing Mental Health Committee's ideas and pressure influence the Ministry's thinking very much?

GG   Yes, they gave support to it, for example, in endorsement of the work that Carse was doing down in Worthing; I remember visiting Carse with Walter Maclay. The thinking of the very good people at the Board of Control – Rees Thomas, Maclay, and Isobel Wilson – was clearly moved by this kind of experience, and their influence was important in getting the Ministry to look again at it.

Then, it came largely into the work of the Royal Commission, which was considering mental illness and mental handicap from 1954. There was a good deal of public concern about some of the facts which were coming to light about the incarceration of the mentally handicapped, and about people who spent their whole lives in institutions, in spite of a capacity to contribute some practical service to the world outside.

HF In the early years of the NHS, was there any political interest in mental health, to try and improve the standard of services?

GG I think it was Iain MacLeod who managed to get Treasury agreement to the Mental Million that was supposed to be used to help rapidly in the development of better provision for the mentally ill.

There were one or two examples of provision for the mentally handicapped too. I recall the Oxford Region, with which I had had pretty close links before I became Deputy Chief Medical Officer, converting a large hutted establishment into a new unit for the mentally handicapped.

That's not quite the same thing, though, as a different approach to the handling of the problem – a serious attempt to do something about a sector of the National Health Service that had been very much neglected. However, if you look at what was done by, for instance, the Manchester Regional Board in some of those really awful units that had been used for the mentally ill and handicapped, probably mixed together, in some of the public assistance institutions in the large Lancashire towns, that was a real advance.

It was a change in the physical basis of treatment, which helped the better handling of patients so much, if they had to go in for short periods.

HF That was entirely a regional initiative?

GG Yes, I remember you going up to study it and asking me whether I really thought that this was a valid contribution to handling the mentally ill.

I didn't claim any special knowledge of psychiatry, but I was convinced of its value, and Walter Maclay, who was my particular confidant on the subject in the Ministry, also became convinced of what could be done by this attempt to cut into what looked like an insoluble problem at an acute and early stage.

We'd had something like that over tuberculosis, right at the beginning of the Health Service. There were long waiting lists for sanatoria, and because of that, people didn't necessarily get admitted at the beginning of their illness, when treatment might be most effective. That was deliberately reversed and, using the new anti-tuberculosis drugs, produced a quite striking change in the outlook for tuberculosis; it stopped people from ever becoming chronic or advanced cases.

I remember talking to Walter about the possibility of going for mental illness in much the same way.

HF Do you remember roughly when that was?

GG I should think it was about 1956. I remember that Walter wrote a section for the Chief Medical Officer's Annual Report in 1958, which presented a thesis for a future of that kind. But of course, the thing was already happening under our eyes, except that it sometimes takes a long time to see.

You will remember the Tooth and Brooke paper about changes in the mental hospital population. I know that the reduction in numbers was facilitated by the drugs that were becoming available, but what the drugs were doing was letting psychiatrists get into real contact with the mentally ill, at a time when something more could be done about it. It became practicable for them to live in the community, given family support.

HF   I suppose that in the mid-1950s, people were still making plans for new mental hospitals, assuming that something like the same pattern as before would be repeated.

GG   That is quite true. I have a particularly vivid memory of one in the Birmingham Region. At Cosford, where the indoor athletics take place, there was a hutted establishment, on a site which was already owned by the Regional Hospital Board, which had been planned for a mental hospital before the War.

The Board had been promised by Ministers that they would be allowed to go ahead with this, as one of the earliest of the hospital building schemes. But it seemed to me quite ludicrous to have a policy of providing acute early treatment at general hospitals, and then to go out and build another large mental hospital in the countryside. The reaction in the Ministry was 'Yes, we know all that, for Ministers have been committed to this for years, and if we go back on it, there'll be hell to pay'.

So I offered to go and try to convince them, and with Isobel Wilson and an administrative colleague, met the Regional Board. We put the idea to them that instead of having this one new mental hospital, they should think of the four general hospitals that were in the catchment area, and consider whether they couldn't rather provide an acute psychiatric unit at some or each of those. At the end of about an hour and a half of discussion, the Chairman of the Board said 'Well, you see, we don't agree with you. What are you going to do? Give us a direction'.

And I gave the answer that I had been authorised to give if I couldn't persuade them, and said 'No, it's your job – it's your mistake if you make it, and you've got to live with it'. So they looked a bit surprised and said 'Well, thanks very much', and we had lunch and all went home. About a couple of months later, I got a letter from the Chairman, saying that they'd really been convinced, and were not going ahead with the new mental hospital.

I'm not giving you that as an example of how I was clever – I was simply the channel through which the idea was being communicated. But people were persuadable; they simply needed the argument deploying, just as one had had to go some years before to a Regional Board and say 'Look. You don't want to put your hospital building resources into a new sanatorium. We aren't going to need sanatoria by the time you've got that one built'. But to do this, you've got to carry conviction with the local people, about the service they are going to have to provide.

HF   By then, the Ministry itself was convinced that there would be no further mental hospitals on the traditional pattern?

GG   After that episode, I don't think there was any prospect of anybody building another of those large establishments. They had sometimes been described as being simply personal estates of medical superintendents.

HF   There was, I think in 1953, a report by an Expert Committee of the WHO on The Future of Mental Health Services, which was a surprising, far-looking document. Do you recall that it had any influence on thinking in the Ministry?

GG   It certainly did. There were two British people in that Committee, I believe. It was certainly read in the Ministry and seen as a possible blueprint for the future. But you know, in a Health Service like ours, you can't say 'It shall be thus and thus', and the Regions are going to do it. You've got to carry conviction to the country with your policies.

HF   From the time it was decided that there were to be no more new mental hospitals, presumably Ministry thinking was in the direction of basing psychiatric care increasingly in general hospitals and in other extramural services. Can you say if there was a point at which it was decided that the existing mental hospital system would actually have come to an end?

GG   You may remember the Annual Meeting of the NAMH which Enoch Powell addressed. He had just seen the Tooth and Brooke paper, which said that the long-term mental hospital population was going down, and it really was happening on a very considerable scale. That did have a very considerable impact, because his presentation, as has been shown in other fields, can be very incisive.

HF   Would you say Enoch Powell's 'water tower' speech represented the thinking at that time, or had he gone rather ahead of your planning then?

GG   I would say that he was reflecting the Ministry thinking at the time, but he was giving it publicity in a way that really took us aback.

When he'd done it and got away with it, that was fine, but civil servants tend to be a bit nervous about how to handle the public. It's the politicians who know how to do that. I wouldn't say that he was by any means ahead of his Ministry's thinking when he did that; it was just that he knew the moment to present it and we did not.

That brings me to something else. One of the things that happened in the Health Service generally from 1952 on was that there was control of consultant establishments. Everybody was asking for more psychiatrists, because the speciality was far too small for the number of patients who had to be handled. I had to chair the Central Advisory Committee on consultant establishments, and we were quite determined that the relatively small annual number of trained psychiatrists should go to the places where they would be properly used. So the Region that just proposed one extra psychiatrist in a hospital with a thousand or more beds, which perhaps had two or three consultants and no real plan to handle the problem as it was now beginning to be handled, so as to get people back into the community – they didn't get their extra consultant.

HF   The Powell speech was followed the next year by the Hospital Plan. It seems to me that the Hospital Plan is really the first time that you see in official documents the idea that there would be psychiatry throughout the country in district general hospitals. Is that right?

GG   I think it's the first presentation of a comprehensive plan for doing it that way, but remember Walter Maclay's 1958 essay.

The Hospital Plan was again an Enoch Powell initiative. The idea of setting about this, region by region, was being worked out when he came to the

F

Ministry, but what Enoch did was to say, 'The way to get this over is to put it together so that we can go to the Treasury for the resources that we're going to need, and for us to publicise what we are trying to do'. He knew very well that this Five-year Plan, to roll forward and be revised regularly, could be wrong in the first presentation; it would have to be adjusted.

At least it was giving us something to adjust, instead of just doing bits and pieces here and there. Every Region had got to produce its own plan, subject it to Departmental scrutiny, and then a national report was produced, which was very much Enoch Powell's personal responsibility. He sat through all the preparatory meetings of that Report and, perhaps even more important, said at the end of it 'Alright. We've done that. Now what about the Health and Welfare Services? Because one is useless without the other.'

And the plan that was produced the following year to develop those services is, of course, the indissociable corollary to a hospital service. Health care for a community isn't just what we do in institutions; it's what is done in collaboration between the services, inside and outside.

I think that the Health and Welfare Plan, though it was not revised and up-dated in the same way as the Hospital Plan, was just as important. It made the local health authorities look at what they were doing and if they weren't doing something in, for instance, the mental health field, they had to go back and show what they were going to do.

HF   The criticism has been made of the Hospital Plan that its financial basis was not wholly realistic, and that to do everything that had been proposed would have cost far more than was likely to be available.

GG   That's quite true, because the cost of hospital building was going up and up, but that was a five-year plan, to be rolled forward year by year. So if you look at it as the first stage of a process, and not a definitive or final plan, it was the right way to do it.

When Kenneth Robinson came along, he revised it of course, but really what he did was to update the Plan as it originally had been imagined it would be updated.

HF   Going back to the question of mental hospitals. From, I suppose, the late 1950s, it was clear that they were not going to expand or be developed and, from the Powell speech, it was clear that they were going to be very much reduced, but was there at any point a conscious decision that they would eventually disappear?

GG   I think that you were not quite right when you said they were not going to be developed, because that reflects much of people's attitude toward care for the mentally ill at the time by suggesting that development meant physical expansion.

It didn't; it meant contraction, concentration, and integration with what was being done in the community. True, that means that your big hospital has fewer and fewer beds, though it may have more and more psychiatric staff, medical and other, do more work, and look after more and more patients. Eventually, as you make different arrangements for the relatively small number of patients in long-stay care, you do the logical thing and pull back to the district general hospital unit. But it's a stage-by-stage process.

HF   Was that thought of then, as likely to happen in the very long term?

GG   Yes. Well, we've had the very long term, haven't we? After all, you and I are talking nearly 30 years after the original Hospital Plan.

HF   I'd like to press you a bit further on this point. Did people in the Ministry at that time who were thinking ahead – did they see a time when there would be virtually no mental hospitals?

GG   Not mental hospitals as we'd known them. There might well be places which would have to be under continuing medical oversight, with nursing support, that might be called something else. They'd serve the same function, only a great deal better than some of the pavilions of the old mental hospitals. In psychogeriatrics, obviously there were going to be relatively long-stay patients – some of them are going to stay a few years or more, because their dementia is going to end only with their death.

HF   Looking ahead from that point, therefore, there would have been a vision of acute psychiatric care based in district general hospitals and a network of community services. Now, that would involve first of all very great development of staff training, the employment of many new staff, and, of course, of capital spending on new facilities. When you added up the whole, it probably came to a huge amount of public spending. Were planners confident that it would be possible to do that?

GG   I don't think people were confident that it would be possible to produce a large number of new buildings, but from the very beginning in all respects, not just in the mental health field, the Health Service has had to operate against that type of background.

It's what you do more than the property that you have that determines the outcome of health care.

You were making the point that there had to be much better developed caring staff in the community to work with those who were institution-based.

It's the people that matter a great deal more than buildings, provided the buildings are reasonably human and not those awful old establishments that you and I knew 30 and 40 years ago.

HF   Could I ask you next about the various Ministers that you have known, and you have known many. Obviously I suppose, their attitudes to mental health will have varied a great deal. Some, perhaps, would not have thought about it very much. Could you pick out any particularly influential Ministers?

GG   I don't suppose it's fair from the medical civil servant's point of view to criticise or commend Ministers in detail.

I think Bevan was interested, but I don't think he was deeply informed about it.

Iain Macleod was well aware of its importance. I remember particularly him saying that this was *the* great problem in the Health Service – the management of the mentally ill. He was then, after all, up against a service that thought only in terms of custodial care. This was only at the beginning of the period when we had some psychotropic drugs, and there were only a few psychiatrists of the T.P. Rees or Macmillan turn of mind, who were trying to handle mental illness differently. So what he could see was the rather appalling physical accommodation we provided for the mentally ill in those days, and he tried to supplement this, to minimise overcrowding.

Dennis Vosper didn't have very long as Minister, because of his own illness, but he was concerned about mental health and I think he would have put a good deal of effort into it.

Derek Walker-Smith was involved with the passage of the Mental Health Act, after the Royal Commission, and he felt that this gave an opportunity for a substantial move forward, as it did of course. It reduced the incarceration element of the care of the mentally ill dramatically.

Then Enoch Powell came along, and he was for doing things for the mentally ill by active intervention, as he was in the hospital service generally, and also for ensuring that community services were properly developed.

I suppose Kenneth Robinson's sympathetic relationship with the mental health services of his time as a former member of the North West Metropolitan Regional Hospital board and Chairman of their Mental Health Committee was specifically important. He had a more direct acquaintance with the service when he started, and a feeling for it.

Dick Crossman saw that mental illness and mental handicap were both fields where we needed to make more rapid progress. He had a pretty high profile and started the Hospital Advisory Service to press things forward. He was very shaken by that inquiry in South Wales into the episode in the mental handicap hospital, and he tried to get something done. I don't know whether it was a personal interest of Dick's, but he saw his job as a Secretary of State as one that required intervention in this area, as did Keith Joseph.

I remember accompanying Keith on a visit to one of the mental handicap institutions in the North West Metropolitan Region, and he was very anxious to see more done. In his case, I think it was a consciousness of a problem, more than the kind of personal concern that some others involved have had, but he tried to get something done and to get extra resources into that field. That, of course, ends my direct contact with the Ministers.

HF Going back to the Royal Commission. Do you recall exactly how and why it was set up?

GG I think it followed some of the public reaction to the long-stay retention of mentally handicapped people. There were some people who spent their whole lives in mental handicap institutions and need not have done so, if we'd made reasonable alternative provision for them in the community. It was curious the way those institutions became little, cut-off towns of their own, where the ablest people helped in the kitchen or laundry, rather than being prepared for going outside and living lives of their own.

That was a factor, but the main factor was the perceived need to do something more about dealing with mental illness in its early stages, as well as general public reaction against certification and compulsory consignment of people to institutions behind walls.

HF Was there any particular individual who was influential in the decision to set up the Commission?

GG I don't think I could put a finger on any particular person. I was then DCMO. The people with whom I had most to deal were those on the Board of Control: Rees Thomas, Walter Maclay, and Isobel Wilson. They were influential in the Ministry, of course – Percy Barter was the Chairman of the Board. I don't think I'd be a suitable person to pick out names on that.

HF Were the Board of Control themselves favourably disposed toward the Commission?

GG I think they were, yes.

HF   Are there any further thoughts on this whole story, that you have, looking back from today's perspective?

GG   I think that the Health Service has had less credit than it deserves for the speed at which it introduced reform in the handling of mental illness.

Other countries may have gone further than we have done since, but we were early in the field of trying to handle the problem by acute treatment and community care. I think we could claim to have exploited the initiatives of people like Rees, Macmillan, Carse, and Poole – and you were in that initiative yourself – as well as some people in other countries, like Cameron in Montreal and Querido in Amsterdam.

HF   From your account, it sounds as though most of the new ideas came from doctors, and this is interesting because doctors are often put in the position today of being the obstacles to progress. Do you think that doctors did in fact play the key role?

GG   I think initiatives have come from doctors, but that the push for wider development came from others who were convinced by them. Because I haven't mentioned their names doesn't mean that they weren't at least as important as some of the medical figures. My contacts were medical, but the NAMH was the public crusading body, much more than the RMPA. I would have said it was the more progressive group of the two.

HF   Have you any particular memories about the foundation of the College? I remember you were at the first public dinner, when the College was founded. Were you involved in these negotiations at all?

GG   If you're Chief Medical Officer, you can't avoid having contacts with that sort of thing, and indeed, you wouldn't want to avoid having them, but I think it would be entirely wrong to pretend that I was in any way responsible for that change.

The people concerned, like Martin Cuthbert and Ben Monro, would come and talk to me about what to do. I'd hear about questions that arose over the Charter and that sort of thing, because it was a Royal Charter and raised important issues. But I suppose in a very minor way, I could have been an honest broker, and I must say I was very surprised and greatly honoured to be made an Honorary Fellow of the College in its early days.

I knew well people like Martin Cuthbert, who ran a very good hospital incidentally, Martin Roth, and Aubrey Lewis, while Denis Hill particularly was my friend among the psychiatrists. So my position was only that of being a friend of the people who were actually doing things, and occasionally being in the position of giving a helping hand.

HF   The College had a very sticky initial progress at some points – there was a fair amount of opposition – if not on the surface, then behind the scenes, wasn't there?

GG   Yes. But then the old Colleges are always jealous of any newcomer. They were just the same over the establishment of the College of General Practitioners. We're very slow to move in medical organisations, and the medical establishment is a particularly conservative one.

HF   Have you any comments on individuals in the mental health field – I suppose we should avoid those still living.

GG   I've mentioned T. P. Rees; he was the person I think who really made an early impression on me. There was Jack Rees, and Ronald Hargreaves, who had been with the WHO. I have mentioned Walter Maclay – I think he gets less credit than he ought to have – he was a very important and benign influence behind the scenes. Macmillan I knew well, of course, from when I was in Nottingham in the early part of the War; again, a man for whom I had a very high regard. And of course there was Aubrey Lewis, with all his intellectual qualities.

I suppose among the psychiatrists of whom I have the pleasantest recollections is Denis Hill who set up, after all, the first department in a London teaching hospital, and breaking into them was no easy matter. His was the first London Chair, but he had predecessors outside London, of whom I knew Bill Trethowan best.

Then I have mentioned that group of whom you were one – Poole and others in the Manchester Region, who I've always looked on as pioneers who haven't had enough recognition. There was Tredgold at UCH, who was the Regional Psychiatrist for the South East Metropolitan Region – a very nice man.

Another person who perhaps ought to have a little credit and doesn't get it is Sir Alan Daley, who was the County Medical Officer of London. As I said, he was the first Chairman of the Standing Mental Health Advisory Committee, and an interesting chap. He was able to take on board some of the needs of psychiatry and hold the balance between the warring elements in that Advisory Committee. They were warring, I can tell you, so I think he ought to be in the 'gallery'.

10   Felix Post

Interviewed by **BRIAN BARRACLOUGH** (1988)

Dr Felix Post, MB BS 1939, DPM (conjoint) 1942, MRCP (Lond) 1944, MD 1961, FRCPsych (Foundation) 1971, FRCPsych (Hon) 1981. Dr Post was born in Berlin in 1913. He trained in psychiatry at the Mill Hill branch of the Maudsley and at the Royal Edinburgh Hospital, obtaining the conjoint DPM in 1942 and the MRCP (Lond) in 1944. Between 1945 and 1947, he served as army psychiatrist (Major), and in 1947 he was appointed Physician to the Bethlem Royal and the Maudsley Hospitals, where he remained until retirement in 1978. He was charged by Aubrey Lewis to develop a psychogeriatric teaching unit but continued to work also with younger adult patients. He obtained an MD with a thesis on elderly depressives in 1961. Having been a Foundation Fellow of the College since 1971, he was elected to an honorary fellowship in 1981.

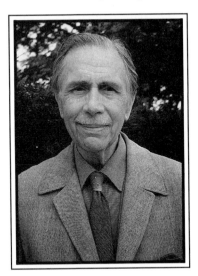

BB *Can you tell me something about your origins?*

FP   I was born in Berlin in 1913. My father and his family were all good Protestant Germans and, as Hanoverians for many years, loyal subjects of Their Britannic Majesties.

My mother's side was entirely Jewish, but she strangely enough, could follow her family back far longer in Germany than my father could.

Theirs was a very happy marriage and my father stuck with my mother right through Hitler and World War II. Unfortunately, I was an only child, possibly because of World War I and its aftermath.

I passed through various German schools. In Berlin, where we lived in a nice house, my father was a director of a Berlin museum, an art historian interested in arms, armour, and costumes.

An interesting thing – when he was a student, in Paris, he bought that etching on the wall behind you. The etching is from the French Revolution; they had a special *Fête Dediée à la Vieillesse*, a festival for the aged. As you can see, there are only about four or five aged people in the whole picture. A bit different from now.

It came to me, prophetically after the War.

BB *You went to University in Berlin?*

FP   I started medicine like my mother's sister. My aunt was close to me, being much younger than my mother. When she married she soon had children and did not carry on with her training. I think my interest in medicine comes from her because of her influence.

I started my first term from her home in Hamburg. Then the next term I moved to Berlin; one did in those days move from one university to another.

BB *Why move around?*

FP   It was the custom, in order to gain experience from various teachers and then to settle down at one university for the last few terms.

Of course Hitler was threatening all the time. I remember I went on the local railway from our home to the centre of Berlin where the University was, and what did I pass but the Reichstag, all burnt out and battered. That was the famous fire of 1933, caused by communists, allegedly. With a Jewish mother, my position was unpleasant, to say the least, even in 1933. Not that anybody was against me, and in fact, I probably could have stayed on. But I have always been on the liberal side of politics.

BB *Under the Nazi rules, you were Jewish?*

FP   I was not an Aryan, but I was half-Aryan. I had cousins in a similar situation who stayed in Germany and survived. In retrospect, I could have stayed, qualifying in 1938, or '39.

BB *What might have happened to you?*

FP   I would probably have been drafted into a field hospital, and it would be unlikely that I would still be alive.

However, I had English connections, which affected my future. My mother's mother had been born in England, in Bradford. Her father had emigrated from Hamburg. They belonged to the large group of German Jews who went to England in the middle of the last century, established themselves in new businesses, and prospered.

In this way, I had an 'English grandmother', and English Jewish relatives; my parents were keen on my learning English. We always had somebody in the house who spoke English to me. When I was 16 or so, I made visits to England, staying with relatives and with one of my father's museum colleagues.

I said to myself, and my parents agreed, that although this Nazi thing can't possibly go on for more than a year or two, because they will crash economically, it would do me no harm to continue my medical studies in England. But it wasn't quite as easy as I thought, because it was so difficult to get into an English medical school.

Fortunately, my father's friend, the Director of the Wallace Collection, had a cousin who was a senior physician at Bart's. Through this connection, I managed to get into Bart's.

BB *Bart's is said to have had a tradition of anti-semitism.*

FP   I don't know about the anti-semitism, but entry to British medical training in those days was restricted.

On the Continent, anyone who passed their higher school examinations matriculated to university. If you had the money or a scholarship and you wanted to get into medicine, you just went to the university, signed yourself in, and started. This is the practice still in Italy, but not in Germany. It has the effect of producing far too many doctors; so that is foolish. In England, it was the exact opposite; only so many places, and competition to get in.

That restricts the number of doctors produced, which is very nice for the doctors who have been produced. Both systems are foolish. But both systems, I think, are coming closer together.

At the time I came here, the British Medical Association spokesmen were against bringing in any except a few chosen refugee German doctors or medical students. Anyway, each year, when I got my permit to stay another year, I was told 'Once you have qualified, you must leave the country'. But once I qualified, I couldn't have left the country because the war had almost begun.

BB *Did you have to start your medical studies again at the beginning?*

FP I had only done a year in Germany. First of all, I had to take the entrance examination – a bit of maths, English, geography – then the first MB. Unfortunately, the tutor didn't teach us how to section plant stems in botany. In the practical, I was completely stranded, but must boast that it was the only examination I have ever failed.

Anyhow, I went through Bart's, very pleasantly, and qualified in June 1939, when I was 26 years-old.

And then, of course, I could not get a job. I was not allowed to work and was unsure what was going to happen. Where was I going to go? Then, one of my fellow refugees got an unpaid clinical assistantship at the Hammersmith Hospital. They were short of staff because everyone had gone off to the War. He mentioned me to them. So I became first, an unpaid clinical assistant for a month, and then house physician at the Hammersmith Hospital.

BB *Were you not an enemy alien?*

FP I was an enemy alien all right. But my father's friend, the Wallace Collection Director, went before a tribunal and swore about my sound background and anti-Nazi views, and so on.

I was a house physician at the Hammersmith from about December 1939. That was a very fine experience. The man in charge there was Francis Frazer, a New Zealander, and his second in command was John McMichael, a Scot. McMichael did his ward rounds, and every patient was examined; he looked at my notes and re-examined every patient and taught me. It was a splendid experience, and I was really keen on becoming a physician.

BB *You were in a sense protected from being called up by the military?*

FP I had volunteered for the Pioneer Corps, but they wouldn't have me. I wasn't called up, not as an alien. Then in 1940, France fell and there was great hue and cry about aliens, and a push to get us interned. The Hammersmith were not allowed to employ me any longer, so I had to leave at the end of June 1940. I had hardly any money, and my parents couldn't send me any. So I said, well, never mind, I will get interned.

So I was, and spent six weeks on the Isle of Man, which was not very pleasant. There were many people together, and most of them were not congenial.

Then, my English grandmother in Bradford and her MP got me out. That was not very good either, because I was not allowed to work. Fortunately, I had belonged to an international student's club run by the Student Christian Movement.

BB   Were you a Christian?

FP   Baptised and confirmed. Anyway, they had a lot of Jewish refugees in the Club. There was a woman there, the Warden, who died only a few years ago, Mary Trevelyan, who was helpful to me and to many others. I got a job to be the porter there, for free board and lodging, in the Club. Having been at one stage the Chairman of the Committee, a man of high office, I became a porter, which really meant sitting in a box making sure that nobody came in who was not a member, and taking messages. I didn't have to do any portering, only take part in the fire watching in our street.

This was early in 1941. Then I was allowed to work again. I got a job at Whipps Cross Hospital, then a kind of Poor Law Hospital. In those days, the worse the hospital, the better the accommodation for the medical staff. It was very nice, having two rooms, after I'd previously stayed in boarding houses.

We had to do almost everything, minor surgery, clearing out abortions, all that sort of thing. But there was not much teaching. From there, I went to the Mill Hill Emergency Hospital, part of the war-time Maudsley.

When I was at the Hammersmith, one of my duties was to take round, and make sure he did not get lost, the psychiatrist, who under the London County Council, came once a week to see patients with any psychiatric problems.

And the psychiatrist was no other than Dr Aubrey Lewis. I had to take him around, watch him, and listen to him taking histories, and I scribbled down notes and then dictated his report. I was very impressed by him.

I had always been, in a vague way, interested in psychiatry. It stemmed from my school-boy days through reading a fashionable book in Germany, one that is also known in this country – *Physique & Character* by Kretschmer. That was my first contact with psychiatric problems, and I was fascinated by them.

BB   What was the fascination?

FP   The mind, and the way people with psychiatric illnesses have certain physiques. And the way the man wrote – extremely well. He was, of course, not truly scientific, as was found out afterwards.

When I was a student at Bart's during the psychiatry course, I had to go out to the Bethlem Hospital. There, a not very impressive psychiatrist would bring out fat case-file books, and the patients were paraded like animals in a zoo, which I disliked very much.

Denis Hill, who was there at a later date as a junior doctor, said he tried to engage Porter Phillips in discussion about the patients, as to whether they were schizophrenic or depressive, and what was the difference, and so on. Porter Phillips said, 'I have sat on the fence for the last 30 years and you are not going to push me off!'

As a student, I had for financial reasons to get qualified as soon as possible. In the MB examination, you were asked about forensic medicine, or public health, or psychiatry. Forensic medicine and public health could be swotted overnight, but psychiatry was quite a complex subject, even then. So I thought, I am not going to bother about psychiatry at all. However, my contact with Lewis at the Hammersmith had changed my view of it.

After I had been at the Whipps Cross Hospital for six months, we had to be re-appointed. So I got in touch with Aubrey Lewis and he kindly arranged for me to be taken on as house physician at Mill Hill, in 1941. That's how I started in psychiatry.

BB *The Maudsley was divided in two by the War?*

FP One part went to Sutton Emergency Hospital, with Sargant in charge. The other went to the public school at Mill Hill, with all its classrooms and dormitories. That had taken place before I went there, in 1939.

BB *To escape being bombed?*

FP Although The Maudsley still had out-patients in Camberwell, there was quite a bit of bomb damage at Denmark Hill, so it was a wise move.

On the strength of my new job, I got married. My wife was English, and it was then possible for Englishwomen to be re-naturalised, within a few days or a week or two, even if they married an enemy alien, which of course I was.

BB *Who was at Mill Hill?*

FP There was the Clinic Director, Lewis, who lived there because his family had been evacuated to America, Elizabeth Rosenberg, who later on married Guttmann, Gillespie, the child psychiatrist, and Maxwell Jones.

I worked for the first few months with Rosenberg in the General Unit, and then in the Effort Syndrome Unit with Maxwell Jones and Paul Wood, the noted cardiologist, who was attached.

BB *Your purpose was to get a training in psychiatry.*

FP It was simply to work in a teaching hospital setting; it was quite difficult for a person of my background to get a really good teaching hospital job.

At Mill Hill, I had a good opening. And there seemed no harm in spending a year in psychiatry, even though I wanted to become a physician. As my year came to an end, I spoke to the administrator, Dr Maclay, who later on became one of the Commissioners on the Board of Control, and asked his advice about my abilities. He gave me an encouraging report and thought I would be a good psychiatrist.

However, they wanted to have Erich Guttmann on the staff. He was one of the many refugee psychiatrists from Germany, who had come to the Maudsley and had worked there in a sort of assistant capacity before the war, being interned later. Guttmann again became available for employment; he was by then a well known neuropsychiatrist and they were very keen to have him. They couldn't have him and me, not because we were both Germans, but because they did not have the establishment.

Lewis and Maclay talked to D. K. Henderson, then professor of psychiatry at Edinburgh, about me, and I was passed on to him. That was a good thing, because although I had been a year at Mill Hill, my experience was exclusively of neurotic soldiers. Anybody who was psychotic was quickly sent somewhere else. That was splendid for anybody who already knew a lot of psychiatry, but hopeless for anybody like me, who knew nothing. The effort syndrome anxiety states following Dunkirk were interesting in many ways, but it wasn't valuable for beginners in psychiatry.

So I went to Edinburgh. First I worked in the private part of Craig House, for about a year, where they had the nobility, the rich, and so on. That's where

I had my clinical experience of psychosis, and then got the DPM and the London Membership.

BB *Why not the Edinburgh Membership?*

FP   In those years, the London Membership was more difficult, more demanding – a different exam altogether.

BB *And what did you think of Henderson?*

FP   He was a martinet, and was well known for that, at least to his 'assistant physicians', who were neither physicians nor assistants. When they married, for instance, they had to leave. He wouldn't have any married doctors there, because he wanted them to be available all day and all night. With the war, he had to give that up.

Then he had to give up something else, through me. I introduced the weekend for staff to the Royal Edinburgh Hospital for Mental & Nervous Diseases. That had been quite unheard of. However, I introduced this very firmly, and because he was short of staff, he had to give in. Therefore, not only did I live out, near the hospital, with my wife, but I also had brief weekends – Saturday midday to Monday morning.

Henderson was in fact a very, very nice, kind, and pleasant man, as was his American wife. But having been used to McMichael, Lewis, Paul Wood, people like that, and having medical ward rounds, when we went round and discussed the patients together, learning all the time, Edinburgh was a disappointment.

Henderson was the man in charge of the whole hospital and spent all his time every day in a different part of the hospital, going round and literally seeing all the patients; going from room to room, because many of them were private rooms, going from bed to bed, and saying 'How are you today', and then mumbling a few words.

There was very little teaching, only a weekly case conference when a patient was produced, with a little discussion with the staff.

Fortunately, Erwin Stengel, as a research assistant on a grant, found employment just before or just after I got there, having moved from Crichton Royal, Dumfries. Stengel wanted to spend his time with the younger people. He was accessible; he and his wife were hospitable and helpful. He would see patients with me, whenever I had a problem, and would spend a lot of time. He taught me psychiatry.

BB *What did he teach you?*

FP   How to take a mental state, assess clinical problems; he guided my reading.

BB *Was he then quite different from anybody you had met?*

FP   I could not say he was the first real psychiatrist; I mean the others were real psychiatrists too, and Aubrey Lewis held weekly teaching sessions, but Stengel's was the first intensive teaching and perhaps the only real teaching I have had in psychiatry.

Your interview recently with Rawnsley was interesting and gave me great pleasure in showing how different the Maudsley training had become from the sort of training that was in fashion when I took up psychiatry. In fact, right up to the time when I became a consultant – you know, this systematic teaching, the consultant taking tremendous time to sit with you and examine the patient like E. W. Anderson obviously did in the presence of his registrar.

This is the sort of experience that I only really had with Stengel.

BB *Stengel was from Vienna?*

FP The tradition there was to mix the psychiatric, the neurological, the neuroanatomical, and the psychopathological. He had been assistant to Wagner-Jauregg, who introduced malarial treatment for GPI.

BB *He brought to England something from Central Europe which English psychiatry did not then have?*

FP Stengel as a friend was a very, very kind man, but he could be a bit cruel and bitchy. He had the greatest disregard for English psychiatry. He used to say to me, 'You know, in Germany, when they have classics – classic books or classic literature, and it's too highbrow for the ordinary person, they bring out a special edition, known as *Volksausgabe*, an edition for the common people. English psychiatry is a *Volkspsychiatrie*.'

BB *Do you think that true?*

FP In those days, it might have been. Certainly, British Psychiatry appeared superficial. There were some good psychiatrists, of course, the Maudsley consultants being among them, who in their own subjects were very searching. But the psychiatry of the majority, I think, was rather superficial, as in Henderson & Gillespie's textbook.

But of course, in those days, the English mental hospitals were run on more humanitarian lines than the continental ones.

BB *Were they?*

FP I think so. But as far as scientific work was concerned, there were few capable people. Look at back numbers of the *Journal of Mental Science*, there are Lewis's famous papers, Anderson's, Slater's, and one or two other people's, but generally, very little else.

BB *Can you say exactly what of value in European psychiatry was brought into English psychiatry by the refugees?*

FP Well of course, they were very much more often woolly and semi-philosophical; one has only got to read the papers written.

Where English textbooks, for instance Henderson & Gillespie, were two inches thick, the German equivalent was eight or nine volumes, written by various experts starting back in 1926/27 or before and going into the 1930s. They were tremendously detailed; much of it, I think, was higher nonsense. That was the irreverent opinion I came to later – a lot of wordiness and going on and on.

The French too, were in my opinion too idiosyncratic and therapeutically weak. Frankly, I opted for the Anglo-Saxon way.

BB *In spite of its apparent superficiality?*

FP I must say that the Continental way of taking time and listening to the patient and getting to know what's going on, how it feels to be mentally ill – that technique I learned from Stengel.

You see, people like Aubrey Lewis were pupils of Adolf Meyer, a Swiss who worked in America. Their method was that you asked the patient something and then you wrote down exactly what the patient said, as if dictated by the Holy Ghost. Every word, you know. You didn't, unless I misunderstood, explore the patient's mind; you just asked a few questions, and wrote down what the patient said. Not the best way of conducting a psychiatric interview, is it?

BB   How long did you stay in Edinburgh?

FP   Until January 1946. As soon as the German war finished, I volunteered. But it took some time before I was actually called up and by that time, the war with Japan was also finished.

I had not wanted to be in the Army earlier because that would mean fighting against Germans and my parents were there still. I took out an 18 months short-service commission. The Army were quite glad to have me then, as so many doctors were being demobbed. After doing some short jobs in Britain, I spent about a year in Egypt, in the military hospitals there. And that again was more neurosis experience, but also some psychosis.

BB   Did you become a British subject before you joined the army?

FP   I couldn't have. You are not supposed to naturalise enemy aliens during the war or immediately after it.

BB   But you had the King's Commission?

FP   And I had been promoted in the Army to Major.

When I left the forces, I contacted Aubrey Lewis and asked if there were any jobs suitable for me. I wasn't under great financial stress, because I had back-pay to come from the Army. Still I had to do something.

He said there was a job as assistant physician at the Maudsley; my predecessor had tragically committed suicide. So I was then interviewed, first by the LCC people and then by the Committee at the Maudsley. I cut a poor figure at the interview, but I was the only candidate, and I suppose that explains my appointment.

At the same time, the Committee appointed two senior registrars. Kräupl-Taylor, many years my senior, and Henri Rey.

BB   And that was 1947, just before the Health Service started, when the Maudsley was controlled by the London County Council?

FP   The Director was Aubrey Lewis.

BB   And the Professor?

FP   None. Mapother, the first Professor, had died before the war. I had not met him. There was a physician superintendent, Arthur Harris, who later on with Ackner did the investigation exploring the value of insulin in the treatment of schizophrenia.

BB   So in 1947, you had finished your training as a psychiatrist?

FP   I never had any training, that is the point. Guttman, some of whose beds I took over because he had too many, said, quite rightly, when I told him about my past, 'Post you are, so to speak, in psychiatry, an autodidact'.

I thought Aubrey Lewis wanted me at the Maudsley, and supported me because of my brilliant promise. Later on, it became clear that he really appointed me because he was thinking of having a department for old age psychiatry, for which he had ear-marked me. He never told me this, which is maybe just as well.

When I was in Edinburgh, on the wards in Craig House, at the end of a round, Henderson said 'See all these poor old people here, Post. Why don't you write them up'. So I did write them up, in the usual way. How many patients there were, how many years they had been there, and what their diagnoses were.

I gave a little talk on this to the local RMPA. Then it was published in 1954, in the *Journal of Mental Science*. That was the first paper I published.

BB *Did you describe something important?*

FP Nothing important. There were two observations and one was a dreadful mistake. This was in the pre-ECT era, and what struck me was that people with dementia came into hospital and within a few months were dead. But the ones who stayed were the 'endogenous' depressives, who went on for years and years and years.

I foresaw that the increase in the aged ill in the population was worrying. But I predicted that the main problem would not be the organic mental illnesses, because the patients quickly died, but the depressions, then untreatable.

Completely wrong, you see, completely wrong. I did not realise that at a place like Craig House and other mental hospitals, most patients suffering from senile dementia were admitted just before they died. They were nursed and looked after at home. Then, when everything broke down, often the result of a terminal confusional state rather than dementia, they were admitted and died rather quickly.

With the depressions, it was a different story. We didn't realise at the time how long dementing mental illnesses can last. It was said to be three years, but we now know it's often over ten. So I made this incorrect prediction.

BB *You anticipated Roth in pointing to the differing outcome of depressions and dementias?*

FP In a sense. Having read quite a bit of the German psychiatric literature, I knew perfectly well that you must not say that because people were old they were dementing. That is a great mistake; many were depressive. Although they went on for a long time, with a high death rate because there was no specific treatment, many ultimately recovered.

In my little monograph on affective disorders, I quoted Gaupp, who in 1906 made this point. So the rule was quite clear. There were dementias, which were organic, and there were non-dementias, mainly depressions. There were possibly some depressions which ended in senile dementia, but not many. There were many elderly depressives who were not really dementing at all.

Roth & Morrissey's paper, very important, an excellent paper, hit me rather by surprise. I said to myself – if I had known that this fundamental observation was not generally known, I could have easily made the point myself.

In my first few years at the Maudsley, I continued with my observation ward studies and there again, showed that the outlook, in terms of life, discharge, and so on was completely different between the obviously organic and those that were not.

BB *Your interest in psychogeriatrics was determined in Scotland?*

FP In a way. But I did not come to the Maudsley thinking I was going to do the psychiatry of old age. That appeared later on at Bethlem. At first, I did general psychiatry only at the Maudsley. When Bethlem, then a private hospital, was joined with the Maudsley in July 1948 at the start of the NHS, there was an exodus of staff from Bethlem, which became short of staff, and I was moved there to do general psychiatry.

BB *The union of the Bethlem and Maudsley was an astute move to provide funds?*

FP It was a marriage between the Maudsley, then an LCC hospital but to become a National Health hospital, and the Bethlem Royal, a private hospital. They were both teaching hospitals. The staff of the private hospitals feared they would be swallowed up by the National Health Service and become District Hospitals, but the Bethlem Governors were glad to join with us. Bethlem had a long history of lecturing, teaching, and studying psychiatry. The Maudsley was a much younger hospital, having been founded in 1912, although it did not start to have psychiatric patients until after World War I, when the Military used it.

BB *It is rumoured that Bethlem had an endowment of millions?*

FP That's no rumour; it's absolutely true and correct. One of the inducements was that both hospitals would enjoy the capital, or at first the income, from the wealthy Bethlem.

I had wards at the Maudsley as well as Bethlem. Aubrey Lewis came out with the idea I should establish a department for people over 60 on one of the Bethlem wards. Old age then began at 60.

BB *What was life like in the late 1940s and early 50s at the Maudsley?*

FP The doctors studied for their DPM; they changed firms every six months. The Dean, Guttman, arranged the posting of the registrars. The ward rounds changed: instead of going from bed to bed, the patients were brought into one's room. We had discussions in the vein in which you yourself were taught. There were various units, a general unit, a psychotherapy unit, and an insulin ward, which had moved to the Bethlem.

BB *Was this largely according to Lewis's plans?*

FP There was a medical committee on which, because of his ability and experience, he had a large voice. The Dean was on it, and all the other senior people – about nine of us I think.

BB *Do you think he had a grand plan at that stage?*

FP I am sure he had. He had, in my view, two great influences.

One was to be critical and scientific in approach to the entire subject. Not to take anything for granted. To be logical and not to live in a fuzzy wuzzy atmosphere that was then so very common with psychiatrists, and still perhaps is. He impressed this on his fellow consultants. The Monday case conference, for instance, was a good training. He would come round, in those days, to every firm, once every few weeks, and patients would be shown to him.

He would go through them with the registrars with precision and thoroughness, and investigate everything. He would have a social worker along, making sure that the whole case was assessed, including the social background, of which, of course, the Germans knew nothing much. I mean the patient in relation to his family background, to his education, religion. These are the things that he clearly impressed on us. An innovation in many ways.

His other great influence was on education. He gradually shaped, with the Dean, who was really his instrument, a system. This saw to it that every person who entered the Maudsley Hospital as a junior doctor, after a tough selection, and who stood the course right through various specialities, passed out as a broadly trained psychiatrist. That was the famous Maudsley training. In my opinion, it was an even more important contribution of Lewis's to psychiatry than his papers on melancholia or his instilling the critical, sceptical, scientific, attitude.

Although he seemed severe and forbidding and austere, he was a kind, approachable man, as other people have told you. He put himself out enormously for many European refugees, and was tremendously kind to me.

On the negative side, he had this idea that people did not learn unless you hit them, not physically but mentally, and he sincerely believed people only gave their best if pushed. That, of course, is why if anybody wanted to do psychophysiological experiments on anxiety, they would choose the half hour before one was due to appear at the journal club or the clinical conference to present a case.

Also, he was a therapeutic nihilist. He didn't believe much in treatment, and it is true, that in those days, treatments were not terribly effective. He was not enamoured of ECT and certainly not insulin coma. Lithium he, and Shepherd too, thought dangerous nonsense.

BB *Why was he such a nihilist?*

FP It was a personality trait. And maybe in the early years of his chairmanship, there really wasn't an effective treatment for schizophrenia, and very little for depression; ECT, perhaps, but nothing fully accepted.

BB *Those were all his achievements?*

FP There were others. For instance, the MRC Social Psychiatry Unit, which reflects his interest in the patient's social background.

Before World War II, he wrote a very good paper on unemployment.

During the War, he published an important paper on old age in psychiatry, writing on people he had investigated in collaboration with a social worker. He did this at the Unit for senile dementia at Tooting Bec, which was a reason for his interest in my little effort.

He was on the Rowntree Committee, looking into old people's homes during the War. He was one of the prime creators of social psychiatry as a subject. The work done, even now, by the MRC Unit goes back to his efforts.

BB *What did he think of his achievements? Did he ever speak of them to you?*

FP Hardly ever, although I saw quite a lot of him. I lived outside London and did not have a car, so I used to come in by train and catch the tram at Vauxhall Bridge Station. Who would be sitting on the tram very often, but

Aubrey Lewis, who came from Barnes by train and then by tram to Camberwell. So we had quite a lot of chats, but I could not say that he ever opened up to me about his thoughts or feelings. But you must remember that I was then a junior person.

He was, however, friendly with Dr Carlos Blacker; they were close. Whether he opened up to anybody like Davies, I will never know. We used to have lunch together in a group of two or three. He was tremendously charming, kind, and interesting in conversation, but I wouldn't say that I ever had a personal experience with him.

Again on the negative side, was his response when one wanted real advice. I tried once, but never again. In those days, abortion on psychiatric grounds was a tremendous problem. Could you, should you, was the patient sufficiently depressed, and so on. I had one patient, who to me was the greatest problem, and I was very worried about her. I asked Lewis, the senior physician, an experienced man, and said please give me some advice. How am I to handle this matter. We saw the patient and talked together. He was of no help whatever.

BB   Did he know you were asking for help?

FP   Yes, of course. In contrast, when I wrote one of my first papers I brought that along to him. He kept it for quite a long time and handed it back, scrawled all over with useful comments. When it came to scientific matters he was tremendously helpful. When it came to human problems, which are after all what doctors' problems are, he was not so good.

BB   You were appointed before the NHS began?

FP   I was an assistant physician before July 1948. Then, there were physicians and assistant physicians. But as soon as the NHS came in, there was no place for assistants. They didn't want to have senior hospital medical officers, certainly not in a teaching hospital. At the Maudsley and other teaching hospitals, either you taught or you were taught. So I belonged, probably wrongly, to those who taught, and therefore I was a consultant. I suppose I did not have any business to be a consultant. I had neither the training nor the experience.

BB   How do you rank Lewis, overall?

FP   Lewis, in my opinion, was the greatest, the most important, psychiatrist this country has ever had. He was in my view far more important than Maudsley himself, who was of course a child of his time just as Lewis was of his own. Aubrey Lewis' influence on American psychiatry and that of other countries was far, far greater than Maudsley.

BB   It was the right time?

FP   That's always the point, the right man in the right time.

BB   There was the money about to pay the people to come and study subjects which were starting to be developed?

FP   He was a very able politician. Very able, and with good connections. He had the ear of all sorts of people. That the Institute of Psychiatry was built is also to his credit, to add to the achievements I have already mentioned.

BB *I find people's responses to questions about him vary considerably, and a lot of it is determined by how anxious he made them feel at the time they were doing their training or working at the Maudsley.*

FP   Of course, he did quarrel on scientific grounds with his senior colleagues: Slater, Hill and Sargant for instance. They were great fights. He dealt with a lot of hostility, and was sufficiently sure of himself not to yield.

BB *Why did he not get on with Stengel, a man of comparable intellect?*

FP   I believe Stengel found the education system Lewis was introducing too scholastic, too institutionalised. There was too little free-wheeling. What else they fought about, I wouldn't know.

BB *Stengel once said to me 'Aubrey Lewis drove me out of London'.*

FP   Lewis made life difficult for him, because Stengel wouldn't do as he was told. He was, as it were, only the assistant professor. He was appointed Reader when he came from Graylingwell Hospital Research Unit to the Maudsley. But he felt that Lewis and Davies were gunning for him.

I suspect that if Stengel had played his cards correctly, and given in when he saw that the other side were determined, they could have lived happily together. He was much appreciated as a teacher, not only by the junior people but also by Lewis.

BB *I would like to turn to the development of your psychogeriatric interests. You described how Lewis suggested you take up psychogeriatrics, and gave you some beds at the Bethlem for that purpose.*

FP   One ward at first. He had a tremendous stand-up fight with the Matron, Miss Robinson, who was against the beautiful, recently private Bethlem being occupied by these nasty old people. But Lewis won. The Matron later became a most fervent admirer of the Unit, and delighted in it.

At first, I had just a few beds in a general ward. But it developed, and by about 1950–51, the whole place was more or less devoted to people over 60. I was fortunate that one of my first registrars was so interested in working with the aged. That was David Kay; he stayed a year, instead of six months.

BB *He went on to Graylingwell Hospital?*

FP   He was passed from me to Roth, and never looked back. David co-operated in a study of our observation-ward patients, where we tried to predict the outcome from the diagnosis. There was a serious disadvantage with this kind of work at the Bethlem Unit, which applied to the Maudsley as well. Both were hospitals for patients likely to recover. Anybody who had a chronic mental illness had to go to one of the area mental hospitals. They couldn't stay at Bethlem or the Maudsley. There was no exact time limit, but there were questions asked if the patient stayed too long.

That, of course, in psychogeriatrics limits you entirely to the affective and neurotic illnesses. If you have dementias, you have to offer long-term care. Each time we did have patients with organic mental syndromes, we hoped they would improve or that other arrangements would be made by the relatives. But again and again, they would occupy a bed for months and months, before the local hospital would graciously accept them.

Therefore, we were restricted in the study of the most important psycho-geriatric condition – dementia. This problem was only more or less cured in the late 1960s and early 1970s, when beds nominally under the jurisdiction of the joint hospital in the area hospital became available to long-stay patients from the catchment area. It is a great improvement, which has helped my successor to develop more interest in the dementias than I could.

BB   What were your aims when you began?

FP   All one knew about mental illness in the aged in 1947 was that their depressions tended to be more severe, more chronic, and recur often. As for paranoid illnesses, we were not sure what they were all about. I soon realised that I couldn't say anything useful about these conditions without following them up in sufficient numbers to draw conclusions about the course of the disease. That had not been done before, and that was what I did, up to a point.

BB   Did you develop these aims on your own?

FP   I wasn't put up to it. For example, David Kay and I confirmed that there were clear distinctions between organic and affective disorders in the short term. Then there was the question, not so obvious, of whether or not a high proportion of the depressive subjects demented.

The study that Roth, Kay & Hopkins carried out at Graylingwell was also a follow-up one. I was doing mine at the same time, but theirs was a bit different in terms of a follow-up period, which varied a great deal, with a minimum of 18 months. I decided that it was necessary to follow-up all patients for the same period of time. That, of course, came out in 1962, based on patients who were in the hospital in the 1950s.

BB   What did you find?

FP   The main point was that, compared with known statistics about the prevalence of dementing disorders in old age, there was no evidence that depressive subjects without brain symptoms subsequently developed them. That corroborated the findings of Roth and his colleagues, which came out around the same time.

Cerebral organic symptoms occurring with depression were of prognostic significance only when clear-cut and definite. Dubious dementia, memory disturbance when patients couldn't do this or that, a little facial alternation, the 'minimal signs' of organic involvement, did not predict dementia.

Sometimes I suppose they did, but very rarely in any sense that would make one take notice of dubious psycho-organic signs. On the other hand there were patients who did have some brain changes. Usually, they would not be of senile dementia, but more of what was then called 'arteriosclerotic dementia'; then, the immediate outcome for the depression may be quite good, but the ultimate outlook, even in terms of the depression let alone the brain, is far less good. That was the most clear thing that came out but there were lots of other things, for instance, a very high proportion of depressives had previous neurotic symptoms. Then, I looked at various possible sub-types of depression and of depressions which had first manifested themselves in the senile period, and compared them in various ways, but really did not find that any of these 'Aunt Sallys' of sub-types of depressive illnesses in the elderly stood up to investigation.

The next question I investigated was the difference between depressions that start late in life and those that begin early but persist into late life.

There is a lowering of arousal, even in agitated depression, as measured by EEG changes during sleep or by sedation thresholds with barbiturates. There is a similar lowering of arousal with dementia. The idea, therefore, was that patients with late-onset depression and minimal brain changes – the result of ageing, will have a lower arousal level, predisposing them to depression. In contrast, those with early-onset depression would not have age-related minimal brain changes, and therefore normal arousal. We did show that this was so in one group, but couldn't replicate the finding, so the whole thing is inconclusive.

The subject has now been taken up by Levy & Jacoby, using computerised tomography to measure brain changes instead of arousal levels. They found that patients who develop depressions late in life for the first time do have more brain changes, more severe brain changes, and a shorter duration of life – all at a statistically acceptable level, but not too convincing all the same. The problem is unsolved.

The notion that elderly patients are more severely depressed is wrong. That's been taken over from previous accounts. In fact, the later depressions are less severe, but longer lasting and more frequently recurring, with a higher death rate. Elaine Murphy found this in a recent study. Incidentally, the main findings on prognosis of depression were confirmed by me, and again quite recently, by Baldwin & Jolley. So apart from the biological mechanisms, the clinical course for the elderly depressives is now a clearer picture.

The other topic I worked on was rather more difficult because there were fewer patients – some had to be collected retrospectively. These paranoid delusional states were not secondary to affective disorders, according to the course of the disorder and response to treatment. Some of them were included because one was not sure at the time about the association of paranoid symptoms with any cerebral organic condition.

BB *Had paranoid states been much studied before?*

FP There was the paper by Roth & Morrissey. Roth described this group, in an observation that was far more innovating than the distinction he made between affective and organic disorders. He described a small group at Graylingwell who had paranoid symptoms of the kind long called 'paraphrenia' – hallucinations and delusions in an otherwise well maintained personality, occurring in later life. He described this group too, and went into speculations about whether this was a late kind of schizophrenia. Kay had followed such patients in this country and in Sweden, so late paraphrenia was a well described disorder.

I started a double-blind trial to compare paraphrenic patients treated at the Bethlem & Maudsley Hospitals before and after the introduction of phenothiazines. But I had to have eye surgery, and could not get back for some months. By the time I came back, the response of paraphrenic patients to phenothiazines was so undoubted that it would have been unethical to leave a large number untreated as a control. It wouldn't have been unethical just for two or three weeks, as one does in depressions, but it would have been for the six weeks to two months required here.

The study showed the results of treatment, and related the symptomatology to the previous personality and to outcome. There are three ways in which paranoid symptomatology shows itself in old age. One is by paranoid ideas, or delusions, or hallucinations in a very narrow field, like thinking that coal is being stolen or that people talk about you downstairs. Then there is one with much more widely spread signs but not of 'first-rank' in the sense that Schneider uses the term. Then thirdly, there are those with classical schizophrenic symptoms. These three types remain stable and respond equally to phenothiazines. Whether they are three separate conditions is unknown. Others have confirmed that these subgroups exist.

Another interesting subject was paranoid disorders which developed in the course of a cerebral organic condition – a stroke or senile dementia. So one has paranoid symptomatology in three forms, occurring in various clinical settings including depression, or in pure culture. But whether this pure-culture condition is a separate illness or a late form of schizophrenia is unknown. Recent investigations have described a genetic marker present in the younger paranoid schizophrenic which is not present in paraphrenics. This suggests that paraphrenia is a distinct condition.

BB *In general, it's not possible for NHS consultants to do as much research as you.*

FP   I don't know; I had contemporaries who were NHS who did. Think of Edward Hare. When I was appointed, it was said that physicians were to teach and to do research. So whenever any duties were distributed, I would say I have to have time for research. But I never took study leave or anything like that.

BB *Edward Hare said he took two days a week, promised by Aubrey Lewis.*

FP   I was allowed to go, for a time, one day a week to Oxford, because one of the geriatricians there was interested to see whether dementia could be improved by suitable stimulation with occupational and social therapies. They had a good community therapist and a good psychologist, who were interested in disorders of old age. I was lent as a sort of organiser to lead them. I went once a week for about a year to do this work. So in a sense, I suppose I did have study leave for about a year.

The aim was to identify the dements who were likely to survive more than six months. We did this, and then ran various occupational and social programmes to stimulate them, with the psychologist monitoring the outcome. And what it showed, not surprisingly, was that whatever you did raised the level of measured purposeful activity. But as soon as you left off, they could not get going again on their own. This was really disappointing to my geriatrician colleague.

Otherwise, all the work I did was on my own patients. They were looked after by the registrars, but I saw them twice, three times, or more often during their hospital stay, in the manner you experienced. I conducted the follow-ups, even when there wasn't any special research.

BB *Where do you think your interest in research came from? Was it the influence of Stengel or of Slater that induced you to think curiously?*

FP   What fascinated me about psychiatry was the human mind; why people develop mental diseases. That would be a big area to work on, I thought. As soon as I was in contact with patients, I began to want to find out a little bit more.

At one time, I was interested in anorexia nervosa and published a paper on it. But then Denis Leigh took this subject over. I was also interested in the type of patient who has an unduly high prevalence of relatives, not only blood relatives, who are affected by some psychiatric condition. We did quite a nice investigation, and found that chronic neurotic patients were especially prone to have other neurotic people in their social networks. A nice piece of work, I thought at the time. I wanted to go on with it, but I couldn't get a grant. I suppose it was quite fair that I shouldn't extend into this area, when other people were beginning to take it up. Besides, I was getting more into my studies of the elderly.

At that time in the Maudsley, I did not have competition; nobody else was doing research on the elderly. It was natural, I think, to try to find ways of predicting which one of these depressive patients was going to do well, which one was going to do badly. It's an obvious goal. So I concentrated on the older patient, and realised that there is no point just following them to the last ECT, sending them out of the hospital, and saying they are cured, but you must look upon an episode of psychiatric illness as a phase in a life. There is no point just looking at the illness. You have to look at the life, not only the life before, which you can do as history, but the life after, which you have to do by follow-up.

It came to me as a natural part of wanting to help patients. You really want to see what good you are doing, what contribution you are making to the life of these people.

BB *When somebody takes up scientific work, then usually they have come from a scientific background or somebody has taught them to look at things in a scientific way. Neither applies to you. Your family were not scientific and you had no scientific training.*

FP   I don't think I agree. I am at present reading biographies of scientists. Many do not come from scientific backgrounds. They are highly gifted people, who get into a certain type of work at an early age. I am not comparing myself with them, of course. At a very early age, they want to find things out. Some have published papers at the age of 15 or 16.

Take Faraday, for instance. He was almost entirely self-taught in chemistry, physics, and electricity; he had no background at all. He was Humphrey Davy's lab assistant.

BB *I think he had Davy as a teacher and model.*

FP   In a way, Davy was his teacher. But I believe the idea of investigating was a natural development. You learn all there is to learn, and then you want to go on from that. That's how it was with me.

BB *Would you like to say something about the contentious subject of leucotomy?*

FP   Aubrey Lewis was involved with the neurosurgeons in evaluating leucotomy – a very ambitious project. They were to use three different operations in a properly randomised way. Linford Rees, Schurr, and Falconer wanted to assess, retrospectively, the results of their work. The trial had ground to a halt. I don't know why.

I think it was because of my expertise, as it were, in follow-up studies that they asked me to collaborate. We got a research grant for a social worker and followed up nearly a hundred people who had had one of the operations. We devised scales with which to score their case notes, retrospectively, their responses to interviews, and their relatives' assessments. This was to measure their post-operative progress, to find if certain types of surgery had done better than others. That was my only investigation.

BB *Was the study intended to evaluate whether leucotomy was effective, or whether types of leucotomy differed in their outcome?*

FP The original study was large and well planned, and its purpose was to compare the clinical effect of different operations.

BB *What is your view of leucotomy now?*

FP The opportunities for it, the need for it, are fewer and fewer. In its time, leucotomy did improve the symptoms which can now largely be controlled by drugs. But the real problems which make schizophrenic people, for instance, socially so often incompetent are not reached by drugs or by leucotomy; in fact, some are made worse by surgery. For depression at that time, ECT was the only treatment, as tricyclics had not been devised. There were patients who did not improve with many ECTs or who, if they did, persistently relapsed. They might be kept going by 'maintenance' ECT. There weren't any drugs, no lithium or anything, and so in those days, leucotomy was an important treatment. Now, there are far fewer patients likely to need it.

In the July 1987 edition of the *Journal*, people from the Brook Hospital report that there are still patients who cannot be managed by non-surgical means and who respond to a tractotomy. This is a much more limited operation than the one which my patients had. In the last few years of my consultantship, I no longer referred any patients for surgery at all. Other treatments were satisfactory, or if patients did not respond and became chronic, they would refuse to give consent to the operation; or they were physically unfit. We did show, in an earlier study, that patients who were physically not fit, not just in their brains, did not do so well after a leucotomy. But this has nothing to do with the difficulties now placed in the way of would-be leucotomists to ply their trade.

BB *You are convinced that it is an effective treatment?*

FP It is an effective treatment in certain patients, who have not responded to other methods. I am quite convinced of that.

BB *But how do you handle a critic who says where is the evidence?*

FP This is in the various publications.

BB *But the critic says there has been no adequate controlled trial?*

FP You can't do a controlled trial of leucotomy. The controlled trial is useful to compare the value of two different drugs or two different treatments, a new against an old. But when the patient has had all the available treatments, and you give a treatment which cures, or improves, then the presumption must be that it is that treatment which caused the change. The probability of the change being due to chance is remote; it can happen, but is highly improbable. I think that is good enough.

BB *There are others who say, for example, that the longer the illness goes on, the more likely it is to reach a point of natural remission.*

FP   Supposing the leucotomy shortens the natural length of the illness by two months, three months, six months, a year, two years or whatever. It is still a valuable thing. I have never been really depressed. To be depressed must be absolute hell, and to be let out of that hell, and it usually is hell for patients who have a leucotomy, is really worth doing.

BB *Another argument is that it is not the cut in the brain but the 'aura of neurosurgery' which effects the change.*

FP   If patients are that suggestible, I am surprised they have not already responded to other treatments.

BB *Can I change tack and ask what pleased you most at the Maudsley?*

FP   My main pleasure at the Maudsley was the wonderful, the excellent junior staff that I had. There were, it is true, very occasionally difficult or impossible, or even incapable people. Very, very rare. As a rule, one worked with people who were tremendously interested, very capable. I suppose about six junior doctors went through my hands annually, three changing every six months. So there are lots of people who came through, and so I can't give you all their names, unless you want me to. There is a phrase "In teaching, we learn". That's what I have done, because I like teaching and I have been told by many people that I was good at it.

I enjoyed having the resonance of capable and interesting people, who put their life's interest into their work. That was a great spur, and what I miss now.

BB *Would you like to reminisce on some of your registrars?*

FP   I always remembered you.

BB *I regard myself as one of the worst students you ever had.*

FP   No, not at all.

It started with Shepherd. When I took over Guttman's beds, Shepherd was the registrar. The poor man must have been very disappointed and sad, because really I had no business to teach anybody. He was very good, very pleasant, obviously an able man. The next one was Storr. Isaac Marks made a mark, if you will pardon the pun, by being the only registrar who ever made me come to the Villa on a Saturday afternoon to help him with a patient. And that was a good mark in my opinion – an excellent mark. Another who stands out is Kreitman. He was the only registrar ever to ask me a question at the end of his term 'What do you think of me, my work, my abilities?'. He was the only one, isn't that amazing?

BB *What did you tell him?*

FP   I told him I had a very high opinion of him.

There were lots of others. Among them was Gerald Russell, he was in geriatrics. And there was Bob Kendell; many very wonderful people to have;

really a great pleasure and joy. David Kay I mentioned already, because he collaborated with me a great deal, as did Bob Cawley as a fellow investigator. And then of course from the psychogeriatric point of view, there are perhaps two people who were most important. Tom Arie, one of the leaders of the subject now, and Raymond Levy, the first Professor in the Department of the Psychiatry of Old Age.

BB   What do you do now, clinically?

FP   I am invited to meetings and conferences. I am going again to Canada in the autumn to be a visiting Professor for the second time; otherwise, I don't do any clinical work.

BB   Writing?

FP   Writing and not being published. In the first few years of my retirement, up until a year or two ago in fact, I had always something to write, chapters on this and that. I did them because I did not want to say no. But it got a bit boring.

Then I also read, for my own entertainment, on the psychiatric aspects of modern biographies of famous people. I found it interesting. To my surprise, there was a lot of psychiatric stuff there. Not interpretations of their novels, plays, and so on; they do not fully explain the problems and complexes that the writer had. But simply accounts of their lives, what they did, what illnesses they had, what people wrote about them, how much they drank, their love affairs, their marital lives.

I decided to investigate these biographies for factual evidence of psychopathology. There is the old idea, now exploded quite satisfactorily, that genius and madness go together. I first took a group who I thought were most likely to be earth-bound, and normal. These were mainly recent dramatists and novelists, people who lived in the past 150 years. I did 55 of those, and found that only one or two had become psychotic. But I did find that they had a tremendously high incidence of minor psychiatric illnesses, some disabling some not, and a very high proportion of abnormal personalities. I mean continuously abnormal in some way, not psychopaths; there were only three psychopaths. But I can't get it published.

The criticisms were so sharp I asked Raymond Levy to read it, in case it showed senile deterioration.

BB   How did you select the sample?

FP   I chose from the names of famous writers or novelists, and because a modern or fairly modern biography was available. I assumed that biographers don't choose their subjects because they are interested in their neuroses, except very occasionally, but in the artist's work, and life, and how that all hangs together. I can't imagine that they just picked up all the ones that were abnormal. It is, however, not a random sample, and publication has been declined because of that.

I am now doing scientists; I have got about 25 so far, and I hope to get 50. I have selected them on the same principles as the writers – being world-famous and with an available biography. There are fewer biographies, and I cannot always have recent ones. I have some where the biographies were written in perhaps the 1870s. Even so, a lot of material is very useful. So far, one scientist is psychotic, and a few are neurotic, one or two severe, but far, far less than the authors, and there certainly are fewer abnormal personalities.

BB *I suppose the Royal Society's Fellows' obituaries would provide a sampling frame?*

FP   Yes, maybe. But I have chosen to have world-famous scientists, because my authors were chosen as world-famous. So I have to have people of international repute, Einstein, Bohr, Rutherford, Faraday, Darwin, Pasteur.

BB *Sounds an absorbing hobby?*

FP   I have found evidence of a lot of minor psychiatric disturbance, especially amongst the authors. Quite a lot of family histories of suicides, more than you would expect. With many of the minor psychiatric disorders, it is difficult to be sure that they are not cyclothymia: I mean the tendency to depression of a mild sort. Not every neurotic breakdown is cyclothymia, although one suspects it is very often.

BB *It's the euphoria that's the interest, isn't it?*

FP   There were very few who were euphoric. They have drive, and that's why they are geniuses. All these geniuses have things in common with world-famous people. They are tremendously engaging, they are going at it and not looking right or left, and persevering when other people would have given up. Tremendously industrious.

BB *Industrious on the right things?*

FP   Not all were successful. A lot have also done things which didn't produce.

BB *Lord Rutherford was pretty normal?*

FP   He smoked all the time to keep himself calm, because he was so tense and nervous. But he didn't have breakdowns, well nothing that you could say. But then you have to be careful. When he was first in London on his own and did not know what to do, he had a lot of migraine, a lot of aches and pains. I don't call that a psychiatric disturbance. I am cautious and conservative. These are some of the self-inflicted tribulations of retirement.

11 Heinz Wolff

Interviewed by SIDNEY BLOCH (1988)

Dr Heinz Wolff, MB BChir 1940, MD (Cantab) 1950, FRCP (London) 1966, FRCPsych 1972. Dr Wolff was born in 1916 in Strasbourg (then in Germany) and died in 1989. He came to England as a refugee from Hamburg in 1936, first to read mathematics at Cambridge but he then changed to medicine. He served as a Major in the RAMC from 1941–46, first as a general physician and then, after three months training, as a psychiatrist. He held various house appointments in medicine at University College Hospital from 1946–59. He was Consultant Psychotherapist at the Maudsley Hospital from 1961–81 and at UCH from 1966–81. Dr Wolff was one of the founders of the Psychosomatic Research Society and was editor and part-author of the UCH *Handbook of Psychiatry*. He was Chairman of the Psychotherapy and Social Psychiatry Section of the College from 1970–73.

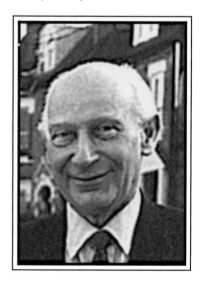

SB   It is almost half a century since you graduated from Cambridge in medicine, and yet I believe that at one point, you might have been a mathematician.

HW   When I left school in Hamburg, and went to Cambridge in 1934, I was still undecided whether to study medicine or mathematics. I therefore started by doing both, and took Part I of the Tripos in the Natural Sciences as well as in mathematics.

I then took Part II in physiology and went to UCH to qualify in medicine.

SB   What determined that it was going to be medicine rather than mathematics in the end?

HW   I think my great interest and enjoyment of pure mathematics, which started when I was twelve, may in part have been reinforced by my having been a rather withdrawn adolescent. I felt more at ease when dealing with abstract concepts and symbols like infinite numbers than with people.

I changed a lot during my years at Cambridge, and preferred contact with people after all. This made me decide to give up mathematics as a career and make medicine my profession, but I can still get fascinated by mathematical problems.

SB   How did you actually get from Hamburg to England as a student?

HW   I was very fortunate, because this was much easier for me and my immediate family than for most other families of Jewish origin in Germany at the time. My father, who was practising as a general practitioner there, was born in Manchester and kept his British nationality, while my mother, whose family lived in Hamburg, was German. We therefore had no difficulty in leaving Germany and coming to England.

I was the first to leave in 1934, after finishing school, and stayed with our relatives in Manchester before going to Peterhouse, Cambridge. This meant that I could spend a few months at a tutorial college in Manchester, to prepare for my entrance examination to Cambridge. This was important, because my schooling at a classical gymnasium in Hamburg had included hardly any teaching in science, so that I had to make up for this. I was also determined to learn to think and write fluently in English; I still remember feeling very pleased when I started to dream in English.

In fact, for me personally, coming to England, felt like coming home because even as a small boy, I used to think of England as the 'land of the angels', a feeling fostered by my father, who always preferred England to Germany in spite of my mother's German background and her family, to whom we were very close.

SB   Was there any impact on you of the Nazi era, even at this early stage in 1933–34?

HW   We were very aware of the threat of Nazi persecution, and I felt this particularly at school. We were especially concerned about my mother's parents, and her sister. It was my father who helped them to join us in London in 1938, shortly before the war. Otherwise, they would almost certainly have died in a concentration camp, although we did not fully realise this at the time.

This move from one country to another actually helped me personally to adapt and relate to people with different backgrounds and nationalities. Perhaps this also accounts for my dislike of any form of rigidity and orthodoxy in politics or religion.

SB   You spent five years in the Services, and most of that in India?

HW   I look back on my time in the RAMC from 1941 to 1946 as a very varied and valuable experience. I qualified at UCH in 1940 and after my two house jobs, including one as house physician to Sir Thomas Lewis, I went into the army and was soon sent to India with the 17th General Hospital.

Suddenly, I found myself in charge of two hundred or so acutely ill British and Indian soldiers in a tented general hospital in Dehra Dun, in the foothills of the Himalayas. I quickly learnt to take full responsibility for patients with all kinds of acute illnesses, including tropical diseases, not to mention having to give anaesthetics, which I found very frightening at first

At the same time, I enjoyed getting to know Indian families and their religion and culture. I also spent two months' leave walking across the Himalayas from Darjeeling, through Sikkim into Tibet, an experience I shall never forget.

My time in India also gave me my first experience of psychiatry. At that time, there were virtually no psychiatrists in the army in India, and they were asking for volunteers. I therefore spent three months to be 'trained in psychiatry' at a European mental hospital in Ranchi, Bengal.

In fact, this has remained my only formal training in psychiatry. I read a great deal and learnt to give ECT without anaesthetics or muscle relaxants, and came in contact for the first time with seriously ill psychiatric patients. As a student at UCH, I had only done one week of psychiatry, mainly lectures and demonstrations at a local mental hospital, I believe at Shenley.

After that, I went back to the 17th BGH, by then in Dacca, which is now Bangladesh, to continue to do medicine, but I also became 'psychiatrist to Eastern India' for about a year and a half. This meant a lot of travelling and I saw many soldiers who had become psychiatrically ill during the fighting in Burma, including Gurkhas who had developed hysterical conversion symptoms. These were often cured by a Buddhist priest, who acted as my interpreter and used exorcism and suggestion, which seemed to be very effective.

After the war, I returned to UCH as a medical registrar to continue my medical career at home.

SB   I have the impression that it was something of a tussle between medicine and psychiatry, and I wonder how you actually resolved it?

HW   I was very happy doing medicine and enjoyed practising it and later on teaching medical students at UCH. I also found that I was more interested in the patient as a person than in any particular specialised branch of medicine. As I enjoyed teaching, I hoped one day to get on the staff of a teaching hospital, but realised this would be difficult unless I decided to specialise in some relatively narrow speciality, and that went against the grain where I was concerned. This also led to my growing interest in psychosomatic medicine, but there were no opportunities to specialise in that subject.

SB   It seems that medicine was winning the day: your MRCP and the influence of eminent figures like Sir Thomas Lewis and Sir Francis Walshe?

HW   They both had an important influence on me, Sir Thomas Lewis particularly. As a physician and a teacher, he insisted on extreme accuracy in history-taking and observation. I still remember that after telling him as his house physician that a patient's attacks of angina tended to come on during a row, he asked me who he had had a row with and about what – a question I couldn't answer.

Ever since, I have paid great attention to detail when taking a history in medicine or psychiatry, and especially during psychodynamic assessment interviews and psychotherapy. I therefore owe a great debt to Sir Thomas Lewis.

I also know that my experience as registrar to Sir Francis Walshe, after the war, laid the basis for my continuing interest in neurology and in the relationship between the brain and the mind.

SB   Psychosomatic medicine as a concept was much in its heyday around this time, in the 30s and 40s. Were you involved in this?

HW   I certainly was, though a little later. In the 1950s, I became one of the early members of the Society for Psychosomatic Research; later on, as president of the Society, I organised several of its conferences, which are still being held annually at the Royal College of Physicians. I also attended many of the European Conferences on Psychosomatic Research in different countries, and made many friends abroad.

I did not, however, go along with the idea that there were a few specific psychosomatic disorders, as proposed by Franz Alexander in Chicago, and by others working in that field. I have always preferred to think in terms of a psychosomatic approach to be applied to every patient, whatever illness he happens to be suffering from.

SB   The Society for Psychosomatic Research continues today. What do you see as its main contribution in the contemporary psychiatric scene?

HW   You are asking an interesting and controversial question. When I originally became interested in psychosomatic medicine, both in my clinical work and in teaching, my main interest was in the psychodynamic aspects. I considered it important to get in touch with the patient's subjective experience, how he felt about being ill and its consequences, and especially how the onset and course of his illness might be related to internal psychological conflicts and interpersonal stresses.

In the early days, members of the Society for Psychosomatic Research shared many of these interests. Nowadays, much psychosomatic research is directed towards the observation of objective and measurable data. Such research is of course essential, as in medicine and psychiatry in general, but I fear that the original purpose of psychosomatic medicine – to pay attention to each individual patient's subjective experience and how this relates to his illness, often gets lost in the process.

Also, the psychoanalytic aspects relevant to psychosomatic medicine are often ignored or overlooked; by this, I don't mean out-of-date classical psychoanalysis, but analysis as it is practised today, with its emphasis on early object relationships.

SB   I suppose that might be a message you would want to convey to the new liaison psychiatry group in the College.

HW   I belong to the Liaison Group but, having retired from hospital work seven years ago, I have only been at a few of its meetings. I do hope that the Group will ultimately be able to integrate both these approaches.

Papers on epidemiological and psychophysiological research tend to predominate at present. These are obviously important, but in actual clinical liaison work and in teaching the psychosomatic approach to students, doctors, and psychiatrists, it is even more important to understand the individual patient's inner world, his relationship to his psychosocial environment, and how these interact and affect his illness.

I hope the Liaison Group will in future pay more attention to these aspects; otherwise, the essence of liaison work will get lost.

SB   How in fact did your interest in psychoanalytic psychotherapy evolve?

HW   In my last year at school, I came across Freud's *Interpretation of Dreams*. I was fascinated by his attempt to understand the meaning of dreams by careful study of the individual's mental processes, including those which were unconscious. The role of symbolism in dreams impressed me particularly, perhaps partly because of my interest in mathematics, where symbols and symbolic logic play such an important part.

I remember writing an essay in my last year at school, on dreams and forgetting, using the concept of repression. This interest did not find further expression until I came to Cambridge, where a psychoanalyst, Karin Stephen, sister-in-law of Virginia Woolf, came to give lectures once a week on psychoanalytic concepts. This refreshed my interest in psychoanalysis, and I began to read some of Freud's papers and case histories and the work of later analysts.

When I started my clinical training at UCH, I therefore decided to have a personal analysis. I think I should mention one important personal reason that made me have analysis myself. My mother had died suddenly when I was only eight years-old, and I had not yet properly recovered from this shock; my analysis helped me a great deal with that. I might add that the influence of losses on human development and on the origin of mental or physical illness has always seemed to me to be crucial.

Freud, in his famous paper on 'Mourning and Melancholia', discussed the process of recovery from losses due to bereavement. Later, Melanie Klein described what she called the 'depressive position', the way in which one has to learn to tolerate feelings of guilt and being sad and mourn, following a loss. I described some of these issues in a paper I wrote in 1977 on 'Loss, a Central Theme in Psychotherapy'[1].

SB   It seems that in the late 1950s, you were having to decide about your future – medicine or psychiatry, and either way you were going to lose something in the process.

HW   I had to make a choice, which meant giving something up and losing something. It wasn't easy.

By that time, I had been the Resident Assistant Physician at University College Hospital for four years. This meant carrying a great deal of personal responsibility for in-patients, acute admissions, out-patients, and the teaching of medicine. By that time, my interest in the psychosomatic aspects and in psychotherapy had also grown considerably, and I had to make a choice.

I think I survived the loss of giving up being a physician by joining the Department of Psychological Medicine at UCH, at first as clinical assistant, under Roger Tredgold, and by concentrating on liaison work and psychotherapy. I had already treated a few patients with psychotherapy in his department, and was extremely grateful to him for offering me these sessions at this critical time in my career. At the same time, the liaison work kept me in touch with medicine and the medical wards where I had worked before.

Following that, there was another important development. Tredgold, Dr Dorothea Ball, and I felt that students might learn more about psychological understanding, interviewing, and the doctor–patient-relationship if they could take on a patient for weekly psychotherapy under supervision.

I gave a paper on this student psychotherapy scheme in the early 60s. It was then that Sir Denis Hill, who at that time was the first Professor of Psychiatry at the Middlesex Hospital, heard me talk and invited me to join his Department as his senior lecturer in psychotherapy. By then, my interest in psychosomatic medicine, analytical psychotherapy, and in the teaching of psychiatry was becoming more widely known.

This, to my great surprise, led to my receiving a handwritten letter from Sir Aubrey Lewis, saying that the psychoanalyst William Hoffer, who was psychotherapist and consultant at the Maudsley Hospital, was due to retire in a year's time; if I were interested in becoming his successor, he would be pleased to discuss this with me.

---

1. WOLFF, H. H. (1977) Loss: a central theme in psychotherapy. *British Journal of Medical Psychology*, **50**, 11–19.

When I met Sir Aubrey, I had a long, very friendly interview with him. At the end of it, he said he hoped I would put in for the post when it was advertised, in about a year from then. To my amazement, at the appointments committee a year later, the few questions on psychotherapy Sir Aubrey asked me were almost identical to those he had asked when we had first met. This is how I became a consultant in the Psychotherapy Unit at the Maudsley.

There, one of my main interests became the teaching of psychotherapy to psychiatric trainees. In building up the Psychotherapy Unit, I was greatly helped by my colleague, the psychoanalyst Henri Rey. We soon became friends and worked together in the Unit for many years until he retired.

SB   It is noteworthy that as one of the most distinguished psychotherapy practitioners in the country, you did not actually have a formal training.

HW   I felt it was only right, during my talk with Sir Aubrey, to mention first that I had had no formal training in psychiatry. To that he replied, 'You can't expect to have done everything.' He also said he had noticed I was not a member of the British Psychoanalytical Society. I told him that my training in analytical psychotherapy was based on my own analysis, supervision, and clinical experience. Although I sometimes regretted not having had formal training in psychoanalysis, I valued my independence. He seemed to be satisfied with this reply.

SB   I see psychotherapy as requiring an eclectic or integrationist viewpoint.

HW   I agree with you only in as far as one must not become constrained by a rigid theoretical model; if one were, there would be no room for originality and new discoveries. However, I think one can practise psychotherapy only if one has a theoretical model in one's mind which one can rely upon, but which is open to change.

What has always impressed me most about Freud was his ability to alter his theoretical model in the light of new observations. The psychoanalytical model has helped me most in my work as a psychotherapist because its concepts, especially those concerned with the influence of childhood experience, inner conflicts, unconscious processes, and re-living the past in the transference, all provide meaningful experiences for our patients and help them to change and recover.

Of course, the British Psychoanalytical Society has had its own struggles and divisions of opinion, especially between the contemporary Freudian and Kleinian groups, and the independent group in between. Although different views remain, the Society has become much more integrated, and, there is now much more common ground between Freudian and Jungian analysts than there used to be.

SB   Are you the sort of psychoanalytically orientated therapist who is willing to take a variety of ideas from within the analytic tradition and integrate them?

HW   I consider myself to be a psychoanalytic psychotherapist, and have always tried to integrate different psychoanalytic concepts and approaches in my work with patients, as appropriate. This has helped me to remain open to new developments and new ideas, and to use these in my clinical work and as a teacher.

G

Openness may also have influenced some of my students at UCH and at the Maudsley so that several of them ultimately became psychoanalysts.

Although I have not gone through formal psychoanalytic training myself, I felt extremely honoured when some five years ago, the British Psychoanalytical Society offered me honorary membership. This now makes it possible for me to mix with many old friends in the Society, and I enjoy and benefit from that a great deal.

SB *You were actively involved in the Institute of Group Analysis and were its chairman for many years.*

HW   My interest in group analysis developed while I was working as consultant psychotherapist at UCH and at the Maudsley, where Michael Foulkes, a psychoanalyst, had introduced the practice of group analysis.

Both Henri Rey and I found that many of our patients benefited from group therapy. Also, we had a long waiting list of patients, and soon realised that time could be saved if some of them were treated in groups.

SB *How did you establish a bridge between working intensely with individuals and in the same day working with groups.*

HW   I think there are many links between individual psychoanalytic psychotherapy on the one hand and group analysis on the other.

When, say, eight patients are treated together in a group, each of them brings his own inner world and past and present experience into the group. Therefore, in order to understand what happens in a group, one must understand individual psychodynamics and psychopathology.

In the Institute of Group Analysis, which is concerned with the training of group analysts, I have always felt it to be important for the trainees to start by getting a proper grounding in psychoanalytic concepts and how these apply to groups. So it wasn't difficult for me at the Maudsley and at UCH, where by then I was spending the other half of my time, to do both individual psychotherapy and run groups.

When I run groups, I think not only of the group as a whole, but also of each of its members and how they interact; after all, it is the individual patient who, we hope, will benefit from the process. Moreover, some patients need individual therapy first, and later benefit from joining a group. Foulkes and I had quite a number of discussions on these issues.

How a group can bring about change in the individual was brought home to me by an experience I have never forgotten. A patient in the open group you observed was extremely schizoid and very frightened when he first joined it. He always came early, took one chair out of the circle, and sat in a corner, hiding behind a newspaper throughout the group, for the first year or so. From time to time, individual group members, and occasionally I, would make a comment to see whether he was listening; gradually, he began to respond to this by lowering the paper and looking at the rest of us, before once more hiding behind his paper. Slowly, he became an active and ultimately the oldest member of the group.

He stayed in that group for ten years and the ending was most moving. He had by now become well established professionally and in his personal life, having previously been a total isolate and a failure. During his last group, all the members and I were very sad at his leaving, and his final comment was: 'It is very hard, but I know it is time for me to go; after all, this is the only family I have ever had'.

SB *I wonder if you could talk about your UCH student psychotherapy scheme.*

HW   I would first like to respond to your question about teaching students early; by that, I mean before they have had too much formal and factual training which can restrict their ability to develop their own ideas, think for themselves, and use their critical faculties. This applies not only to the teaching of psychotherapy, but at least as much to that of medicine and of psychiatry in general.

One has to strike a delicate balance here. Basic factual and scientific knowledge is essential, but all too often, I have seen students being taught in a rigid manner, at the cost of being discouraged to think for themselves, so that they lose their enthusiasm and sense of discovery.

My own experience has been particularly fortunate in these respects. At Cambridge, subjects like mathematics, biochemistry, physiology, even anatomy, were taught by outstanding teachers who encouraged us to discuss and think, rather than remember facts. At UCH, teachers like Sir Thomas Lewis took a similar line, and he gave me, as a student, space in his laboratory to take part in research.

I also believe strongly in learning from taking clinical responsibility as early as possible in one's career. My experience in the RAMC, just after qualifying, taught me more about medicine than the more formal training I received at UCH before and after the war. As I said earlier, my knowledge of psychiatry is largely based on having had to teach myself, and from clinical experience over the years, except for the brief and inadequate period of training at a mental hospital in India.

I had to formulate my own ideas and approach each patient as a new problem to understand and investigate. This does not mean, of course, that I do not value and use established psychiatric concepts. I have learnt many of these over the years from colleagues at the Maudsley and at UCH, especially from Sir Denis Hill, whose clinical approach always impressed me greatly, and who in many ways served as a model for me. Similarly, as a teacher, I have always tried to make students formulate their own ideas and stimulate their interest; this applies equally to medicine, psychiatry, and psychotherapy.

This then brings me to your other question about the student psychotherapy teaching scheme at UCH. Tredgold and I both recognised that some students had greater natural gifts in understanding their patients' emotional problems than others, but during their clinical years, there was little opportunity to help them develop these gifts further. In fact, under the influence of the scientific training, some of them lost their interest in the psychological and social aspects and in their patients' personal problems.

It is now thirty years since Tredgold and I first offered volunteer students at UCH the opportunity during their first clinical year of treating a patient in dynamic psychotherapy for an hour once a week, for twelve to eighteen months. An essential part of this scheme is the weekly supervision of the students in small groups by experienced analytical psychotherapists or analysts. Not only have the majority of patients benefited from the therapy they received from the student-therapists, but most of the students have later said that they learnt a great deal about psychodynamic understanding and how to relate to patients.

I want to make it clear that our aim has never been to train students to become psychotherapists, but rather to help them become better doctors, able to relate to their patients and handle some of their emotional problems. Many of them have later become general practitioners, while a few have become psychiatrists and psychotherapists or analysts. They all agree how essential the supervision groups have been in helping them to work with their patients.

A valuable extension of this scheme has been a joint research project with the Psychosomatic Clinic in Heidelberg, where talks we gave about our scheme led them to start a similar project for some of their students. I managed to get the European Community to fund this joint project. The students and supervisors from UCH and Heidelberg enjoyed travelling between London and Heidelberg, working together and getting to know each other. We have published our findings in a book on *First Steps in Psychotherapy*.

I am sorry that no Department of Psychiatry in Britain has taken up the scheme on a regular basis, in spite of considerable interest expressed by some departments. I suspect that anxiety about letting students undertake such responsible work so early in their training, and antagonism to the psychodynamic approach, may have played a part there.

SB   You sat on the Joint Committee for Higher Psychiatric Training psychotherapy sub-committee, which now has the responsibility for setting down guidelines for training.

HW   My interest in the teaching of psychotherapy to postgraduate trainees in psychiatry led to my getting involved in politics within the College, first as member and then chairman of the Psychotherapy Section, and later, as you say, as a member and chairman of the Psychotherapy Sub-committee of the JCHPT. I have always regarded these political and administrative tasks as an essential part of my work as psychiatrist and psychotherapist; although often hard work and time-consuming, I enjoyed and valued the opportunity of promoting the subjects that I felt strongly about.

This applied particularly to persuading the College to accept that training in psychotherapy should become an integral part of the training of general psychiatrists. This was by no means the case in the 60s, when I first got involved in committee work in the College. I recall how hard we had to fight to have the first Guidelines for the Training in Psychotherapy accepted by Council and the other committees in 1971. For me, it was less important exactly what the guidelines said, but rather that the College should acknowledge the importance of training psychiatric trainees in dynamic psychotherapy.

Later on, my work on the JCHPT, especially the accreditation visits, gave me plenty of opportunity to see how far this was or was not being achieved, and to promote this further. I realise that we still have a long way to go.

SB   When one looks around, there are many psychiatric trainees who do not get to learn how to conduct psychotherapy.

HW   I know many psychiatrists who combine their expertise in general psychiatry with understanding of their individual patients' psychological problems, and use a psychotherapeutic approach to help them.

I believe we must accept that doctors, psychiatrists included, are bound to differ in their particular interests and skills. There are those who are more interested in the biological basis of psychiatric illness, while others are more interested in the psychological and psychodynamic aspects, and some are able to combine the two to a greater or lesser extent.

I have always retained an interest in the biological aspects, but as you know, my main interest and expertise are directed towards psychological understanding and psychotherapy. What concerns me is that the different groups should have more respect for each other than is often the case. Some biologically orientated psychiatrists fail to recognise the value of the psychodynamic approach, and some psychoanalysts, even those with a medical background, overlook the importance of biological factors and the functions of the brain and body. I find this surprising, because Freud himself always stressed that our ego is a body ego.

Making allowances for these differences, I would like to feel that I have helped some psychiatrists to acknowledge that their patients, whatever biological, genetic, or biochemical factors may be relevant to their condition, also have a mind, and that their mental processes and personal experience profoundly affect their illness and need attention in their own right. I believe it is both possible and essential to integrate the two, and to teach at least some basic psychotherapeutic skills to the majority of psychiatric trainees.

SB *Some would argue that the establishment within the NHS of consultant psychotherapy posts has perhaps served to obstruct this development.*

HW   I don't think so. On the contrary, many patients require highly skilled psychotherapy from experienced analytical psychotherapists; those who provide such psychotherapy and teach or supervise others need to have had specialised training and experience in their subject in order to teach psychiatrists and other professionals at a high academic level. Only the existence of a specialist consultant grade of psychotherapists can ensure that these aims are achieved.

I should like to add that in my view the most important part of the training of a specialist psychotherapist consists of his having had his own personal analysis or analytical psychotherapy.

SB *Do you think personal analysis or some form of therapy is required of just the specialist psychotherapist or of all psychiatrists?*

HW   Definitely no. I think no one can or should be *made* to have personal psychotherapy or analysis. That can only come out of a personal wish of one's own. To make this a necessary condition of training for all general psychiatrists would be quite impossible. It wouldn't work, but the position is different for specialist psychotherapists.

If someone decides to train as a group analyst he needs to have the experience of being a patient in a group himself. And, similarly if someone decides to become a psychoanalyst or analytical psychotherapist he needs to have the personal experience of having an analysis. But to expect every psychiatrist or general practitioner who uses psychotherapy with his patients to have his own therapy as a condition of training would be inappropriate and counter-productive. It depends on the individual person's motivation and on the level of psychotherapy at which he wants to practise.

SB   Is the Australian & New Zealand College of Psychiatrists' requirement that all examination candidates wishing to join that college have to conduct an individual psychotherapy case of at least fifty sessions not sound?

HW   I think that is a very sound idea, and I have always been envious of the fact that their College, unlike our own, takes that view. But to expect every psychiatric trainee to have some experience of conducting individual psychotherapy under supervision is quite different from expecting every psychiatrist in training to have personal therapy.

What it does mean is that the trainees should see at least one patient regularly in psychotherapy once a week, for a year or longer, under the supervision of a trained and experienced therapist. It is the supervision process that is fundamental here.

My experience in the student psychotherapy scheme at UCH, and as supervisor of psychiatric trainees at the Maudsley and at UCH, has taught me that. The weekly supervision by a trained psychotherapist helps the trainees to recognise the role of unconscious mental processes, and to understand what happens in the relationship between them and their patients, or in technical language, to recognise and use the process of transference and counter-transference.

It is the supervisor's task to put the personal experience of the patient and of the student, and of their interaction, into the very centre of the supervisory process. This is how trainees learn to conduct psychotherapy. The majority of them are, of course, not in therapy, unless one or other of them has chosen to do so for personal reasons or because he has decided to become a psychoanalyst.

SB   Many of these ideas about training emanate from your many years of leadership in the Maudsley Psychotherapy Unit, but through this time, you were also still at UCH, and conducting a different sort of practice.

HW   I used to say that I had to make a daily transition crossing Waterloo Bridge. At UCH, I was both a general psychiatrist and a psychotherapist, and I looked after psychiatric in-patients and out-patients. Ultimately, I became Head of the Department of Psychological Medicine and started the Academic Department of Psychiatry.

At UCH, we did not have this problem of a split between biological psychiatry on the one hand and dynamic psychiatry and psychotherapy on the other. My predecessor, Roger Tredgold, like I and most of our colleagues, took it more or less for granted that these aspects of psychiatric practice should be integrated, both in clinical practice and in teaching.

When I crossed Waterloo Bridge to go to the Maudsley, where the Psychotherapy Unit largely functions as a separate unit, the split between psychotherapy and general psychiatry was much greater than at UCH. This meant that at the Maudsley, I functioned almost entirely as a specialist psychotherapist. In a sense, I felt more relaxed at UCH, where I could function in both roles, but my missionary zeal was greater at the Maudsley. There, I felt the need to bring about more integration between the two approaches, especially when teaching psychiatric registrars who came to the Unit, and at case conferences and staff groups on the wards.

SB *Why didn't they create a Chair at UCH and why didn't you become the first incumbent?*

HW There were several reasons for it. First of all, as in many other medical schools, it took a long time before psychiatry was given full recognition as a major subject to be taught in the undergraduate curriculum.

When I was a student at UCH in the late 1930s, we only had a few lectures on psychiatry and about a week of demonstrations of patients with major psychiatric illnesses at a mental hospital. After the war, this changed and by the late 1960s, the psychiatric clerkship had grown to three months full-time, largely as the result of Roger Tredgold's efforts. I think the introduction of liaison teaching on medical wards and the importance we attached to the close relationship between psychological medicine and the practice of medicine as a whole led our non-psychiatric colleagues to value and support our efforts.

But this was still a long way from the establishment of an Academic Department and a Chair in Psychiatry. I fought that battle in the Medical School for many years and got a good deal of support, but there was a great deal of competition for University funds and whenever it came to the crunch, preference was given to academic posts being established in other disciplines.

Ultimately, I was asked to start an academic department and was appointed its Honorary Director. In essence, this meant that my salary did not have to be paid by the Medical School, but by the NHS as before. I did, however, succeed in getting funds to appoint a senior lecturer and a lecturer. In a sense, this arrangement suited me because if I had been appointed to a Chair at UCH, I would have had to leave the Maudsley Psychotherapy Unit, which I was very reluctant to do.

As you know, a joint Chair in Psychiatry has been established in the new Joint Academic Department of the University College & Middlesex Hospital Medical School. This evolved out of the Chair at the Middlesex Hospital Medical School, originally held by Sir Denis Hill, before he went to the Institute of Psychiatry.

SB *It seemed a puzzle to me that UCH didn't set up its own Chair earlier, like many of the other London schools did in the 60s or early 70s.*

HW I might be a bit provocative in my reply to that. In a way, UCH may actually have benefited from not having a professor appointed earlier. For many years, it has had a high reputation for its under- and postgraduate training in psychiatry, and the number of our students who ultimately became psychiatrists was higher than in most other medical schools. Our emphasis on the close relationship between medicine and psychiatry and on integrating a psychodynamic with a biological approach when working with each individual patient has, I believe, contributed a good deal to this.

We often feared that this tradition might be disturbed if a professor were appointed who held very different views, and might impose these on the department. We therefore valued our relative freedom, but we undoubtedly paid a price for this, especially where research and the expansion of the academic department were concerned.

SB   One of the trademarks of that school of psychiatry must be the textbook that you and Roger Tredgold wrote.

HW   The new *UCH Textbook of Psychiatry*, has developed out of the much smaller *UCH Handbook of Psychiatry*, published by us in 1975. It has, however, been written in the same tradition as the earlier book, emphasis being placed on the individual patient's experience in the context of his personality development and the life-cycle, and how this interacts with social and biological factors involved in the causation of psychiatric illness.

In the new book, this integrated approach also finds expression in detailed accounts of the various forms of dynamic psychotherapy, and the need to combine these with physical treatments and social rehabilitation when appropriate. The new textbook is much more comprehensive and has been written for psychiatric trainees as well as for medical students.

I think what distinguishes it from other textbooks is the integration of the descriptive, biological, social, and psychodynamic approaches, and the detailed consideration of psychosomatic medicine and liaison psychiatry. I hope that for these reasons, it will be at least as popular and widely read as the earlier book.

SB   It is seven years since you retired. I know that you are still as busy as ever. What occupies your time these days?

HW   For me to retire has meant changing my work, rather than giving it up. I knew before I retired that as far as possible, I would want to continue doing what I had done before. However, it is a relief no longer having to administer two departments, one at UCH and one at the Maudsley. This gives me much more time to continue my psychotherapeutic work with patients. I enjoy that a great deal.

What I enjoy most is knowing that if I work in the right way with a patient for long enough, he will mature and grow. It is that process of growth through therapy that I value most, and I now have much more time for that than I had before.

But in more personal terms, something very similar plays an important role in my life nowadays. I have seven grandchildren between the ages of one and thirteen. I thoroughly enjoy seeing most of them on Sundays for lunch; playing with them and seeing them grow and develop is a great source of pleasure for me.

The other thing I value is that I am still teaching students and watching them develop. I continue once a week to supervise a student psychotherapy group at UCH, and similarly, once a week at the Maudsley, I run a supervision group for psychiatric registrars.

I think the common denominator which makes my retirement so enjoyable is that in my family and by continuing to teach and to treat patients, I can help and watch many young people develop.

SB   I have always known that you had an interest in nurturing young people, and indeed I felt much like a sort of son to you, even throughout my period at the Maudsley. It also wasn't a surprise that when we organised the first AUTP conference on teaching dynamic psychotherapy in Oxford, in 1982, we invited you to give the keynote address. I remember on that occasion that we all saw you as pater familias, and indeed still do. This discussion reminds me of another paper of yours, which I would group with the one on Loss as a contemporary classic; it is the one on the 'Therapeutic and Developmental Functions of Psychotherapy'[2]. It is another paper

---

2. WOLFF, H. H. (1971) The therapeutic and developmental functions of psychotherapy. *British Journal of Medical Psychology*, **44**, 117–130.

which I often recommend to my students. It is something within that paper, and related to what you are now talking about, which suggests that the nurture of young minds is really what gives you the greatest pleasure?

HW   For me to help people to develop their own potential and to facilitate that development, is crucial.

That reminds me that the psychoanalyst who has had most influence on my work as a psychotherapist was Donald Winnicott. He started as a paediatrician and then became a psychoanalyst, always emphasising the importance of providing a facilitating environment in which children can mature. If, after growing up, they still have problems of a serious nature, it becomes the task of the psychotherapist or analyst similarly to create a facilitating environment in which such further development can take place, even much later in life.

This is the developmental function of psychotherapy, which I have emphasised in the paper you refer to. In that sense, this is very much a unifying theme in my life.

SB   Do you feel that the British psychoanalytic tradition has something to offer to the world?

HW   I think I can best answer this by saying a word about my visits to the United States. I was very fortunate in the early 1970s to be asked by Professor Peter Whybrow, then Chairman of the Department of Psychiatry at Dartmouth Medical School, New Hampshire, whether I could spend some time there teaching dynamic psychotherapy. Many years earlier, he had been a medical student of mine at UCH, before he became a psychiatrist and went to the USA. I was therefore delighted to spend several weeks teaching in his department, and did so for several years running. I also visited and gave lectures or seminars on psychotherapy in many other psychiatric departments in the United States.

It was a pleasant surprise for me to find that we did, in fact, have many contributions to make to psychodynamic psychotherapy in the States. For example, the concepts of the British school of object-relations theory were of great interest to psychiatrists, psychoanalysts, and psychotherapists in the USA when I first started to teach there, especially the findings of Fairbairn, Melanie Klein, Balint, and Winnicott.

I thoroughly enjoyed teaching in the USA and made many friends among colleagues and students over there. I also learnt a great deal from them, which in turn helped me in my work back home.

I found too that there was considerable interest in recent developments of psychodynamic concepts in several countries on the Continent, especially in Germany, but more so in departments of psychosomatic medicine and among psychotherapists than among psychiatrists.

I hope that the need to integrate the psychodynamic with the biological aspects will continue to gain recognition among psychiatrists, both in this country and abroad, so that patients can benefit from this wider approach.

12   Alex Baker

Interviewed by HUGH FREEMAN (1990)

Dr Alex Baker, MB BS 1944, DPM 1946, MRCP Lond 1971, FRCPsych 1971. Alex Baker was born in a Hertfordshire village in 1922. He had no family background of medicine and became interested by chance. He entered St Mary's Hospital on a Kitchener Scholarship and qualified MB, BS in 1944. Following experience as house surgeon on Sir Alexander Fleming's Pencillin Unit he trained at the Maudsley (then at Mill Hill) and later at Dartford with Maxwell Jones and Sargant at Belmont. He became Deputy Superintendent at Banstead in 1955 and later Medical Administrator. In 1967 he was appointed Senior Principal Medical Officer at the DHSS and in 1969 the first Director of the Hospital Advisory Service. In 1973 he returned to clinical practice in psychogeriatrics in Gloucestershire and retired from whole-time psychiatry in 1977.

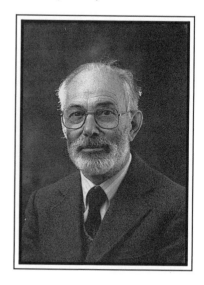

HF   Can I ask about your early life, your education, why you went into Medicine?

AB   I was the first in the family to do so, and I believe this gave me both considerable advantages and disadvantages. The advantages were that I looked at a lot of medical situations afresh, with no previous idea of what was possible or impossible. On the one hand, I missed the background many doctors had – the easy entry into the old-boy network; I've no doubt that at times, this limited my effectiveness. On the other hand, at times it's been an advantage to be quite independent, without feeling any need to be influenced by previous practice or old loyalties.

I became a doctor by accident. I was working for the equivalent of A levels and had a very good biology master, who was encouraging two or three others to go into medicine. One day, he arranged for three of them to spend a day at Charing Cross Hospital, to see what it was all about. At the last minute, one of them became ill and the master persuaded me to go instead. I didn't really enjoy that day – I was distinctly put off by operations and pathology – but there's no doubt that it stirred something inside me. Eventually, as the same master had a link with 'Mary's, I went for an interview there, and was accepted. Certainly, once in medical school, I found the work so interesting, that it wasn't a problem to learn. I read text-books for the fun of it!

HF   As a student, did you have any teaching in psychiatry?

AB   I remember 12 lectures which, if anything, put me off. I thought that if this is what psychiatry really is, I'm not impressed. We also had one or two visits to mental hospitals, but these were disillusioning: sometimes patients were put on display – rather like some television programme – and I felt that this was wrong, demeaning to both patient and interviewer. On the other hand, though, I had become very interested in psychosomatic medicine, after reading Katharina Dalton. At the end of my time at St Mary's, we had end-of-term competitions, with small cash prizes; I was terribly hard up, I suppose as many students are, so I had a go at them just for the money.

I won the prizes in paediatrics and psychiatry, and this probably reinforced my feeling that psychiatry might be a field for me.

HF   What happened when you qualified?

AB   My first house job was partly orthopaedics and partly ENT, and there is hardly any mixture that could be more off-putting to a young doctor. But I was extraordinarily lucky, because in June '44, I was suddenly removed from the job to Park Prewett Hospital, Basingstoke, where a surgical service for D-Day casualties had been set up. There, I volunteered to work on Alexander Fleming's Penicillin Unit and had some of the most interesting, exciting work any young doctor could possibly want. Seeing the early results of penicillin in battle casualties, experiencing the difficulties involved, and working with people who were very stimulating made me think hard about surgery. However, all good things come to an end and when this post finished, I had to look round again.

I met Professor Stokes – he was Dr Stokes then – the Deputy Superintendent at the Maudsley. He thought I should apply for a job there, and so I did.

HF   What was your experience of the Maudsley?

AB   When I was accepted, I went to Mill Hill, where one half of the Maudsley had been evacuated. Again, I was very lucky in being appointed houseman to Eric Guttmann, who was a neuro-psychiatrist. As a person, he was so helpful and supportive to a young doctor, particularly one like myself who was naive, incompetent, and ignorant. I was indebted to him and always will be.

I was keen to take a training analysis in those days, but when I told him about it, he said to me, 'Well, you may have decided, but think about it for another week, and during that time, carefully observe your colleagues here who are themselves analysts or have been analysed'. So I did, and I must admit that a study of fellow psychiatrists, all of them very senior of course, was very interesting!

At the end of it, I decided I would not have an analysis; most of those who had been analysed seemed to me too detached from their patients. If something went wrong or a patient disappeared or committed suicide, there was always an intellectual explanation.

HF   What did you do next?

AB   After Mill Hill and Guttmann, I went to Dartford with Max Jones, treating ex-POWs. Again, this was a very different experience and some of my early attitudes to group therapy were developed there, but I was still very green and naive and didn't understand a lot of what was happening.

As a complete contrast, I then went to Belmont, where I was registrar to Sargant. I was very impressed – not by his polypharmacy, which I think one had some reservations about even under his immediate mantle and in awe of his personality, but by the care he took over individual patients, the interest he showed in them, and the detail he would go into to understand their lives and how medication would influence them.

I learnt a lot from him, not so much about polypharmacy as about relating to patients and how to help them. I was then conscripted and went into the Army.

HF   How did you find that?

AB   To my surprise, I enjoyed it and found a lot which was useful from the point of view of gaining psychiatric experience. I became Area Psychiatrist at Aldershot and from there, curiously enough, learned a great deal about family psychiatry, about running an out-patient clinic, and about organising my time. The pressure of work – I was the only Army psychiatrist for a large area – was tremendous. So I learnt that I had to know what the priorities were, how to get a quick history, who to contact, and how to make a decision. I also became involved in Army Apprentices Schools, wrote two or three papers on their problems, and became quite interested in the difficulties of adolescents and how to distinguish between adolescent reactions and illness in adolescents.

I also visited a number of Army 'glasshouses', and did a paper on the relationship between deserters and civilian crime. This was at a time when there was interest in an amnesty for Army deserters, and I was able to show that a proportion of them who had previously been honest citizens, went on to commit crimes while on the run, because it was the only available way of life. If there had been an amnesty, they would have returned home to ordinary work.

This paper was not acceptable to the Army, and I was told I was still bound by the Official Secrets Act. I applied for permission to publish every year for ten years, and eventually got it, by which time, of course, the whole thing was irrelevant.

HF   You were then demobilised?

AB   I returned to Belmont, and worked on Max Jones' unit, which was now dealing with psychopaths. He was away for a year, and I enjoyed it more then than when he was there, because we didn't always see eye to eye. I was now beginning to feel much more self-confident and had a better idea of what psychiatry was about. The unit helped me to understand my own behaviour in a group, as well as group and staff interactions, but I was unimpressed by the actual results. In hospital, many patients seemed better, but with follow-up for a year, their outcome was generally poor.

I was then senior registrar, and it was pointed out to me by Walter Maclay that since my experiences were limited to neuroses, groups, and psychopaths, I must get experience in mental illness.

HF   How did you do that?

AB   I went to Netherne with Dr Freudenberg, and again, how lucky I was. What a nice man to work with and how helpful and supportive he was to me, being green in that field. I remember my first day there. I started off on the ward for neurotic patients with a ward round and a group session, spending about an hour and a half.

I was then told I would have to spend the next hour on a long-stay ward. So I went there and said to the sister – it was all locked up of course – 'What do I do here?' She said 'Well, there are 50 ECTs waiting for you'! They were laid out in rows, with a screen between each: you just went from one to the next. There was no anaesthetic; you just pressed the button, waited until they finished convulsing, and went on to the next.

I learned a lot at Netherne from the mistakes I made – such as the errors in judging what long-term psychotics might do if you let them out.

Another stroke of luck was in 1952. Freudenberg had been to the Continent and had brought back some chlorpromazine, which he gave me to try. The first patient I gave it to was an elderly lady with dementia, who had had an operation and was tearing at her stitches. Since she seemed moribund, I thought at least I could do no harm, so I gave some intramuscular chlorpromazine and to everybody's surprise, her restlessness ceased, she stopped tearing out her stitches, recovered from her pneumonia, and proceeded to live for some time longer.

Thus encouraged, the next patient I treated had an acute early schizophrenic illness – a young woman who had attacked the psychiatrist in the out-patient clinic and had been admitted in a very disturbed state. Again I was fortunate, because this young girl responded so well that two days later, I was able to demonstrate her at a clinical conference, to the surprise of all.

I then treated a series, gave a paper to the Divisional meeting of the RMPA, and wrote it up in the *Journal* in 1954. So as far as I know, these were the first British psychiatric cases in which chlorpromazine had been used, and the first paper on it in this country. So Netherne was a rewarding experience.

HF *What came next?*

AB   I had a short spell at St Ebba's, and then became a consultant and deputy superintendent at Banstead. Dr Charlton was the superintendent, and he said to me on the first day, 'If you do *anything* it must lead to improvement'.

HF *What did he mean by that?*

AB   Conditions were very bad there. It had been grossly overcrowded during the war, when patients from other hospitals had been put in to clear their beds for casualties. I was told it had been the cheapest of any of the London lunatic asylums, and evidence of that was widespread.

I was the only consultant on the female side, which had 1500 beds – seven wards of over 100 a piece, and almost all of them locked. At this point, I felt quite bitter about the training I had had.

Nothing, except at Netherne, had prepared me in any way for working out the logistics of the service, of how to allocate time, where to give priority, or how to devise the best way to create a service for the maximum number of patients.

HF *Your training had really been on an apprenticeship basis?*

AB   Yes, on the whole. At the Maudsley, I was taught how to diagnose; in fact, there used to be an old crack that if you wanted to have a diagnosis, you went to the Maudsley, but if you wanted to be treated, you went to a mental hospital!

A little exaggerated perhaps, but I had to solve some pretty awful problems at Banstead. There was a waiting list for admission, grossly overcrowded wards, and many patients going from the admission ward to a back ward after about a week or two of arrival, because there just wasn't time to work out their problems and try to treat them.

So instead of having one ward which took all the female admissions, I split it into three. In a three-storey block, I had the patients aged up to 40 on the top floor, the middle ward had the 40–60 year-olds, and the ground floor had the over-60s, which must have been one of the first psychogeriatric services.

Then, in the ward for younger patients, I set up a research programme on first-admission schizophrenics, which compared the results of ECT (giving 20 as a routine course), insulin coma (which was still in use), and chlorpromazine. I used fairly heavy doses of chlorpromazine, to give something like the experience of a coma. Then, I compared the end-results after three months, and followed the patients up for a year.

I rapidly abandoned insulin coma, as too many patients did not complete the course and in any case, the results were not good – many patients were still left with emotional flattening. The results of chlorpromazine and ECT at the end of treatment were very similar, but a year later, those who had had ECT experienced far fewer relapses.

I also did research on the treatment of long-stay patients, comparing habit training with ECT and other treatments, and wrote a series of papers with Dr Thorpe, a psychologist.

Some of these early papers compared different drug treatments, but others were on the theory and philosophy of double-blind trials, which were certainly not blind to the nurses – some thought the only people who were blind were the doctors!

HF   In your paper on the ECT regime, I wondered at the time why you chose 20 as the standard course? It seems rather high.

AB   It does now, but I have no doubt it was effective. I know from bitter personal experience that to give six or eight treatments to patients with schizophrenia would often relieve the symptoms, but relapse was almost certain. On the other hand, more intensive ECT – if need be administered daily for a week, or certainly three times a week for two or three weeks, and then twice a week and then once a week, up to about 20 treatments, produced very good results, while the relapse rate was dramatically lower than with fewer treatments.

Using chlorpromazine and other drugs as maintenance treatment helped to maintain a good remission, once it was obtained.

The other thing that made me feel ECT was a valuable treatment in schizophrenia was that the patients had a better affective response at the end of the course, whereas many of them now on long-term medication are somewhat 'flat'. I think this is overlooked in the current feeling that the drugs ought to cure everything.

HF   Do you feel now that ECT was depended on too much at the time?

AB   Yes, but now it is used too little, partly because of the complications involved in anaesthesia.

I followed-up a series (from Netherne and Banstead) of young mothers who had schizophrenia, and found that after a year, not one was looking after her baby. I thought that a very bad end-result, so I started a small ward for mothers and babies at Banstead, specialising in those with schizophrenia, and those mothers all received approximately 20 ECTs. I admitted there a number of young women who had been in other hospitals, including good teaching hospitals, and who had been referred to me as chronic patients, but if I gave them an intensive course of ECT, they emerged bright, able to care for their babies, and with a very different prognosis.

In the years of running the unit, every mother left caring for her baby herself, and that is not a bad record over some years. We followed-up all patients ourselves, which makes a tremendous difference.

HF   How did you manage to do that?

AB   Since we took patients from our own catchment area and also, by a gentleman's agreement, from other parts of the south of London, we could offer an out-patient appointment and follow-up for everyone. They nearly all managed to come regularly, but I would not take a patient from further afield. I was able to show that the relapse rate of patients I didn't follow-up personally was roughly double.

This work led to a book, *Psychiatric Disorders and Obstetrics*, which was the first based on British practice.

HF   Could I ask you to describe what the atmosphere was like in a mental hospital in the 1950s?

AB   Dreadful. At Banstead, there were several wards which *only* took disturbed patients rejected by other wards; this was a very bad system indeed. One of these had 100 or more patients, and when I went round, the hair on the back of my neck would stand up for fear of what would happen: it was not unknown for missiles to fly across the room, or for quite blatant assaults to occur.

There was no occupational therapy, and patients just stood or sat around the outer edge of the ward in a state of apathy or tense frustration. The smell of paraldehyde filled the air and some patients were persistently drunk and disorderly on it. Many were in strong clothes – very strong garments which in theory, they couldn't tear, but the reality was that it acted as a challenge to the more destructive ones, who just tore them up the more.

On the female side alone, there were 50 or more patients every day who were secluded the whole day, some having been so for months or even years at a stretch. I remember one who had been in seclusion for three years in a padded room – dreadful conditions. Time did not permit going round and assessing everyone.

All I did was to ask that before a patient went into seclusion, the nurse should write out a paragraph to explain why, and when the patient would come out again. As a result of this, the number secluded went down dramatically in two or three months to four or five a day, which was manageable and meant they could be individually assessed and treated as needed.

At the other end of the scale was a ward of over 100 patients who were active and ambulant; all had useful jobs about the hospital, in the laundry, the bakehouse and similar places. Many of them had pets, and with only one sister running the ward, it was a very easy, relaxed place; these patients had the benefits of an enormous television screen of about 6 ft by 6 ft – an absolute gem. I went to this ward and had an open meeting and explained to them that I was willing to help contact relatives or friends, to find accommodation, to find work, to make sure they were financially viable, and offer follow-up in the outside world. I asked for volunteers, and had none. So a week later, I did the same again, but suggested that if they were reluctant to talk to me, would they talk to the ward sister? There were still none. After the third such visit, the ward as a whole did a 'round robin', which they sent to the Minister of Health, protesting that I was trying to discharge them! They certainly weren't oppressed or imprisoned.

This particular block was needed for development, so, over a year or so, all the patients on that ward were transferred to others. Without any further effort on my part, many of them left the hospital; they seemed to find relatives that they didn't know existed before, and found jobs. Some were undoubtedly helped by the occupational therapy and factory work we provided, but of the series I followed-up, not one was actually doing work for which he had been trained.

They had found a wide variety of jobs, though. One was running a restaurant and wrote me a pleasant letter, thanking me warmly for all the help given her and for allowing her to leave. It was quite clear from the letter that she retained her paranoid delusions unchanged, but a social worker reported that she was functioning efficiently and offering a good service to the public in her restaurant. One of the former patients wrote references for others! Some, of course, were still unemployed and one or two relapsed, having to come back into hospital.

At the time I'm describing, though, the system of treatment in psychiatry generally was changing. Out-patient clinics were gaining importance, so that the one I began fortnightly became twice weekly and the availability of treatment there, including out-patient ECT, made a a big difference.

HF   Did you have any other professional activities at this time?

AB   Yes. In 1957, I worked for the WHO in Geneva with Llewelyn Davis, a very able architect, and Professor Sivadon from France. We produced the first WHO monograph, called *Psychiatric Services in Architecture*. Again, I was fortunate at that stage in my career to meet Sivadon, a very modest man, who introduced concepts which helped me to understand the basic principles of providing a service to meet the needs of patients.

For example, small spaces encourage close relationships. If the patient is severely disturbed, a one-to-one human relationship is needed in a small area, with feeding by the person undertaking care, and very elementary occupation, almost at baby level. But with progress, patients can begin to deal with a small group of people and form a variety of relationsips. They then need less personal care, can develop choices, and later emerge from the small family grouping into a wider sphere of perhaps a whole ward of people.

This was described in our book and the early chapters are still worth reading; it formed the basis of the work I did in the Department of Health later on. It also taught me how essential it is to involve an architect in early discussions when planning to build.

HF   What was your next assignment?

AB   I was writing quite critical articles at that time about the way psychiatry was organised and the defects of the mental hospital system. The Regional Board approached me and said that as some money was available, would I be willing to advise on and if need be run, a psychiatric admission service at St Mary Abbot's, Kensington? This was a very nice opportunity.

With an architect called Harry Smith – young, alert and quick to pick up what was needed – the present unit there evolved. I think we had something like £60,000, out of which that prefabricated unit was built, and a little was left over to develop another building as a day hospital. It helped me to see how a properly designed building made treatment and the development of good relationships relatively easy.

HF   What were the special features?

AB   There were a small number of single rooms for very disturbed patients, near to the nursing station, where close contact and individual care by nurses was easy. To follow this were small cubicle-style dormitories for four, five or six people, where the patients moving from individual care could enter an area in which they began to form relationships with a small group of others. The ward as a whole had 30 or so patients, so there were natural groupings in which they could progress from complete dependence and maximum nursing care to a situation of increasing independence, and move eventually into the community.

I was also able to show that if this was closely linked to the day hospital, with patients moving from one to the other, both follow-up and admission became easy: you could see some patients at the day hospital and admit them to the ward, or discharge them from the ward to the day hospital. The chief problem for psychiatrists is dealing with patients' anxieties of one sort or another, and the more you can do to relieve these by your attitudes, in the buildings you provide, or the way you run the service, the better.

During the four years I was working there, no patient of mine went on to Banstead. It was possible to admit, treat, and discharge a very wide variety of cases, but in those days, one-third were brought in on an Order of one sort or another, a fair number by struggling policemen.

HF   What happened to those patients who had chronic handicaps?

AB   An old saying I used was that you don't have chronic patients, you only have chronic staff. There are certainly patients with long-term disabilities, and you need to adjust your service to make the best use of that part of the patient's personality which is still functioning well. It was at this stage that I found the day hospital invaluable; day hospitals should be willing to carry a proportion of very handicapped long-term patients.

HF   In the late 1950s, it was said by a number of people that the day hospital is really only for short-term cases, while long-term patients should be in day centres.

AB   There is certainly a group with long-term handicaps who are better placed in a day centre and managed by social services, but there is also a group of quite severely handicapped patients, still needing skilled management, who have their best chance of maintaining social competence on a day hospital basis.

Sometimes it was almost impossible to find accommodation for them until we realised that the people who know best where to find accommodation for patients are other patients. We would say to the group, 'Mr or Mrs so-and-so is leaving hospital with nowhere to go. Can you help?' They'd almost always know who had a spare room, which hotel would tolerate bizarre behaviour, or other relevant information. Patients were often more successful than a trained social worker.

We need to look at the assumption in this country that only the professionals have solutions. Sometimes the ordinary public or people with their own handicaps know best. We need to listen to them.

HF How did your next assignment come about?

AB   After writing up the St Mary Abbot's experience, I wrote a series of articles with rather provocative titles like 'Breaking up the Mental Hospital' or 'Pulling Down the Mental Hospital'.

I was at a social function when Dr Tooth approached me, saying that since I had been so critical of the Ministry of Health, would I be willing to have a go and see if I could do any better!

Eventually, I agreed and went to the Department of Health as their Senior Principal Medical Officer.

HF You came to the Ministry in 1967?

AB   I had no previous experience of civil service life or the sort of work expected, though some of it had been explained to me. But I think anyone going there had to learn the hard way, by finding out how things are done. I was told my first duty was to protect the Minister, i.e. to make sure that any advice, or anything the Minister said, was in keeping with accepted policies and would not lead to criticism in Parliament.

I found to my surprise that there was very little, if any, forward planning for psychiatric services. At first, much of my time was spent either dealing with the problems surrounding addiction or problems of the Special Hospitals.

I must be frank now and say that I felt I was wrongly employed.

HF In what way?

AB   To set up a drug addiction service based on the NHS was a political decision and one not necessarily based on any medical evidence that I knew. Personally, I feel drug addiction is primarily a social problem with some medical complications, rather than primarily a medical problem.

The Special hospitals were then administered from the Ministry of Health and I felt that trying to run a hospital from a distance, without day-to-day involvement, was a mistake. Also, I had to express an opinion on the release or admission of patients to Special hospitals from the documents alone, and this was against my better judgement; I thought I should see a patient before I expressed an opinion.

On the other side of the coin, I found a singular lack of planning for future psychiatric practice, an absence of any up-to-date physical plans for new buildings, and an absence of policies to go with them. Eventually, we got together a team to look at future planning for psychiatry and at some point, this got labelled 'Mainstream', because I said that we needed to look at the mainstream of psychiatry and not what I regarded as the frills and outside activities like drug addiction and special hospitals. I don't mean any disrespect to eminent colleagues working in these fields, I am just explaining how I felt personally.

It was only after I had been in the Ministry for some months that I found there was an architectural section, which was also very interested in planning buildings for psychiatry and once we got together, things went ahead very rapidly. We were able to produce a draft building note and draft plans to go with it; with very little modification, these are the basis for current planning for admission wards and the policies that go with them. It has been very interesting indeed to see the psychiatric wards at Worcester, Chase Farm, and elsewhere based on those plans.

HF *It was in 1961 that Enoch Powell first proposed a very drastic reduction in the size of the mental hospital sector to half or less. What was the response from within the Ministry; did they prepare plans for a future service as an alternative for mental hospitals?*

AB No. The Worcester Project should have been initiated in 1961. There was a statement of intent, but none of the detailed planning that was needed to make it possible to close the big mental hospitals. New admission services with day hospital support were not being planned in the numbers that were needed, nor were the policies to go with them. The higgledy-piggledy production of new admission services, without adequate co-ordination, was a recipe for failure.

HF *That was what happened?*

AB That was how I saw the development at the time, and of course, in the mental handicap field, it was even worse. There was singularly little forward planning of any kind, either at the Ministry or at Regional Board level.

The two years I spent at the Ministry of Health were difficult ones. I certainly didn't have universal approval from some civil servants, though I had a lot of support from Sir George Godber, the Chief Medical Officer, and some others. However, the Department wasn't primarily a planning organisation. It didn't see the need to solve problems of the future in the way that I did; it was more concerned with covering the day-to-day problems.

The situation did begin to change, though, when Mr Crossman came. He was then the Secretary of State for Health and Social Services in the new DHSS – a big, powerful, man, quite willing to express a vigorous opinion on any subject. People either liked him or disliked him; luckily, we got on well. He was very critical indeed of senior colleagues in the Department – sometimes publicly and certainly tactlessly by any standards. There is no doubt whatever that he did the cause of psychiatry, and mental handicap in particular, a great deal of good. He was the only politician I saw who was willing to challenge civil servants on their own ground and argue with them on the need for improvements in the service.

For instance, he asked for a list of expenditure on the mental handicap services, and went through it with the senior staff. Much less was spent on these patients than on others. It was said they needed less doctoring, fewer nursing staff (there's a lot of supervision, so they don't need many nurses) and so on, but when it came to diet, he said 'Stop! They eat, don't they?' And I think that this insistence on looking at the resources allocated to the under-privileged section of medicine made an impact on the Department.

He could be quite frightening when he got into a combative mood, and I think civil servants either had to find good reasons for what was happening or accept that sometimes he was right. Understandably, he put people's backs up, and that also made problems for him. I have no doubt he did begin to change policies significantly and made very senior people in the Department think about their priorities.

HF   How did the Hospital Advisory Service come about?

AB   There were the scandals within the mental hospital service, and particularly the one for mental handicap in Wales, when Crossman said that instead of sweeping it under the carpet, he would use it.

The report was published and one of the recommendations was for some sort of inspectorate. This eventually became the Hospital Advisory Service, of which I was first Director. The proposal was vigorously rejected by the Department, which didn't like the idea of any sort of organisation looking at the mental health service having the right to go direct to the Secretary of State. They wanted to feel they were the only channel to give advice to the Secretary of State.

The post of Director was advertised, but I didn't apply. Crossman was not satisfied with the applicants, and so he took me aside privately and asked me to do it. I had already been told not to apply by a senior colleague in the Department, but the job interested me and I could see its potential. I knew it was possible that at the end of the day, I wouldn't have a friend left in psychiatry, but on the other hand, that there was a real need for something of this kind.

Crossman thought that in the past, people had said they didn't know what was going on and therefore didn't do anything. If we provided an effective assessment service, people couldn't use that excuse anymore.

So I took on the job, and had four of the most exciting and busy years I have ever had. My only regret is that I didn't do it earlier in my career, because there was so much I learnt in those four years which would have been absolutely invaluable earlier.

Mr Crossman was very supportive, keen to make it work, and organised all sorts of meetings, including a vast one with the press; they were very interested and excited. I said that I was very willing to give them a daily review of what we were doing, but it would contain only the good things I found in the service. After that, there were only two who remained – Mr Wilkinson, who maintained contact and did very responsible articles, and the *Times* correspondent, John Roper.

The same thing happened to television. We had a television crew turn up, but when they found they weren't going to see something horrible, they went away and we never saw them again.

So those four years were spent visiting every mental hospital, psychiatric service, and geriatric service in England and Wales. I set it up on a multi-disciplinary basis with a consultant, an administrator, social worker, administrative nurse, ward nurse, and at times a GP, occupational therapist, or physiotherapist.

HF   When you started this, it was completely new?

AB   Absolutely. I developed it entirely in accord with my own ideas. I was appointed in November and had the first team out in February, 1969. I was very lucky with the staff I was able to recruit; only one consultant was a disaster and one to two other staff unsatisfactory, but most of them could see the value of the work they were doing, and found it very interesting and very stimulating. Many of them said, as I have, that if only they'd been able to do it before, what a difference it would have made to their professional lives.

I tried deliberately to recruit a wide variety of opinions among consultants; some were superintendents and some were known to be hostile to the superintendent system. Again, with administrative nurses, some were progressive, and some were old-fashioned, so I tried to make sure I didn't produce a stereotyped approach.

In the HAS, I tried to make sure the teams had the right variety and that there would be somebody on the team that any hospital staff would talk to. I had five or six teams working, so that visiting them all and looking after the final meetings, was very intensive work indeed, but I enjoyed it enormously, though I had some very disillusioning experiences.

Some eminent colleagues who wrote in the Journals and spoke widely at meetings were found to be running very poor-quality services. On the other hand, some modest consultants that one had not heard of were running a very good service indeed.

HF   How effective was the HAS, do you think? What difference did your recommendations make in terms of what actually happened?

AB   I think changes happened at all levels. Certainly at Governmental level, ample evidence was provided for the Secretary of State to use in discussions with the Treasury, as increasing amounts of money were directed towards the longer-stay services. Perhaps more important, though, was the fact that because of these endless reports going through the DHSS, some of them with horrific information, the Department as a whole began to see that there were major problems that couldn't be ignored.

So a large number of people at both Departmental and Regional Board level changed their attitudes. For example, when I started the HAS, out of 15 Regional Boards, only two or three had forward plans for their mental handicap services, but by the end of the first year, they all had them.

Even before visiting, a lot of things began to happen. In my first report, I quoted a letter from a charge nurse in a hospital which said, 'We hear that you are coming next month and already have' – and he listed – 'toothbrushes on the ward, better food, fresh clothing for the patients', and so on. To some extent, this may have been the most valuable result – that people began to think about what they did, why they did it, how they co-operated with other professions, and things of this kind. Hospital staff knew we were multi-disciplinary, and so they had to begin to ask themselves about the quality of their own inter-disciplinary co-operation.

Of course, as we were an advisory service, we couldn't make anyone do anything; we never tried to and wouldn't want to. The thing that pleased me most was when I revisited a hospital and somebody would come along and say, 'of course, we're doing so-and-so. It wasn't your idea, we worked this out for ourselves'. Now it gave me more pleasure to hear that someone *had* accepted my ideas, and thought they were their own, than the feeling that I had put something over on somebody and they had taken it on board just because I'd said so. It's the old story – a man convinced against his will is of the first opinion still.

I think we worked as yeast in the dough – by encouraging ideas and development generally. Even hospitals which had had a bad press in the past, always had some good features.

HF   What about national political changes?

AB   After the 1970 election, Sir Keith Joseph became Secretary of State, and although a totally different person from Crossman, I found him equally supportive. I think he had quite unjustified criticism in the press; he did a great deal for the Health Service while he was there and for psychiatry in particular, but this had been little recognised.

When I left the HAS, to my surprise, I found I had more friends than I had ever had in my life before! I have a large correspondence from that time which I still keep because it was quite heartwarming – the goodwill that I personally and the service generally received.

I think it was indicative of the reluctance the Department showed over the whole function of the HAS that after I left, they failed to appoint another Director for some months. I found this sort of delay and procrastination too common.

HF   What did you do next?

AB   After leaving the HAS, I was in the pleasant position, domestically as well as professionally, of being able to choose where to work and what to do. I decided I didn't want to live the rest of my life in London and its suburbs, but that I would like to take on a psychogeriatric stint to see what I could make of it.

HF   Why psychogeriatrics?

AB   I thought it was an underprivileged area of psychiatry – there was the opportunity to do fresh work, something new. I had fairly strong ideas of what I wanted to do, and when a post came up in Gloucestershire, which is a nice county to live in where the way of life is so much pleasanter than Greater London, I couldn't resist it.

So for four years I worked in Gloucestershire, developing a psychogeriatric service, and by the end of that time had four day hospitals running, two very active admission wards, some community nurses, and very good support from social services.

My policy was to see all admissions before they came in and in general, to admit for a maximum of two weeks. I think that dementing elderly patients begin to become dependent on hospital life after two weeks and find going back home again difficult if they stay longer. So I also agreed with relatives, GPs and others the date for discharge *before* they were admitted.

In general, negotiations for discharge are much easier if you make them before admission, rather than when the patient is inside.

We also planned, in detail, exactly what programme would be provided for the patient and what improvement could be expected. I would assume that the day hospital would always have some patients coming in, perhaps daily, who were doubly incontinent and very demented. Those patients sometimes benefit from the service more than the apparently 'easy' ones that the staff were more likely to welcome.

HF   What about those patients who were on their own?

AB   Sometimes this was a real advantage, because there were no relatives complaining about the nuisance to their own lives. Even those with no relatives always have a supporting group: there are always neighbours, the local Salvation Army, or somebody going in to see old people living alone.

Very often, you can mobilise this support and I was able to demonstrate that with an effective community psychiatric nursing service linked to the home helps, we could always get the old person up in the morning and get them to the day hospital, where we could give them a bath, redress them, feed them, and see them home at night. The most disorientating thing for the elderly is being away from their home base overnight and waking up in strange surroundings. So with day hospital support, we could manage the most difficult of the elderly dementing patients if we wanted to, but many were admitted.

I was admitting 400 patients a year, as well as dealing with a lot of patients in the day hospital service. I was also doing up to 500 miles a week, visiting various places on a fairly routine basis, and knew I simply couldn't keep this up indefinitely.

HF   What was to come next?

AB   I had thought about taking retirement at 55 for some years and the more I thought about it, the more appealing it looked. I realised I was beginning to burn myself out – the work with the HAS had been very intensive indeed – probably the hardest period of work in my life – and in Gloucester I was the only consultant doing psychogeriatrics for the whole area.

The end-result was that I decided to retire. I also began to take some of the holidays which I hadn't done over the years, and to indulge my interests in gardening and fishing.

The first year after retirement did not work out as expected, because I found as soon as you are retired, everybody begins to say 'Ah, now you are retired, will you please do a locum, a lecture, or something or other'. That year was very busy indeed, but after that, I took a more positive line and cut my working time to about five sessions a week. This was mostly for social services and particularly giving advice on the management of children and adolescents, which is a very old interest of mine that resurfaced when the opportunity arose. After some years, we decided for domestic reasons, to retire to Devon, and for the last few years there, I have worked two sessions a week and done occasional medico-legal work. I feel I have been a singularly fortunate and happy man in my profession.

HF   From your present position, what do you feel about the ways things are going now – how psychiatry has developed in recent years, and the way it seems to be going at present, with Griffiths and the other changes?

AB   Personally, I'm optimistic and hopeful. In 1984, with Dr Reardon and Dr Rogers, we did a series of visits to psychiatric units in general hospitals. This was written up by the HAS and called *The Changing Pattern of Care in Psychiatry.*

It demonstrated very clearly that there are a lot of young, energetic psychiatrists with both new ideas and the ability and the courage to implement them, and that many interesting new services are developing. I've no doubt that psychiatry has changed dramatically and is still changing; it is necessary for the young men and women in psychiatry to have the courage of their opinions and to produce new ideas and to implement them.

I was lucky in my career, and could do this. I have no doubt that there are many other, more able people who could do the same and better. I'm well aware of the current frustrations with money shortages, the need to fit in with management policies, and managers who may not even understand psychiatric needs. But I still think there are ample opportunitieis for someone who is willing to look for them, to convince people and to talk their way into a situation where things can be done.

This is certainly the case in developing a service to general practice, and community work generally.

HF   Do any trends worry you?

AB   I am uneasy about a number of trends; in particular, I think the legal threat which hangs over doctors nowadays makes them practise defensively. I am sure this is one reason why ECT is not used as frequently or as freely as it should be, and I think this deprives many patients – schizophrenics as well as depressives – of their best chance of a good-quality recovery.

The present tendency to assume that every patient must have a detailed plan on leaving hospital doesn't make allowance for human nature. All these plans need to be flexible and particularly flexible in response to the patient's wishes, as opposed to what staff may feel is good for them.

I still think psychiatry is a Cinderella profession and runs the risk of being outvoted and out-manoeuvred by other professionals. This, of course, holds true for geriatrics too. Yet I think psychiatrists complain too readily about their difficulties in relationships with other professions, particularly social workers. As I see it, a psychiatrist's job is not just to make good relationships with patients, but also with other professionals. If he can apply his skills to one, he should apply them to the other. I think that makes life much easier and much more interesting.

13 John Howells

Interviewed by HUGH FREEMAN (1990)

Dr John Howells, MB BS 1943, MD 1950, AKC 1943, DPM 1947, FRCPsych (Foundation) 1971. Dr Howells was born in Anglesey, Wales, in 1918. He trained at Charing Cross Hospital, University of London. After war service as an infantry Medical Officer, he trained in psychiatry at the Institute of Psychiatry, Maudsley Hospital and in neurology at the Institute of Neurology, Queen's Square. He became a WHO Fellow in 1961. He was Founder, Director and Research Director of the Institute of Family Psychiatry from 1949 until 1983. He was a member of the Planning Committee and Faculty Board of Clinical Medicine, University of Cambridge from 1974–77 and a recognised teacher at the University from 1974–83. From 1965–74 he was a member of the East Anglia Regional Hospital Board and was Regional Adviser in Psychiatry from 1965–80.

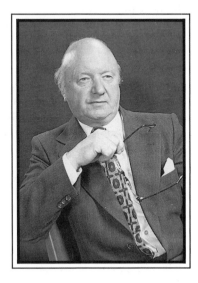

HF   I would like to ask you first about your early life and particularly about anything which may have influenced you in your later career from that time?

JH   Well, to ask a dynamic psychiatrist that question to begin with seems very appropriate. Perhaps I ought to mention, though, that I am a Celt, and we Celts are a little 'melancholic'. I should also add I am a North Walian, and there are significant differences between us and those from the south; we are much more tranquil and our big city is not a Welsh one; it is Liverpool.

I was brought up in Anglesey, and lived for many years at Holyhead. You may know that Anglesey is dominated by Holyhead Mountain; as long as man needed a vantage point, that was it, looking out immediately over the Irish Sea. As a child, I would fish off the 'Rocky Coast' below it, and climb its cliffs for birds' eggs. If you look away from Holyhead Mountain, you confront the mountains of Snowdonia.

I find myself more comfortable with that kind of country, and sometimes find a need to return to the mountains of Wales.

HF   What about your parents?

JH   In my formative years, the biggest influence on me must have been my mother. She was the intellectual one in our family. Her father, my grandfather, was originally a farmer, but as soon as his boys could handle the farm, he became a lawyer, a politician, and a chemist – he actually made an ointment from local products. He was a man of many interests, and I think this influenced my mother.

She was a person who felt strongly about causes, particularly about the underprivileged, and her special interest was the plight of black people in the United States. Now this may seem a strange interest for a woman in North Wales, but I can recall her sending my father off to the bookshop to buy me a book on the life of Abraham Lincoln. To her, Lincoln was the nearest thing to a saint. When my father came back with *Uncle Tom's Cabin*, her scorn that he could confuse the two things was enormous.

You may see a link between her and my interest in psychiatry, because in a sense, psychiatric patients are a minority and an underprivileged group.

HF   And your father?

JH   In a way, my father may also have contributed to my interest in psychiatry, because he was a gregarious, sociable, eminently likeable man. My children called him *taid*; you only had to mention that word and a ready smile would come to their lips.

HF   What does 'taid' mean?

JH   It means 'grandfather' in Welsh. Almost as soon as I could walk, he would take me fishing and shooting. He had a cousin who was a patient in a mental hospital at Talgarth, near Brecon, and occasionally my father would visit him, and I would go with him. He would park the car just down the road from the hospital and instruct me that I was not to talk to anyone who approached the car, was to keep the door locked and the window shut. He would then disappear through the big gates and after a while would return.

He would make no comment on his visit; it seemed to be a taboo subject, but I naturally wondered what was going on behind those gates. And this may well have fired some interest or curiosity about psychiatric patients.

HF   What was the atmosphere of your childhood?

JH   The atmosphere, I suppose, turned around the chapel; as a child, I looked forward to the long sermons, which were often oratorical efforts rather than religious contributions.

Occasionally, to enliven things, they would bring in a local singer, and this would have been my first introduction to music, which may have precipitated my interest in opera later on. There were not many big choirs up in North Wales, though they were a feature of life in the south.

There were a lot of eisteddfods, and I suppose these would have influenced me, because I am very much interested in poetry and particularly that of Dylan Thomas.

This has led to an analysis of his writings, which I have lectured about in America a number of times.

HF   What about your school?

JH   It gave me a good grounding in scientific subjects – especially in chemistry, almost despite my disinterest.

My history teacher was an eccentric Irishwoman, with whom I had a special relationship. I can recall her impersonating the Younger Pitt in the House of Commons when they derided the way he pronounced 'sugar'. She stood erect and declaimed over our heads 'I said sugah, Mr Speaker. Sugah'.

Welsh interests were prominent there, but not excessive! I was very taken with cricket, and was captain of the school team in an indifferent year.

Any real accomplishment I had was in the direction of the academic. I couldn't sing and couldn't compose poetry, as many other Welsh children could, though of course, I could speak Welsh.

It's of interest that two Scottish medical superintendents of Welsh mental hospitals learnt fluent Welsh – Ian Skottowe and P. K. McCowan.

Then a sad thing happened. In my adolescence, I lost my mother. It was a major loss and I sometimes think I have never really sufficiently grieved her death.

HF   How old were you then?

JH   I must have been 15, and the blow was such that I sometimes think my melancholy isn't so much due to the Celtic temperament, but is a throw-back to that moment of stress.

Indeed, I can recall once suffering a severe disappointment and immediately after it, the death of my mother came to my mind, and I burst into tears, which was an additional moment of grieving.

HF   What brought you into medicine?

JH   Oddly enough, it wasn't my mother who ordained my going into medicine, but my stepmother. She was a singer who married my father about 18 months later.

Like all adolescents, I wondered what I should do in life, and in fact, my first interest was in trees. At that time, there was a great deal of government activity to train people in forestry, presumably because of the depletion of forests during World War I.

After discussion between myself and my father and stepmother, my thoughts were turned greatly towards a helping profession. Becoming a veterinary surgeon came to mind as a possibility, to which my stepmother said, 'Well, why not go the whole hog? Why not go into medicine?' I caught on this avidly, because I realised that it was the longest university course, and a lengthy period at university was, above everything, what I desired.

HF   Why did you feel that?

JH   Because at that time, I was curious about so many things and it seemed to me that university was the gateway to knowledge. But in particular, the gateway to London. Happily, our general practitioner, who was consulted at this point, had trained at Charing Cross Hospital. The obvious place to go would have been Liverpool, which is where North Walians generally study medicine, but to me the place was London.

HF   Why were you drawn to London?

JH   Because it seemed to open so many doors to so many things, and when I did go to London, I had metaphorically to eat it all up. There was so much to fascinate one.

I was also vaguely interested in politics. The reason is that one of the saints of North Wales was Lloyd George; he was very active at that time and I saw him on two occasions. Once he was in Holyhead, when he came to support his daughter in an election campaign; he was a very impressive figure, very charismatic, and an orator to his fingertips. The second time was at the start of the war; he made a speech in the House of Commons in which he advocated an effort to make peace with Hitler. This was not well received, and someone dared him to go back to his constituency and make the same speech.

HF   Did he?

JH   He took up the challenge, and my father and I went to the meeting, which was held in Caernarvon, in the old building for the National Eisteddfod. They were so pessimistic about his attracting an audience that they only put seats in the first ten rows, but in fact, the place was packed.

Lloyd George came on stage, and he first of all invited the audience to sing a few hymns and in so doing, he created the *hwyl* – the atmosphere. Then he painted a word picture of the dove of peace flying over the flooded water between the Siefried and the Maginot lines and of course immediately, he had the audience in the palm of his hands. He did repeat what he said in the House of Commons, and he did get away with it.

HF   Did you pursue your interest in politics?

JH   There was a moment during my medical training when I did actually wonder whether I should beg an interview with Lloyd George, and see if he could somehow or other introduce me to politics. But there was a conflicting thought – during my early spell in London, I studied many things, including logic. I began to discern that politics was really something which came after the event, that the great trends were in fact precipitated by the creators, the innovators, and it was afterwards that politicians came along and applied them by regulation and law.

So I felt it was really more important to belong to the innovators than to the politicians, and that curbed my interest in politics.

HF   Where were you studying then?

JH   I was at King's College. In those days, Charing Cross pre-medical students joined the students from King's College Hospital and also from Westminster and St George's at King's College.

One of the privileges of being a student at King's College is that as it was founded as a religious college, you could take a free course in theology for the AKC – a theological qualification. This was of great interest to me, because having been brought up in a non-conformist milieu, I was interested in theology. One of the things I had done when I got to London was to study all the different types of religions; I went to meetings of Christian Science, the Ethical Movement, the Humanists, the Quakers, various types of non-conformists, and to the Catholic cathedral. During my holidays, I did a bit of lay preaching.

I was also reading logic and the result of my theological training, far from bringing me closer to religion, was to take me further away. I found myself happy with Christian ethics, but very unhappy with the nature of God and of the deity. So I ultimately came to be a humanistic agnostic – that may be the best way I could describe it.

HF *What other matters fascinated you?*

JH Another privilege of a student at King's is to take a course in another faculty, again free; in my case, I wanted to take it in philosophy, but when I went to enrol for it, they told me the course was full.

However, there was a vacancy on a psychology course, which was in psychopathology, by J. A. Hadfield, who had written a bestseller on *Psychology and Morals*. There was another, allied course, on developmental psychology, actually taken by his wife, and I booked up for both. He was a fascinating lecturer, introducing many case histories from the First World War. I think we tend to forget that there was a British school of psychopathology, really emanating from the First World War; people like Crichton Miller, J. A. Hadfield and J. R. Rees; they were founders of the Tavistock Clinic. That movement, with a careful basis of research, could have been the basis of a sound British psychopathology. But psychoanalysis was introduced and choked the local product, so that British psychopathology disappeared, and we have yet to resurrect it. It was Hadfield who introduced me to psychiatry.

Later on in my medical training, my nickname was 'Psycho'; it was very unusual for a medical student at that time to be interested in psychiatry or abnormal psychology.

HF *I had the opportunity of seeing Hadfield in action with patients a couple of times in 1958, through the RMPA's Psychotherapy Training Scheme. He used hypnotic techniques, but his appearance and personality were enormously impressive. What other interests did you have then?*

JH Art galleries, theatres, music – my interest then was in orchestral music, but later it became operatic and after that choral.

I also had two other particular interests – one was the Law Courts. King's is, of course, very close to the Law Courts, and after lectures in the afternoon I liked to go along, and through the good offices of the porter, could find in which court there was a summing-up. I loved to sit there and hear the judges marshalling the evidence, and coming to a conclusion.

The other was politics, as I mentioned before. I lived at that time in Pimlico and I would often walk to and from King's – in those days, one did a lot of walking. On the way I passed the House of Commons, and I would pop up there to the Gallery and listen to the debates.

HF *Where did you live then?*

JH In a Toc H Mark – a mark is something like a club. The Toc H movement was founded in World War I as an inter-denominational movement. The idea was that people from diverse backgrounds living together, would get to understand one another.

I had the privilege of meeting Tubby Clayton, who founded the movement. He was the sort of chap who, though there might be 50 people in a room, gave you his undivided attention while he spoke to you; you felt he was just interested in you. It was a remarkable quality.

This was a rich experience for me, because these people were very diverse indeed. On the one hand, we had a compositor from Fleet Street who was a communist, and at the other extreme we had the son of a well-known family, who really did nothing every day except the *Times* crossword. I used to rather look down on this guy, but once you really got to know him, you realised that he had something worthwhile to tell you.

To live there, one had to perform some social service, which was led by someone called the 'pilot', but it was done without any publicity.

HF   What happened when you finished the preclinical course?

JH   Almost as soon as I got to Charing Cross for the clinical course, World War II started, and the hospital was evacuated to Ashridge Park, in Hertfordshire, with the medical school in a large house nearby. Part of the hospital was still functioning in London. We had less lecturing than pre-War medical students, but I think we had a great deal more practical experience. We were expected to help with the bombing casualties in London, and with the wounded when they came into Ashridge.

HF   How did you divide your time between London and Hertfordshire?

JH   Every so often, we had a spell in London; during the bombing, for instance, one was virtually a stretcher bearer. The Casualty Department was in the basement, sandbagged all round, but we lived as students on the first floor. Any patients who came in would be evacuated in the next day to Ashridge Park.

The bombing during that period was really intensive, and many casualties were brought in. I remember the night when a bomb went down the stairway of the tube station at Trafalgar Square, which was very close to us. It finally exploded down at platform level, so that many casualties were brought in. I also remember when they brought the casualties in from the *Café de Paris* bombing.

Our first task was to go down the row of stretchers, take out the dead, and then try to identify those cases which needed immediate operations. There was a gasp from a fellow student, and he said 'Snakehips'. Sure enough, there on the stretcher, dead, was Snakehips Johnson, who was the dance band leader of the *Café de Paris* and a very prominent musician at that time.

Possibly our most disagreeable task was at the end of the evening, when the dead had to be taken to the mortuary on the first floor. We had no lift that would take a stretcher, so each body would be tied to a stretcher, which would go vertically into the lift. One student would go up with the body, holding the stretcher vertical, while the other ran up the stairs to meet the lift; that, in the dark, with the body tending to fall on you, was a very disagreeable task.

HF   Who were the most important figures at the hospital?

JH   One who had a considerable influence on me at that time was Norman Lake, the senior surgeon. I met him in a curious way. At that time, one had to make one's own amusements, and the 'Brains Trust' was very popular. So the hospital had its own, and it consisted of a consultant, in that case Norman Lake, representatives of the junior medical staff and nursing staff, and a medical student, who happened to be me. When people asked questions, I tended to take a psychological slant, which at first bewildered Lake.

He was a very remarkable man, the senior examiner for the Mastership of Surgery in the University of London, as well as having a degree in engineering and another one in music. He kept a little notebook with him always, and recorded any unusual event or information in it; that evening, it would be read up in his reference works, and in that way, he accumulated a vast amount of knowledge about all sorts of subjects.

I imitated him in this habit and ultimately, over 25 years, collected enough material on psychiatry and abnormal psychology to make a two-volume Reference Companion to its history.

He was curious about this student (myself), and became more and more interested in psychology and abnormal psychology himself. Ultimately, he made the monumental statement that no surgical out-patient clinic was complete without a psychiatrist in attendance.

HF   Did you do house jobs at your teaching hospital?

JH   I did two house posts before going into the army. The first was to the firm of Sir Gordon Holmes, who was the senior physician, and E. C. Warner, who was the editor of *Savill's Textbook of Medicine*. Warner was a very fine clinician, but of course, the dominating influence was Holmes. He was a formidable man to work for – tall, iron-grey hair, tremendous fluency of thought and rapidity of speech, and impatient with people who couldn't keep up with his pace. He kept a patellar hammer by his side and when impatience was too much, he would use this on you; his edict was 'Maybe I have to bang it into you'.

HF   On what part of you?

JH   He always went for the head. It could be hurtful, but one did learn neurology from him. I recall a patient who had been admitted from out-patients, where he had been seen by Warner, and the diagnosis was anxiety state. When I did my examination, I could find no abnormal physical signs. When Holmes came round, he said 'Boy. Have you examined the patient?' to which I replied 'Yes Sir'. 'Pray, what is your diagnosis?', Holmes asked. I said 'anxiety state'. Later, people told me that this was like a red rag to a bull. Holmes said nothing, but examined the patient, and then turned to me and said 'And what do you observe?' I had followed his examination and could see no abnormal physical signs of any kind. I said 'No abnormal signs, Sir'. To which he said, 'You're not very observant today, Howells. I will concentrate your attention on the abdomen'. And so he did the reflexes of the abdomen. He then said to me 'Now Howells, what do you observe?' I was a little bewildered and said 'Four reflexes, Sir'. 'Howells you're very inattentive today; I will repeat my examination for you' came the reply. So he did them again, and said, 'Now, what do you observe'. By then, I was completely bewildered and said 'Four reflexes, Sir'. 'Howells I will make it easy for you. Have you not noticed that the right lower abdominal reflex tires before the left?' He did them again, and with the eye of faith, you could argue that possibly this was so. He said 'Now Howells, I'm not impressed with your performance today. You will examine this patient every day for the next week and will then tell me what you observe'.

HF   And what happened?

JH   Sure enough, during the next week, all sorts of physical signs appeared. When he came the following week, he said 'Have you done what I told you?' I said 'Yes, Sir'. He said 'What is your diagnosis now?' 'A frontal lobe tumour,

Sir'. 'Quite right. You've wasted a week Howells. Now get hold of a surgeon'. This was exacting stuff, but very good neurology, so I was really very fortunate in having that sort of apprenticeship.

HF   What was your next job?

JH   House surgeon to Norman Lake. This was as pleasant as the other experience was, in a way, personally unpleasant. He was a very gentle, modest person. One inevitably made mistakes, but he would point them out with a little smile and then would add something encouraging like 'Of course, you will soon put that right'. Not only was he a general surgeon but also a neuro-surgeon, which was quite unusual in those days. He did his brain surgery on a Sunday morning, with the advantage that things were quiet in the hospital then. There would be a mix of cases – bullets and shrapnel in the brain, and the occasional brain tumour. This made the weekend very busy for me because I would have to prepare the cases for operation on Saturday and look after them on Sunday afternoon and evening. What I liked so much was the intimacy of the occasion. In the theatre, there was just Lake and me and the nursing staff. For shrapnel and bullets, one had to try to estimate the position from X-rays, done from various angles. Then, we had to try to discern the best approach to the problem, so that I learned a great deal of brain anatomy. I developed an interest in neurology then, and later on did a neurological job at Queen's Square.

HF   Did you meet the psychiatrists at Charing Cross?

JH   I attended the psychiatric out-patients at Charing Cross whenever I could. There were two psychiatrists there – A. A. W. Petrie, a well-known superintendent and an ex-President of the RMPA, and Clifford Allen, whose special field was sexual pathology. Allen was an interesting man and was very helpful to medical students; we were allowed to take case-histories from the patients, most of whom were war casualties.

HF   What did you do next?

JH   I went into the Services. I had toyed with the idea of going into psychiatry, and consulted Petrie. He said 'How old are you?' I was 24. He said 'I think you are too young to specialise. Furthermore, if you want to go into psychiatry later on, you ought to look around first, and if you decide to do it, your military experience will be invaluable to you.' I think this was probably right. So after training at the RAMC Depot at Crookham and a short period in a field ambulance, I found myself with an infantry battalion. I still go to their annual reunions.

It was through this battalion that I came to practice in Ipswich. Before D-Day, many troops were moved over there, to give the impression that the attack was coming from East Anglia to the Low Countries; then overnight, they were switched in a magnificent logistical effort to the south coast. So for three weeks we were in this area, the sun shone every day, and I remember it as a fine place to be.

HF   What was life like in an infantry battalion?

JH   Sir Richard Doll has given a good picture in a series of articles in the *BMJ* recently. With the regiment, one learned about life, how to look after oneself, and a little psychiatry of a sort. For instance, just a few minutes after the battalion was told they were going on active service, a man was brought in with a self-inflicted injury to his foot – a nice clean hole.

There was also a certain amount of marital and other similar problems. A regular attender was the battalion butcher, who had a very tiresome wife; after every leave, he would come back upset and would have to come and talk to me about it. As a matter of fact, at every reunion since the war, he has still consulted me about his wife.

HF   Any curious episodes?

JH   Human nature exerted itself. I once had a message from the commander of D Company, who said that a strange thing happened to his men; they all seemed very phlegmatic and exhausted. So I went along and found these men were guarding a pontoon bridge across the Rhine; I examined a number of these 'exhausted' men, and could find no physical cause, but there was no doubt that they were exhausted. So I said to my batman-driver, 'I want you to circulate among the men and tell me what's going on'. He went to the cookhouse and after about an hour, came back; I could tell that he had obtained some information. The top and bottom of it was that no one except military personnel was allowed to cross this bridge, but many Germans wanted to do so. So at night, they were allowed to cross if the women slept with the guards, and this was happening so frequently that the men were exhausted. So I drew the company commander's attention to the need to be more in touch with his men.

Ultimately came the time when I left the Regiment because the European war had ended, and I found myself in a field ambulance, but was very unhappy there, feeling like a caged bird! Then, they put me in charge of a reception station, which was a hospital of about 20 beds, with a couple of medical officers, a dentist, and a number of medical orderlies. I quite enjoyed that; we were at an attractive part of the Rhine.

HF   This was when you attended a course at Göttingen?

JH   I was selected by the Army to go on this course, which was a partnership between German and British professors, and one saw their different techniques. For instance, the Germans placed much greater reliance on laboratory findings, whereas Professor Tunbridge asked us to make an estimation of the degree of anaemia in a patient by physical examination, looking at the lips and eyes, etc. When we looked at the laboratory findings, they were identical with our clinical estimates. An impressive feature of life at that university hospital was the post-mortem meeting at 12 noon every day, which everyone attended, and learned about the mistakes they had made.

Something comparable in psychiatry might be possible; when a patient is discharged prematurely or commits suicide, the psychopathology could be thoroughly explored – a kind of post-mortem.

HF   What happened when your demob came?

JH   I was so happy to go that I arranged for an ambulance to come behind my truck, with instructions that should I have an accident, my body was to be put on the train anyway! After the actual demobilisation, there was a short period when one gathered breath and wondered what one should do. At that

H

time, the National Health Service was coming in and it wasn't clear what the role of the general practitioner was going to be. So my thoughts turned to psychiatry.

HF   How did you start in psychiatry?

JH   The Maudsley had set up a training scheme at St Ebba's, Epsom, which was run by Linford Rees; one became a supernumerary registrar in the NHS, with a view to taking the DPM. Then he suggested that I should think of training at the Maudsley.

So I had an interview there with William Gillespie, who was a child psychiatrist. I still remember that he started off the interview, as you have today, wanting to talk about one's early experiences, and looking back, this was absolutely right. He was a very quiet, modest man, but I think a first-class clinician; later, he was one of my supervisors in the children's department. Presumably through his good offices, I was selected for the Maudsley, where some of my contemporaries were D. L. Davies, Trevor Gibbens, Desmond Pond, Michael Shepherd, David Stafford-Clark, and Anthony Storr.

HF   What did you feel about your time there?

JH   I am delighted to have had a Maudsley training, which I regard as one of the best in the world. But nothing is perfect, and certainly there were problems there in my time.

One of the things you noticed was the tremendous tension about the place, and this even resulted in trainees occasionally committing suicide. There was a curious formality, that led to distancing between people. If you passed a senior colleague in the corridor, you never acknowledged him and he never acknowledged you. But one trainee, passing Eric Guttmann one day, was moved to say 'Good morning' to him. Guttmann passed by, as he always did, without acknowledging him. The trainee ran after Guttmann, stood in front of him and said 'Good morning, Good morning' to which, with surprise, Guttmann replied 'Good morning', politely. Clearly, he didn't regard it as his role to communicate with people, and this seemed to apply to the staff generally.

HF   I remember this atmosphere very well myself. What was the cause of the tension?

JH   I think one has to mention the personality of Aubrey Lewis, because he dominated the place. On the clinical side, it was very similar to the continental system – Herr Professor and no-one else counting for very much.

He was brilliant intellectually, but at the same time, I thought he was basically an anxious person – his anxiety didn't allow him to drive a car for instance. And of course, he was abysmally shy; at a party, you could see his torment. It seemed to me that his defence against anxiety was his intellect; he struck first, before anyone could possibly hit at him, and I think this created tension around him.

I well remember the Monday morning conferences. I was on his firm and we used to meet in the Villa, around a table covered with a green cloth. Lewis would come in, pick up a ruler, start tapping the table, turn to the presenter and ask him to start. It was a harrowing experience. When my turn duly came, he said 'Well, who is presenting this morning?' I said, 'I am Sir'. Then he said to me, 'This whole exercise is getting rather tedious, isn't it? I think this morning, for some relief, you should give us your presentation reversed'. I was immediately in a panic state and thought he literally meant that I should start at the end of a sentence. Then I collected myself and realised that the part of the history that normally came last should now come first; somehow or other, I got through it.

HF   Presumably others suffered too?

JH   There was one of us who decided that he was going to put Aubrey Lewis on the spot by presenting the 'history of all histories' without a flaw. So he took a two-week holiday to work through it, and arrived cock-a-hoop for his Monday morning stint. Well, he got about six sentences along, when Aubrey stopped him and said 'Dr so-and-so, am I to understand that you *really* mean that?' The fellow managed to answer, but a dent had been made in his self-confidence. He then got another few sentences along, and Aubrey stopped him again in the same way. Ultimately, he was like jelly, and could barely finish his history. A few weeks thereafter, he left.

I think that sort of thing is not good teaching. There were very few people interested in human relationships on the Maudsley staff at that time.

HF   Was there a positive side to him?

JH   Aubrey did a great deal; he put the Maudsley on its feet after the War, and created new departments, though when you consider his creative output, one is bound to say it was rather small.

The person who impressed me very much, though, was Eric Guttmann, whose short textbook with Curran was a very sound introduction to psychiatry. He was a clinician to his fingertips. When I joined his firm, there were three cases of anorexia nervosa on the ward. One proved to be Addison's disease, another pulmonary tuberculosis, and only one was a true anorexic. But Guttmann was completely at ease with the situation; he could examine these patients and make the differential diagnoses.

HF   Was Aubrey Lewis a good clinician?

JH   In the observation ward, I had immediate clinical contact with him. One usually had to make a diagnosis within three or four days, so that the patients could be classified and moved out to wherever they needed to go. But at the end of my presentation of cases there, Lewis's stock reply was to find some investigation which I hadn't carried out, and therefore he couldn't express an opinion until this had been done. Well, of course, by the time he came the following week, the patient had moved on anyway.

Guttmann, though, seemed to be able to make patients emphasise whatever symptomatology they had, so that one could come to a ready diagnosis.

HF   Did you have much personal contact with Aubrey Lewis?

JH   I noticed that in his reminiscences, Felix Post mentioned how he used to travel by tram with Lewis from Vauxhall in the morning. Well, I sometimes did the same. I travelled in from Epsom to Vauxhall Station, and I used to pray Aubrey wouldn't be on the tram. But quite often he would be and then, when we left the tram, we had to walk up Denmark Hill together. In preparation for this, I thought of a subject almost every morning, which I hoped I could put to Aubrey and maybe get a response. It never worked, though. One began to feel an utter fool.

But at the same time, once we lapsed into silence, we seemed to have some sort of companionship as we walked up the hill. I had noticed that he was always very kind to someone who was religious, of whatever denomination.

HF   Did you ever consider returning to The Maudsley?

JH   Some years after I had left, Aubrey and I met at a conference in Cambridge. He indicated that he would like me to return, and in fact gave me some advice on how I should proceed. Kenneth Cameron, head of the children's department, who was also a close friend of mine, suddenly died. I was just embarking on a round-the-world lecture tour when the post was advertised, and I decided to apply. I thought I would be in Hong Kong at the time they would be sending out the papers, and asked for them to be addressed to me there. Well, these arrived in Hong Kong alright, but they went by surface mail and were returned to me some months later! So I never applied for the post. Perhaps a happy escape for both parties – who knows?

You benefit from Maudsley training; it gives you self-confidence and in Aubrey Lewis's day, it also taught you history-taking, which I found invaluable later on. If one was bewildered by a patient, one would do a Maudsley-style history and then quite often the diagnosis emerged.

HF   After you left the Maudsley, what did you do next?

JH   I think I know the exact morning that I decided to leave. I had gone temporarily to Queen Square for neurological experience, and then went back to the children's department. One morning, someone asked 'Why is this child disturbed?' The answer seemed to become constitutional, genetic factor. But I felt that very little attention was being paid to the patient's emotional environment. Part of the problem was that the division of labour was for the social worker to see the parent and the psychiatrist to see the child, so that the psychiatrist was largely ignorant of stresses emanating from the parents. I became very upset by this situation, and felt that a great deal more attention should be given to the management of the parent/child situation as part of the family. So I decided that I would try to study family psychopathology systematically on my own.

HF   Where did you decide to go?

JH   I was just 30 at the time, so the only possibility would be a consultant post outside London. Two of these were going – one in Swansea and the other in Ipswich. I remembered the nice weather in Suffolk when I was in the Army, so I applied for that post, which was an unusual one in that it was at a general hospital. I think my Maudsley training was mainly responsible for my getting the appointment at such an early age.

HF   How did your writing career start?

JH   The Regional Board had given me some financial help towards research – a full-time secretarial post – and after the end of ten years in 1960, as agreed, I sent a report on my work. They said it was rather interesting and ought to be published. So this was my first book, *Family Psychiatry*, ultimately published in 1963.

In the meantime, I was given a WHO fellowship and had gone to the States to survey all the family centres there. It became clear to me that, in fact, there were three quite distinct trends in the family field. One was family therapy, founded by Nathan Ackerman in New York, another was the study of family and schizophrenia, of which Lidz was a representative, and then there was family psychiatry from the United Kingdom.

HF   What are the differences?

JH   There is still a great deal of confusion about these quite different approaches. I got to know Nathan Ackerman very well. He was an analyst by training who discovered by accident that he could help the individual patient better through conjoint family therapy than he could by individual psychoanalysis. But this is not family psychiatry – it's individual psychiatry – using the group to restore health in an individual.

In family psychiatry, you regard the sick individual as an index of a sick group, a sick family, and all your efforts in diagnosis and treatment are geared to restoring health in the family group; then, of course, health is restored to the individual patient also. Through being part of a healthy family, the index patient then remains healthy: the primary focus of effort is always the family and not the individual.

The field of family work in relation to schizophrenia is also an individual approach; again, the idea is to restore the individual schizophrenic to health. But the thing that struck me in visiting these US centres, was that none of them were treating schizophrenia. They seemed to me to be treating severe neurosis or personality disorder. Later, with a colleague, I surveyed the literature on all this work and wrote a book *Family and Schizophrenia*, in which we came to the conclusion that it had certainly not been proved that family psychopathology is responsible for schizophrenia. But that did not mean that the family is not important to schizophrenia. Just as a spastic child in a disturbed family will have more restlessness and more abnormal movements than he will in a tranquil family, and an epileptic child will have more attacks, so the schizophrenic is certainly assisted by being a member of an emotionally tranquil family. In fact, if you look for reasons for admissions of schizophrenics to hospital, it is often because the family can't manage, and it can't do so because it's disturbed. I don't think the disturbance causes the schizophrenia, but it causes the admission.

My Chairman's Address to the Child Psychiatry Section of the RMPA in 1961 was on 'The nuclear family as the functional unit in psychiatry'. Again, I was trying to make clear that family psychiatry is not only for child psychiatrists, but is for all psychiatrists. The index, presenting, patient who is indicative of family disturbance can be of any age-group. The family is sick, and it follows that one has to examine and treat the psychopathology of the family, so that the true 'patient' is the family unit. It also means that one has to have a diagnostic system for the family. In this field, I think that far too much attention is given to treatment and too little to diagnosis: many films on 'family therapy' are in fact about family diagnosis. A few years ago, another colleague and I wrote a book on *Family Diagnosis*, to emphasise its importance.

HF   How did your postgraduate teaching programme start?

JH   After I had been in Ipswich for a number of years, a Ministry Memorandum came out, suggesting that post-graduate teaching should develop in district hospitals; the idea was to attract good clinicians to these hospitals, by giving them a teaching role and to bring the trainee to where most of the material was to be found. Shortly after, another Memorandum suggested that where the climate was right, research units should also be created in district hospitals.

The Regional Board seized on this and founded our Institute of Family Psychiatry. This was defined as having four roles. First of all, to construct a clinical service in family psychiatry; secondly, to undertake research in the subject; thirdly, to arrive at useful preventive measures; and fourthly, to teach. The Board made me director of the unit, and increased our permanent administrative research staff to five.

HF   How did you organise your research?

JH   Our research was of two main types. Firstly, clinical. An example is our exploration of the whole field of play therapy, which at that time was a centre of interest, but since, for some mysterious reason, has ceased to be so. As a result of that, we created a department of child therapy, run by occupational therapists who had a two-year, full-time training programme with us, and that is still going on. Then we explored new techniques of treatment by analysing tapes, and this produced 'family group therapy'. We developed new procedures for family assessment and family diagnosis. Again, clinical research resulted in the evolution of 'vector therapy', involving a systemic repatterning of emotional forces.

Secondly, there were formal studies. An example would be our study on separation, exploring the hypothesis that the experience of separation was responsible for much mental ill-health in children. We found that it was not separation itself that was responsible, but rather the deprivation consequent on separation; the results were published in *The Lancet.*

Then we evolved the new technique of the Family Relations indicator, which has been published in a number of languages, including Russian. We did a large study of hard-core problem families, and its findings were published in the *American Journal of Psychiatry.* In another formal piece of research, we undertook a 1,000-family survey in the Ipswich area to explore the pattern of relating in the family. Analysis of the data from this survey has revealed some significant findings for social life and clinical practice, but so far they are unpublished.

HF   What of your teaching programme?

JH   First of all, we had our senior registrars to teach, then registrars doing their Membership, and we ran a two-year course in child therapy. We had four annual courses: for general practitioners, for psychiatrists, for social workers, and for nurses; each was of a week and usually residential. The GP course ran for more than 30 years. Each winter, there was also a ten-week course for local professional groups.

HF   Can you comment on the differences between family psychiatry and family therapy?

JH   Over the course of time, misunderstandings arose about family psychiatry. The common one was not to understand the basic philosophy, which became confused with family therapy, particularly when that came into the UK in the 1970s.

In family psychiatry, the principle is that an individual who becomes sick is an element in a sick family. If, for instance, mother is depressed, then if you look at the family, you may well find that the father has migraine and personality disturbances, the son has got asthma, and maybe his sister is failing at school. This is a total situation, and if you are able to bring harmony to it, then mother's depression clears up, father's migraine clears up, and the children return to normality. You restore health to the whole group.

In conjoint family therapy, the principle is to use the family to get the identified sick person well. But if you concentrate simply on improving the health of one member, then others can get worse or someone else can become ill. Once conjoint family therapy was developed, it became a sort of cult – it was said that one could only help the family in a family group.

In fact, there are a number of techniques which are useful for helping families: sometimes an individual approach is appropriate, sometimes a dyadic one, sometimes a family group approach, or an inter-generational one. Bringing the previous generation into the family treatment situation was our most potent discovery in family treatment. Just occasionally, multiple family therapy might be appropriate. One uses whatever tools are right for a given clinical situation.

I described these developments in a series of books – originally *Family Psychiatry* and later *Theory and Practice in Family Psychiatry*, which went into a number of foreign editions, including Japanese. These were followed by *Principles of Family Psychiatry*, which again went into several foreign editions, then *Advances in Family Psychiatry* and finally the Society of Clinical Psychiatrists report on *Family Psychiatry for Child Psychiatrists*.

HF   *How did your 'Modern Perspectives' Series start?*

JH   In our teaching programme, concentrating on the child as the identified patient, it seemed appropriate that our registrars should learn about current developments in child psychiatry in this country. So I got together a book called *Modern Perspectives in Child Psychiatry*, which passed into American hands and the publisher thought that this idea would have worldwide interest. So we then produced *Modern Perspectives in World Psychiatry*, which was followed by others, ultimately making 13 volumes. The most exciting one, I thought, was *Psychiatry in Surgery*, which appeared to be a very neglected area. More recently, I continued with *Modern Perspectives in Clinical Psychiatry*, then in *Modern Perspectives in Psychosocial Pathology*, *Modern Perspectives in the Psychiatry of Neurosis*, and *Modern Perspectives in the Psychiatry of the Affective Disorders*.

HF   *How did your preventive programme develop?*

JH   In our programme at Ipswich, the disappointment was in relation to our efforts at preventive psychiatry or health promotion. Originally, I had a notion of trying to do a 'Peckham Experiment' – having an establishment where families could attend and be given a model psychiatric service, as well as other family benefits.

The local council went so far as actually to pinpoint a building and start negotiating for its purchase. But, unhappily, that fell through and then local authorities lost the right to undertake medical ventures, so that was that.

Another opportunity came when a new Director of Education arrived and seemed very interested in these ideas; we pinpointed a small town where we could set up a model psychiatric service, but again nothing came of it.

I think the preventive side has been the weakness of the whole National Health Service. But one aspect we did concentrate on was that of child abuse. I had long felt that the gospel of 'no separation' and of a child's own home being better than any other home was basically wrong; there are times when a child is sorely deprived in his own home, and I think that can constitute an argument for separation. In surgery, you don't lightly remove someone's leg, but on rare occasions it is life-saving. I felt very strongly about the Maria Colwell case, and wrote a book called *Remember Maria* as a sort of protest and to try to clarify the situation.

HF   We should talk now about your role in the foundation of the College. I remember very well the original RMPA debate at the RSM. I was sent by The Lancet *to report it, and was told beforehand that, in general, they were not in favour of more colleges being established. But I remember particularly the opening of your speech, when you said 'We can have our College now'.*

JH   Yes! Well, the reason for saying that was that I had been in touch with a psychiatrist called T. Moylett, a member of the Society of Clinical Psychiatrists, who had an encyclopaedic knowledge of legislation in this country. Just before that November meeting, I wrote to him, asking if there was a way by which the RMPA could become a Royal College without a new Charter and without an Act of Parliament. I got his reply the day before the meeting, saying – Yes.

It was very simple, and he quoted precedents. The RSM had changed its name in 1921 to the Royal Society of Medicine by a Supplemental Charter and the Glasgow Faculty had changed its name about 1926 by the same means. So he said emphatically that all we needed was a Supplemental Charter, which was very simple legally. That was why I was able to assure people that it was possible to do this.

Later, I checked with the Privy Council. As a citizen, it is one of your privileges to be able to write to them and to the Lord Chancellor's Office on any legal question, and they have to reply to your letter. So I asked, 'Am I right in thinking that it is possible to effect a change of name of a Royal body by a Supplemental Charter?' After a couple of weeks, they wrote back to say, 'You are correct that this is possible'. Later, just to confirm this, I wrote to the Lord Chancellor's Office and got precisely the same reply.

HF   Why did it take so long to get the College actually established?

JH   Bearing in mind that the whole thing was legally simple, it is a good question, why it was so difficult to execute in practice.

That takes us to the realm of the opposition to the College, which came mainly from the Royal College of Physicians, but more particularly from its Psychological Medicine Committee. Throughout their history, the RCP had been obstructive – to the general practitioners, the obstetricians, and the pathologists, and they were certainly going to obstruct us. There was a reason for this. They regarded themselves not just as a Royal College for physicians, but as covering every aspect of medicine. This, of course, had always been denied by the surgeons and the obstetricians through their own Colleges.

Within the Psychological Medicine Committee, there was a powerful group who felt that they had a privileged position within the College of Physicians and they had no desire to lose this. The guiding light there was Desmond Curran, who was violently opposed to the College's foundation. It was also opposed by Aubrey Lewis, but I think that although he was against the idea of the foundation of a College derived from the RMPA, he might have been happy to have had one separate from the RMPA. He regarded the RMPA as a second-class body and took no part in its activities himself. He was also opposed to the College because he had established the London DPM, and felt that this would be challenged by the foundation of a new body.

Yet again, within the RMPA, there was a focus of resistance in that delightful person, Alexander Walk. Now, I had the highest regard for him; in a sense, he 'was' the RMPA. He was a very able person, a true scholar, and a very loyal servant to the RMPA, but unfortunately, regarded the move towards a college as a threat to it. He could not be persuaded that a College would be the culmination of his own work. He fought against the idea right down to the last meeting of the Petitions Committee. We had a letter from the Privy Council conceding everything, and saying, 'Well, we agree with you that you are ready to launch a College, so please petition immediately'. But he twisted the letter around to mean the exact opposite, advising us to have no truck with the Privy Council and to cease negotiations. Happily, although he was supported by Eliot Slater, the Committee thought otherwise, and we petitioned shortly after that.

HF Can you describe the course of events?

JH The College quest really occurred in two phases – the 'open' one, when people had to persuade themselves that they needed or wanted a Royal College, and the 'closed' one, consisting of a number of steps towards the actual formation of it. I had come on to the RMPA Council at quite an early age, because I was Secretary and then Chairman of the Child Psychiatry Section, and their representative on Council. Someone asked the Council whether we should be thinking about founding a College, and immediately he was set upon by the remainder, who insisted this wasn't an appropriate moment and in any case, we might be upsetting the Royal College of Physicians.

Your *Bulletin* interviews with Sir Kenneth Robinson and Sir George Godber both pinpointed the opposition as being centred there. A couple of years after this first discussion, T. P. Rees raised the matter in the Psychological Medicine Committee of the BMA, but they didn't regard themselves as an appropriate body to pursue this, so they referred it to the Council of the RMPA. I'm sure that Rees intended this to happen from the very beginning. I contributed to the discussion, and when Council decided to set up a committee to explore the whole thing, they put me on it.

HF What happened?

JH Alexander Walk was the chairman, and we took evidence from a number of bodies. I was pretty naïve in those days, and didn't realise that the easy way of settling any dispute is to set up a committee to explore it, but to constitute your committee in such a way that they will give you the reply that you want! Walk had in fact cleverly constituted this particular committee in such a way that it would never, ever ask for a Royal College. Well, ultimately came the moment of preparation of its report, and Walk asked for an expression of opinion. A third of the Committee wanted no action, a third wanted a Faculty within the College of Physicians, and another third wanted the Royal College. In effect, this meant a stalemate, and it was going to be difficult to write a report.

So a compromise was put forward, which was that maybe the College might be a desirable aim in the future, but it wouldn't be appropriate at the moment. When it came to voting, there were 11 members in favour of the proposition, which really meant 'no action', and I opposed it. However, before the meeting, I'd had a word with T. P. Rees, because I could see what was happening, and he said 'Now look here, my boy. You know you've got the right to write a minority report if you want to'. So I then asked whether I could write such a report, and they had to concede that.

As a result, two reports should have gone to Council, but I then went off to the States, and when I came back and looked at the minutes, I discovered that my minority report had never gone to Council. Had it done so, had a hearing, and been turned down, I would probably have let the matter rest.

HF   What did you do next then?

JH   I read the Byelaws of the RMPA, though normally, people simply consulted Alexander Walk! I discovered that it was a right of a member, if he wanted, to move a motion at the Annual General Meeting, but that was the only time during the year that one could do this. That right is still maintained in the new constitution of the College. So I put down a resolution for the next AGM, and this caused great upset in the office. They were deeply offended that any member should exercise this right, and particularly that it should be on the issue of a College. I was told that this was inappropriate, that it wasn't the right time, that I would be causing offence, and that in any case, I would be disrupting the AGM. I had to insist.

Then I met Monro, the Secretary, and Curran, the President, and we made a deal. If I would agree not to raise it at the AGM in July, they would defer the business part of the AGM to the quarterly meeting in November. I readily agreed to this, because I realised that the AGM was being held in a remote hospital somewhere, and there might not be a very good attendance. But the November meeting was being held in London. I think they realised later that perhaps it was a mistake to have deferred it. So came the meeting at the RSM that you mention – and reported for *The Lancet*.

HF   Can you describe what happened on that occasion?

JH   When the day came, Council had invited two other people to speak. The speaker in favour of maintaining the *status quo* was Leslie Cook, Superintendent of Bexley Hospital, while the speaker on having a faculty within the College of Physicians was Denis Hill. After a lively discussion, Alexander Walk, who was of course a master of procedure, moved an amendment to my motion which, being an amendment, was voted on first. Not only that, but if it was carried, then the motion would not be put. This amendment in a sense was a negative, but not a complete negative. What he was saying was 'Members, leave this in the hands of your officers'. Then he made a promise that there would be a postal vote, which appealed to the audience, as it seemed reasonable. So they voted and, on a recount, they carried the amendment.

It looked as if there wasn't going to be a direct vote whether or not we should have a college, but happily, Curran and Walk made a miscalculation. They thought the vote meant that the people present were against a college. Curran then said 'Although it's not strictly necessary under the constitution, it still would be rather nice to have a vote on the motion'. I'm sure he was confident that it would be turned down, but in the event, there was a handsome majority in favour. So the whole thing ended most happily, because there had been a vote in favour of a college and we got a promise from the officers of a postal vote. Your account in *The Lancet* ended with a phrase to the effect that 'This matter must now be pursued with greater urgency.'

HF   What happened next?

JH   The next step was the postal vote, which was to take place the following January. The difficulty was that there had to be a clear question on the ballot paper, or otherwise, one might get an ambiguous answer. The wording of it was left with Walk, and his first effort at this was absolutely masterly: there were a number of questions, but it would not have been possible to get a clear answer from them as to whether or not the members wanted a college. Of course, we were dismayed by this. Three of us put our heads together – John Hutchinson, Clifford Tetlow (who recently died), and myself – to see if we could contrive one unequivocal question on the ballot paper, and if possible it should be the first one. We did ultimately gain our objective.

Then, to our consternation, we heard the Council had deferred the postal ballot until May. They hoped that by then, the RMPA would be physically within the new building of the Royal College of Physicians, and that members might find it difficult to oppose our hosts. The other reason was that the College of Physicians had decided to resurrect a ploy which they had used to obstruct the obstetricians back in 1926. Then, in order to make it unnecessary to have a College of Obstetricians and Gynaecologists, they founded an examination for them. So they were now going to frame a new examination, which they thought would be suitable for psychiatry. In fact, it wouldn't have been, because the first step was to be an examination in general medicine; it was only in the final part that one could have elected to take psychiatry as a clinical subject.

HF   How did the ballot go?

JH   The papers went out to members in May 1964. For the Society of Clinical Psychiatrists, it seemed most important that members should reply to them, because, only a short time before, the RMPA had sent out a questionnaire on the subject of remuneration and less than 10% of the membership responded. That would have been a catastrophe, because the other Colleges would not have been impressed by a turnout of that sort, nor would the Privy Council. So the SCP asked me to compose a leaflet to inform every psychiatrist in the country of the importance of the occasion, and we told them 'We don't mind how you vote; all we ask of you is that you vote and that you vote immediately'. The next week, RMPA members received a communication from Council, giving background to the whole thing in rather pessimistic terms, and *The Lancet* had a leader advocating a faculty in the Royal College of Physicians, as well as a letter from the RMPA President, inviting people not to vote before considering carefully the offer being made by the Physicians. However, reacting to the SCP, most people had already voted, and as you know, there was a handsome majority in favour of the College.

HF All this was taking time?

JH Yes, but it was just the beginning of the delay. Under the constitution of the RMPA, no action could be taken in its name without it being approved at an Annual Meeting. This was set for Basingstoke in July, and again, it was a critical moment, because it was necessary to have a handsome majority to impress the Privy Council and the other Colleges. So another 'For your information' leaflet was prepared by the SCP and went to all psychiatrists, pointing out the importance of the occasion. Traditionally in the RMPA, very few people turned up to the business part of the Annual Meeting, but members of the SCP got busy all over the country, getting people together in carloads, to come to the meeting. We from Ipswich had a contingent of three cars and we arrived in the car park at Basingstoke just after nine; the meeting was to start at 9.30, but there wasn't a car in the place. However, at about 9.25, they came pouring in and in fact by 9.30, you couldn't get in the car park! When we finally got to the hall, the place was packed. The motion was put – that the RMPA should now petition for a Royal College – and was carried by a very handsome majority.

That was really the end of what you might call the 'open phase', when everybody knew what was going on and the efforts were there for everyone to see. During this time, I'd been stumping around the country talking at divisional meetings, and the President had been stumping round the country saying the opposite. Most of the contributions from the floor at these meetings were against the College, but this taught me that often, when there is an expression of opinion, people who are opposed to something will get up and express it, but those who are in favour keep to their seats.

HF That brings us to the 'closed phase', does it?

JH From now on, everything went on behind closed doors, as it were. Council had to set up a Petitions Committee to undertake the negotiations with the Privy Council, as well as another committee on the Higher examination and the Byelaws. The Petitions Committee consisted of the officers and two members, of whom I was one.

Remember that from that moment until we successfully petitioned, six years went by, despite the process being so simple legally. The reasons for this were really within the RMPA itself. The only officer who had any enthusiasm for the venture was A. B. Monro, who had a great loyalty to his members; he regarded himself as their servant. However, he was under enormous pressure from the other officers and from what you might call the College of Physicians faction; they went so far as to offer him a Membership of that College, which in time would have gone on to a Fellowship, but he declined it. Alexander Walk, the Librarian, was violently opposed to the College proposal, as indeed were Eliot Slater, the Editor, and William Sargant, the Registrar. So in the Petitions Committee, it was very difficult to get movement forward.

Ultimately, a meeting was set up between the Committee and the Secretary of the Privy Council. Monro, Slater, myself, and our solicitor represented the RMPA. But it was a frosty meeting, as Sir Geoffrey Agnew clearly wasn't interested. We talked about various matters, and he indicated there was opposition to what we were intending to do and that other colleges would have to be consulted.

HF The Royal College of Physicians' support was clearly crucial. How did you get that?

JH After a heated dialogue in Council, it was agreed that a letter should be sent to the Royal College of Physicians, inviting their support, but when it reached there, they decided to temporise. Nothing was heard from them for months. At a second heated dialogue in Council, it was agreed to write an open letter to the College of Physicians which stated that if we did not hear from them by a certain date, then we had to assume that they were not supporting the formation of a College of Psychiatrists.

This caused consternation within the College of Physicians, but led by Lord (Robert) Platt, who had become President, they grasped the nettle and wrote a handsome letter of support.

HF Was there still delay?

JH Matters should now have been smooth, but in the event, they were not. The easy road was to petition for a Royal Charter and then, when it was granted and the College had been founded, to undertake a leisurely revision of the Byelaws. Opponents to the College managed to sell the idea that the Byelaws and the petition should go in at the same time.

As years of work were needed to negotiate with the Privy Council on the Byelaws, this led to endless delay and with each passing year there was always the prospect that members would lose interest, the issue would be forgotten, and the whole thing would peter out. You yourself were a member of the committee of the Society of Clinical Psychiatrists, and know that without the continual pressure by the SCP over the years, the matter would, indeed, have petered out and there would have been no College.

However, the final agreement of the Privy Council on the Byelaws ultimately came, with the invitation to petition, and so the Royal College of Psychiatrists was founded.

HF I understand that you stood for President of the College on one occasion.

JH Indeed I did, immediately after the formation of the College. There were four candidates of whom three, including myself, had been pro-College. My presidency would have made me even more unpopular than my advocacy of a College, but I would not necessarily have been wrong.

My central aim would have been to change the course of psychiatry and psychiatric practice. Let me explain.

HF In what way?

JH Throughout psychiatry, there has been a widespread tendency to accept a viewpoint put forward by Szaz and others which asserts that medicine is concerned only with organic pathology. But, in fact, it is concerned with illness, deviation, abnormality, in other words, all pathology – both organic and psychopathology. Indeed, they are indivisible. You can worry and develop a gastric ulcer and you can have cancer and worry about it. But neuropsychiatry and biological psychiatry are really a branch of neurology.

This has been the only truly successful field of psychiatric practice, but the whole continent of emotional experience behind the unhappiness of people is neglected. Psychiatry's inability to get to grips with this field has led to frequent disparagement from general practitioners, who feel we are remote from their interests, to remoteness from our specialist colleagues, who find we give no help with their major problems, and ultimately to divorce from the public, who often feel we are impotent in helping them.

Psychoanalysis has to be replaced through systematic research by realistic psychopathology. Nosology, which is based upon the two big divisions of organic psychiatry and psychological psychiatry, has to be completely re-written.

HF   What else would have been in your programme?

JH   I would also have made every effort to pull the psychiatrists away from the team concept. This crept in, in a most unfortunate period of British history, that of pseudo-democracy. We failed to see that it was simply a means by which related professions crept to power on our backs. They all have laudable aspirations and should be supported, but should establish themselves in the light of their own achievements. The psychiatrist should be an individual who is highly trained in psychopathology and related organic pathology, capable of the highest standards of practice, and depends on no-one except his own judgement.

I should also have been trying to relocate public funding so that psychiatry and the quest for the mental health of its people should have a far higher priority than in the present scheme of things.

HF   How do you find retirement?

JH   I am as busy as I ever was, but now able to choose my targets and able to proceed according to my own inclinations and timing. Age brings with it a new area of experience – the lives of one's grandchildren.

I continue researching and writing. I lost my research team when I retired, and so moved into private practice; this enables me to retain some help. I am writing on psychopathology and nosology. History was always an interest since I edited *World History of Psychiatry* in 1975. As I mentioned earlier, for 25 years, I collected material for *A Reference Companion to the History of Abnormal Psychology*, published in 1984. It took seven years to write and three years for the publisher to produce. The two volumes are always alongside me on my desk, but their considerable cost must deter others from having them. I am now editing *Concept of Schizophrenia – Historical Perspectives* for the American Psychiatric Press. As Chairman of the History Section of the World Psychiatric Association, I am much involved in that organisation and with historians worldwide. I have now started a new 'Clinical Psychiatry Series' for Brunner/Mazel.

On retirement, I was given a video player, which makes it possible for me to indulge in one of my strong interests – Italian opera. I have studied Verdi in particular. He was a man of a massively strong personality, which is projected into his music. You will find him confronting a mob in the council scene in *Simon Boccanegra*. The love for his foster-father is found in the bass arias of his early operas, but they died with this man. His touching tribute to his 'other woman', Guiseppina, who later became his wife, penetrates the whole of *La Traviata*. His feelings for women always make the most melodious music of each of his operas, expressed particularly in a father–daughter dialogue. I read Dylan Thomas and have made a particular study of the art of Salvador Dali. A new interest takes me into horticulture. I sit on the Council of the International Clematis Society, edit its journal *Clematis International*, and have just finished a book for Ward Lock on clematis.

HF   What advice would you give young people?

JH   I would suggest that they try to advance on a narrow front; you can only penetrate in depth in that way. Even so, the further you move towards truth, the more change you will advocate, and the more difficult life will become. Secondly, test your theories with daily experience; discuss them with an intelligent and creative layman. Thirdly, steel yourself to being unpopular. The insecure and the deprived in particular seek for approval and appreciation; they find unpopularity intolerable. The search for truth has to mean change; this creates insecurity, the insecure will defend themselves, and your unpopularity is an inevitable consequence. Fourthly, avoid picking up too many of the 'golden balls'. You can never reach the truth if you stoop to pick up too many committee memberships, marks of public approval, chairmanships, visiting professorships, public addresses, etc. You may end up 'very distinguished', but sick with yourself for lack of real achievement.

14   Michael Shepherd

Interviewed by GREG WILKINSON (1991)

Professor Michael Shepherd, CBE, MA, DM, FRCP, FRCPsych(Hon), DPM, PAPA(Corr), FAPHA, Emeritus Professor of Epidemiological Psychiatry, Institute of Psychiatry, London. Michael Shepherd was born in 1923. He began his psychiatric career at The Maudsley Hospital in 1947. In 1956 he joined the staff of the Institute of Psychiatry as a Senior Lecturer and then Reader in Psychiatry: in 1967 he had conferred on him a personal chair of epidemiological psychiatry – the first of its kind in the world. He established the General Practice Research Unit at the Institute of Psychiatry in the late 1950s and continued to direct its activities until his retirement in 1988. He is the founder editor of *Psychological Medicine*. Michael Shepherd delivered the Maudsley Lecture on 'Changing Disciplines in Psychiatry' to the Royal College of Psychiatrists in 1987.

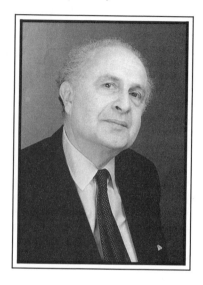

GW *It has been said of you that you are Sir Aubrey Lewis's intellectual heir and this country's best-known social psychiatrist. Your name is attached to some 30 books and 150 papers and a Festschrift has been published in your honour. You also have a distinguished international reputation. Nevertheless, you are not very well known in this country. Why should this be so?*

MS   It's attributable partly, I suspect, to my own temperament and partly to the way in which my career developed. From the public standpoint the high point of my reputation was attained some years ago, when I was introduced at a meeting as the man who wrote the preface to Anthony Clare's *Psychiatry in Dissent*.

GW *How would you outline the development of your professional career?*

MS   The time-honoured method is to sub-divide a professional career into four phases: 'learning', 'doing', 'directing' and 'advising', to which I would add 'reflecting' as a fifth category.

The first two phases, 'learning' and 'doing' extend roughly over the first half of my career, and fall in turn roughly into two halves. In the first period I was employed by the National Health Service, with breaks for military service and a Fellowship in the United States. During this time I underwent a thorough apprenticeship in clinical psychiatry and neurology. In the second period I joined the University staff, becoming first a senior lecturer and then a Reader in Psychiatry.

GW   Where did this take place?

MS   Firstly at the Maudsley Hospital and the Institute of Psychiatry. I did a long stint at Queen Square in neurology and was attached to a general hospital for a time. I spent two years in the Air Force as a specialist in neuropsychiatry, then came back to the Maudsley and worked there for another spell as a senior registrar, during which time I began to develop my interests in research.

GW   Were the interests in research stimulated by your clinical experiences?

MS   Very much so, often stimulated by discussion with the people with whom I was working at the time. Initially, I was learning by example, and I learnt to recognise the difference between good psychiatrists and not-so-good psychiatrists. Some of the senior people at the time were knowledgeable and very helpful. Apart from Aubrey Lewis there was Eric Guttmann, who was a very sound clinician, D. L. Davies, Kräupl Taylor, Erwin Stengel and Eliot Slater.

GW   What about the not-so-good psychiatrists?

MS   From them it was possible to learn what not to do. At that time, during the first post-War decade, practically anybody of any significance would come to the Maudsley sooner or later, either to teach or give a lecture or to provide a clinical demonstration. This provided the junior staff with a very useful bird's-eye view of what was going on and who was who.

GW   Do you have any comments on the typology of psychiatrists?

MS   As a group, the general psychiatrists sub-divided themselves into two broad groups. There were those who might have been general physicians or neurologists and there were those who might have been general practitioners or community doctors. The two groups were quite different in their outlook, in the way they approached the subject, in their thinking, and to some extent in their activities.

For example, if you were dealing with a ward that was full of acute psychotic patients, like the old observation ward at St Francis Hospital with which I was associated for a long time, you were very much a hospital doctor. But in a setting like that of the Air Force a medical officer was much more like a general practitioner and the sorts of problems that came up were very much more similar to those confronting a GP. Both groups, of course, contained good and bad examples.

GW   What about psychotherapists?

MS   They are in a class apart.

GW   Did you play a part in teaching?

MS   Very much so, and in a number of ways. The teaching role of senior registrars was very heavy at the time and I was involved in the running of the MPhil(Psychiatry) examination. This was not the attenuated degree it has since become, but a clinical, theoretical and research examination which enabled trainee psychiatrists to obtain a university-type education without having to take the DPM which was very much a union-ticket to a job in a mental hospital.

GW   *Who was responsible for setting up the MPhil?*

MS   Aubrey Lewis. The thinking behind it was set out in his paper, 'The Education of Psychiatrists'[1]. The research component of the examination was central to the procedure. Many of the people who now occupy senior positions cut their research teeth on the dissertation that they prepared for this examination.

GW   *You introduced seminar teaching at the Maudsley, which was quite novel at the time. On what model?*

MS   It was simply an adaptation of the type of tuition that I had received as an undergraduate at Oxford, where the tutorial system held sway. Lectures were not always well attended and you were encouraged to think for yourself by writing essays and engaging in tutorial discussion. The method is based ultimately on the established fact that active learning is more valuable than passive learning. Unfortunately, I gather that the system withered when the MPhil (Psychiatry) was needlessly discontinued.

Teachers as well as students can learn from this type of instruction. In my own case I recall particularly a group of seminars that I conducted on Karl Jaspers's *General Psychopathology*, which had not then been translated into English. I'd come across it by chance, and was so intrigued that I went through the text with the help of a German dictionary, mostly no more than a few pages ahead of the next class!

GW   *What type of research did you undertake at this time?*

MS   At first, it was principally clinical research, writing up case-histories of particular interest. Then I settled on the large topic of morbid jealousy and I began slowly to develop interests in other aspects of research. One of them arose during my time in the Air Force when, by the merest chance, I was stationed near a mental hospital, St John's Hospital, Stone, near Aylesbury. I knew one or two people working at St John's and with the help of Dr Vera Norris, a lecturer in medical statistics at the Institute, who died tragically young, I worked out a method of using the records of the hospital to mount a large-scale investigation.

GW   *This was while you were in uniform?*

MS   Yes, the routine duties of a medical officer were not too onerous and there was plenty of time to engage in other activities! This task led me to read round the subject, and to realise that the study of mental hospital populations would qualify for epidemiological inquiry, provided that non-infectious disease was covered by the term.

GW   *What other fields of research did you enter?*

MS   I became intrigued by the whole question of the evaluation of treatment. This was prompted by a request to look at the properties and effects of reserpine, which was just coming to attention. I realised that the only way to do this scientifically would be to use the formal principles of clinical evaluation and with D. L. Davies I organised what I think was the first formal clinical trial

---

1. LEWIS, A. (1947) The education of psychiatrists. *The Lancet, ii*, 79–83.

of a psychotropic drug in this country. The climate of opinion bearing on somatic treatments was then overshadowed by the empirical spirit of Sargant and Slater's *An Introduction to Physical Methods of Treatment in Psychiatry*. My concern, by contrast, was with how to try and evaluate whether treatment X was more effective than treatment Y or a placebo. Such questions were rarely posed at that time.

GW *You also developed an interest in follow-up studies?*

MS Yes, I collected a large number of patients with schizophrenia and with alcoholism who could be traced by the follow-up clinic of the Maudsley Hospital. Through those studies I became interested in the natural history of mental illness which was a curiously neglected field at the time.

Carrying out such inquiries as a senior registrar I moved gradually into the academic field because this type of activity is much more suited to the academic life than it is to the work of a busy NHS senior registrar or consultant.

GW *What was the state of academic psychiatry at that time?*

MS After the War the British Postgraduate Medical Federation was created. It contained a number of teaching hospitals which were designated as postgraduate centres within the University of London; The Maudsley Hospital was the chosen centre for postgraduate psychiatric research. This step had been recommended in 1944 by the Goodenough Committee on Medical Education which also proposed a parallel postgraduate centre in Edinburgh and the creation of undergraduate chairs in psychiatry at all medical schools.

GW *How did things turn out?*

MS Very little outside Denmark Hill. There were one or two small undergraduate departments and for various reasons the situation in Edinburgh did not materialise as it ought to have done. By contrast, the Institute got off to a very rapid start, but virtually without any buildings! Visitors who asked the whereabouts of the Institue of Psychiatry were told that it had no physical existence. A few huts, a few converted rooms, some laboratory space – that was all. The Institute really existed in the mind of Aubrey Lewis, whose influence was dominant. None the less, if you were designated an academic worker you joined the academic staff, you were paid on a different scale, and your duties were different. And, of course, there was a much stronger obligation to undertake research than if you were a member of the NHS.

GW *You hinted that the word epidemiology had a certain connotation in earlier times. I always thought that your work had a very strong clinical flavour to it. It was dignified by the word 'epidemiological'. Could you comment on the difference between clinical and epidemiological, as it relates to your work and the themes that you have been talking about.*

MS The word epidemiology, from the Greek, means literally 'on the people'. Briefly, epidemiological research is essentially population research as distinct from the study of individuals which is the traditional pre-occupation of clinical workers. The two approaches are, of course, complementary.

It should also be emphasised that the epidemiological method is common to investigators from a number of disciplines, including statistics, sociology, medical geography, psychology and ecology as well as clinical medicine or psychiatry. The methods are similar but the perspective will often be different.

Personally, I have always felt that if the clinical contribution to epidemiological research is to keep its end up, it is necessary to maintain contact with clinical work because many of the hypotheses that go into epidemiological research derive from clinical observation. For this reason alone I never relinquished my clinical commitments. On the other hand, you could, for example, be a biostatistician and spend a professional life-time calculating rates and numerical indices, without ever seeing a patient.

GW   What prompted your thinking in this direction?

MS   Much of it crystallised in the course of my year in the United States during 1955–1956. There I was attached not to a Department of Psychiatry but to the Division of Mental Hygiene within the Department of Public Health at The Johns Hopkins University, where I learnt a great deal about the theories and principles of epidemiology. It was a very stimulating experience to talk to people who were edging their way towards the same sort of things that interested me. Interestingly enough, they included very few clinical psychiatrists. Even those psychiatrists who were concerned with epidemiology undertook little, if any clinical work.

GW   It sounds as if you felt at home in this environment.

MS   During that time the most sympathetic groups that I encountered belonged to the Mental Health section of the American Public Health Association. This contained a diverse collection of people who were interested in public policy, economics, statistics – almost everything except clinical psychiatry. This went hand in hand with my feelings of alienation from the orthodox standpoint of American psychiatry, which in the 1950s was strongly dominated by the psychoanalytical movement, though even then there were signs of dissatisfaction.

GW   So you felt simultaneously 'at home' and 'a complete outsider'.

MS   Yes, I tried to sum up my impressions in an article entitled 'An English View of American Psychiatry' which I wrote for the *American Journal of Psychiatry*. The whole situation was symbolised for me at a meeting of the American Psychiatric Association in 1956, the centenary year of Freud's birth. A centenary lecture was delivered to a huge audience by Ernest Jones who, as you might expect, gave a hagiographic account of the master and all that he represented. The very next day, at the same time and in the same place, the same audience reassembled to hear a lecture by Percival Bailey, the distinguished neurosurgeon, on 'The Great Psychiatric Revolution' which turned out to be a full-scale attack on Freud and everything he stood for. And the same people applauded Bailey just as warmly as they had Jones the day before!

GW   What did you make of it all?

MS   I learnt a great deal from listening to the multiplicity of viewpoints, but I was particularly impressed by the work going on in the field of psychiatric epidemiology, in which the Americans were well ahead in their activities. In particular, I became familiar with the large-scale surveys that were going on in Baltimore, New York, New Haven and Nova Scotia. At the same time there seemed to me something flawed about this approach to case definition and case detection, which was often based on self-reports or questionnaires.

It was from thinking about the possibilities of how one might improve on the method that I began to wonder about the prospects of using the primary care network in Britain as a means of case identification. This would have been impossible in the United States because the primary care system had been virtually abandoned in favour of a hospital or office-based mode of fee-for-service medical care.

GW *In America you say they were psychiatric epidemiologists, whereas you were interested in epidemiological psychiatry. Who were the main characters involved?*

MS Among the psychiatrists I would include Ernest Gruenberg, Alexander Leighton, Thomas Rennie, Paul Lemkau and Ben Pasamanick. There were also sociologists like Sandy Hollingshead and Leo Srole, psychologists like Joe Zubin and bio-statisticians like Morton Kramer.

GW *What about your interest in psychopharmacology?*

MS Because of the early studies that I had been carrying out with reserpine and then chlorpromazine, I became involved in the other great 'revolution' of the time, namely psychopharmacology. This was just starting in the United States and I met practically everybody active in that field at the time. Again, relatively few of them were psychiatrists.

GW *Who were they?*

MS People like Seymour Kety (neuropharmacology), Louis Lasagna (clinical pharmacology), Ralph Gerard (neurophysiology) and Joe Brady (psychology). Many workers were beginning to focus their attention on the possibilities that were opened up by the prospects of effective drugs for mental illness. And this almost meaningless word, psychopharmacology, gradually expanded and sucked in a mixed bag of people who talked a different language from that employed by the epidemiologists. As they still do.

GW *Did you have any other formative experiences in the States?*

MS At Hopkins my office was across the road from the splendid medical library and the Institute of Medical History. The Professor of Medical History at that time was a very distinguished scholar, Professor Owsei Temkin, who had worked with Henry Sigerist in Germany.

I used to go to the seminars and discussion groups that he organised. They confirmed my long-held belief that there was a great deal more to medical history than the standard textbooks indicated. Its relevance to psychiatry seemed to be especially relevant.

GW *What did you do when you returned from the USA?*

MS I entered the academic stream first as a senior lecturer, and then as a Reader. During this time there were a number of activities that I began to develop. I was now 'doing' rather than 'learning'.

My interest in education continued and a few years later I went back to the United States for some months on a fellowship from the Association for the

Study of Medical Education, to study psychiatric education in depth in the United States and compare it with the system here.

On the research front I began to build on the possibilities of using general practice as a framework for epidemiological studies. The earliest investigations began in 1957–1958 on a very small scale.

GW   Was there anyone else working in this area at that time?

MS   Not to my knowledge. Indeed, I was certainly not encouraged by most of the people with whom I discussed the prospects. They simply did not believe that there would be anything to find out about psychiatric illness in general practice.

GW   What, then, induced you to investigate the matter?

MS   First, because it seemed to me that in principle the field was worth investigating since there was a pre-existent statistical framework. GPs were keeping routine records for administrative purposes and the first National Morbidity Survey had shown that one could count consultations and patterns of morbidity.

Secondly, I had put a toe in the water by approaching a local GP to request that I be allowed to sit in as a 'fly on the wall' for a number of his surgeries. I was introduced as another doctor, and listening to what was going on convinced me that there was certainly enough to merit a more systematic investigation. I had no idea, of course, of just how much morbidity we would detect, but the notion that all you would find in general practice was what was left over from the designated mental health services in hospital was clearly absurd.

None the less, so widespread was this belief that the publication of our monograph,[2] *Psychiatric Illness in General Practice*, in 1966 attracted little serious attention. In retrospect, it has proved instructive to ascertain why so many people should have been so biased against primary care psychiatry.

GW   So that was one area of activity. What were the others?

MS   I initiated a large-scale epidemiological study in Buckinghamshire to do with the mental health of school children.

I also began to extend my work on therapeutic evaluation and became secretary of the newly-formed MRC Committee on Clinical Trials in Psychiatry. As a result I had the great good fortune to meet and work with Sir Austin Bradford Hill. The committee's first project was to organise a large multi-centred trial of treatments for depression. This was the first study of its sort that had been mounted and it showed that the principles of the randomised clinical trial could be applied to the treatment of mental illness, making allowances for the special difficulties, if the will and the means were available.

---

2. SHEPHERD, M., COOPER, B., BROWN, A. C. & KALTON, G. (1966) *Psychiatric Illness in General Practice*. Oxford: Oxford University Press.

GW   To what extent do you think that people have gone on to use this tool to its best effect in psychiatry?

MS   Most clinicians must surely be aware of its existence and should be better placed to assess for themselves the value of the new drugs that continue to flood the market. Whether the average practitioner takes more notice of the findings now than he did remains an open question. Clinical psychologists have cottoned on to the method and applied it to behaviour therapy. Unfortunately it has had a rougher passage with the psychotherapists.

GW   Your career thereafter did not follow what has now become a standard pattern.

MS   I think that was due to what politicians call events, and partly to my response to them.

Having held a Readership in psychiatry for some years, I ran into a patch of turbulence in the form of opposition to the conferment of the personal chair for which I had been nominated by the Institute of Psychiatry in the early 1960s.

This is not the place to go into the details and eventually the matter was resolved satisfactorily. At the time, however, I was fortunate in knowing a 'mole' within the university from whom I learnt a great deal about the innards of academic politics and human sequacity. He also drew my attention to a splendid essay which helped explain much of what had been going on and which indirectly influenced my subsequent career.

GW   What essay?

MS   This is Francis MacDonald Cornford's[3] *Microcosmographia Academica –Being a Guide for the Young Academic Politician*, a minor classic published originally in 1908 and since reprinted many times. I strongly recommend it to all aspiring academics.

GW   Can you indicate its content?

MS   Cornford was a Greek scholar who begins his booklet with a quotation from Plato's *The Republic*.

> 'Any one of us might say that although in words he is not able to meet you at each step of the argument, he sees as a fact that academic persons, when they carry on study, not only in youth as a part of education, but as the pursuit of their maturer years, most of them become decidedly queer, not to say rotten.'

On this premise the argument is essentially a polemic against the corrupting influence of academia and its environment. The style, however, is as important as the content. The best of the television *Yes, Minister* series catches the tone in a more genial key.

GW   Can you give me an example?

MS   Cornford points out that academic politicians are not so much dishonest as fearful, displaying what he refers to as 'genuine, perpetual, heartfelt, timorousness'. He continues by pointing out that the most important branch of academic politics is connected with Jobs – he always spells jobs with a capital J – which, he says, fall into two classes, My Jobs and Your Jobs:

---

3. CORNFORD, F. M. (1908) *Microcosmographia Academica – Being a Guide for the Young Academic Politician* (11th impression, 1983). London: Bowes & Bowes.

'My Jobs are public spirited proposals, which happen (much to my regret) to involve the advancement of a personal friend, or (still more to my regret) of myself. Your Jobs are insidious intrigues for the advancement of yourself and your friends, speciously disguised as public spirited proposals.'

This may convey a touch of the essay's spirit. But what also impressed me at the time was Cornford's conclusion. While assuming throughout that his argument will be rejected by the would-be ambitious academic politician, his final paragraph reads as follows:

'If you find that I was right, remember that other world, within the microcosm, the silent, reasonable world where the only action is thought, and thought is free from fear. If you go back to it now, keeping just enough bitterness to put a pleasant edge on your conversation, and just enough worldly wisdom to save other people's toes, you will find yourself in the best of all company – the company of keen humorous intellect; and if you have a spark of imagination and try very hard to remember what it was like to be young, there is no reason why your brains should ever get woolly or why anyone should wish you out of the way.'

Those words express very well the sentiments that I was forming at the time and which helped make me decide to concentrate the second half of my career on directing and advising in the spheres of clinical work, teaching and research rather than in those of medical politics and administration.

GW *Would you say, then, that you opted for the ivory tower?*

MS If you want to call it an ivory tower you can, but I assure you that the ivory comes from just as many wild elephants inside the tower as there are outside. The advantage resides more in the increased possibility of spending at least some time in Cornford's 'silent, reasonable world'.

GW *Let us move on to the second half of your career.*

MS First of all came the setting up of the General Practice Research Unit. This took some doing because it was not a very popular subject at the time and I had to obtain money from various sources until the Department of Health assumed financial responsibility. The Unit continued until my retirement in 1988. Some 30 books and 400 papers attest to its productivity. I think that it has helped to establish primary care psychiatry as a major area of research and practice.

GW *Has primary care psychiatry become as successful internationally as it has in this country?*

MS That is very difficult to assess. The subject is now recognised as a top priority by WHO. It appeals to many individual workers, in many other countries but they are often handicapped by the fact that their system of medical care does not lend itself to this type of investigation. In this country it has been creeping into the system rather than coming in with a bang and it has had to overcome opposition from both hospital psychiatrists and general practitioners for quite different reasons.

GW *What about the relationship between research and policy?*

MS This question raises a general issue. If you engage in epidemiological research, the very nature of the work tends to carry policy implications, unless it is of a purely abstract nature like, say, a new statistical technique. There is an understandable temptation therefore for workers in the epidemiological field to want to become decision makers and try to implement and promote their own findings. This tendency introduces bias and can vitiate the value of much so-called health-services research. The history of 'deinstitutionalisation' illustrates the theme only too well.

All the early studies that we carried out were focused entirely on the nature and amount of psychiatric illness in the community identified via the GP. I never regarded the practical implications of the data as our primary concern, though as the subject attracted increasing attention during the 1980s we became much more involved in such considerations.

GW *The Unit also provided a training ground for rather a lot of doctors, many of whom achieved professorial status. How do you account for this?*

MS Although the Unit was never numerically very large I was always of the opinion that one of its principal objectives was to train its members in research methods with an academic career in mind. Not all alumni took this direction: they include a research-director in a pharmaceutical company, a private practitioner and even a psychoanalyst.

The Unit was always multidisciplinary and we also helped train workers in non-medical fields – statistics, sociology, social work, psychology. I should like to have included more GPs on the staff, but the career-structure of general practice made this difficult to achieve.

GW *What about other activities during this phase of your career?*

MS There were several topics of research which may be covered briefly. I maintained close contact with St John's Hospital throughout this period and have collaborated with the former medical director, Dr David Watt, on a number of projects. The most recent has been a large-scale study of the natural history of schizophrenia.

The MRC Committee for Clinical Trials in Psychiatry, of which I became chairman, initiated the prosecution of a number of studies which were carried out over a period of about 20 years.

Then there was the setting up of a psychopharmacology research unit with Professor Heinz Schild, who was Professor of Pharmacology at University College. This was, I think, the first of its kind and included Hannah Stein, a psychologist who became the first professor of psychopharmacology in this country, J. D. Montague and Malcolm Lader. Much of this work was multidisciplinary and stimulated me to write *Clinical Psychopharmacology*[4] with Professors Lader and Rodnight; this turned out to be the first textbook on the subject.

I might also mention the MRC-funded project on noise as an environmental pollutant. This had to do originally with the adverse effects of aircraft noise on mental health, but was extended to incorporate experimental work.

At the same time I was involved with the US–UK project, which I helped to direct for a while.

---

4. SHEPHERD, M., LADER, M. & RODNIGHT, R. (1968) *Clinical Psychopharmacology*. London: The English Universities Press.

In addition, I was invited to take some responsibility for various WHO programmes, particularly those connected with the International Classification of Diseases. I think it is fair to say that this work played a large part in reviving the international community's concern for psychiatric diagnosis and nosology. When the programme commenced in the middle 1960s, no more than three or four member countries of WHO out of more than 130 were using the ICD. By means of a two-pronged approach based on diagnostic exercises and education, we generated a great deal of interest in the field.

GW *Do you think that – thinking of the United States in particular – it is possible to say that certain elements might have gone too far in an apparent obsession with diagnosis and classification?*

MS In the United States there has been something of a conversion phenomenon. In the 1960s it proved difficult to persuade the Americans to participate in the WHO programme. They had virtually abandoned the notion of diagnosis in favour of the 'dynamic' formulation. Now what they call neo-Kraepelinian psychiatry is all the rage, with DSM as its foundation. This is probably better than the earlier diagnostic nihilism, but it becomes stultifying when so many of the categories are both logically and clinically suspect.

GW *Returning to your activities, what of 'Psychological Medicine'?*

MS I have tried to indicate elsewhere why and how this journal was set up. It has sometimes been compared mistakenly to the *British Journal of Psychiatry* but they have very little in common. The *British Journal of Psychiatry* is an association journal, an official publication of the College which comes to Members and Fellows automatically. *Psychological Medicine* is an independent journal, international in scope, dependent on subscriptions and concerned primarily with research in psychiatry and cognate disciplines. After 20 years it remains a quarterly, but it has greatly expanded to more than 270 pages an issue and carries a variety of special features; for example, commissioned editorials, research reports, and monograph supplements.

Our original aim was to further the continuing education of professors of psychiatry, but it was soon pointed out that in too many instances they are rendered ineducable by a carapace of omniscience. We therefore aimed at creating a journal which would contain the best work available and help set standards and create incentives, especially for younger workers. One of the hallmarks of any well-established professional group is the existence of flagship journals that represent the group's aspirations and achievements. How far I have succeeded is difficult to judge: it is hardly possible for an editor to assess the quality of his own journal since he has no way of knowing who reads it or how it is regarded. Perhaps the most judicious comment was made by the editor of the *Archives of General Psychiatry* who remarked that *Psychological Medicine* led the field in respect of 'intellectual fortitude'.

GW *Is it true that you have written many of the short, anonymous book reviews yourself?*

MS Unfortunately, yes. Not out of choice, but because of the difficulty in persuading colleagues to undertake the task and to do it quickly. In my view a journal with the objectives of *Psychological Medicine* must have a comprehensive book-review section.

GW *There were other activities concerned with editing and writing?*

MS Indeed there were. Perhaps I might here refer to translation which seems to me to be an area of particular importance. I am a believer in having the original text in other languages, and have always tried to have as much of my own work, and that of my colleagues, translated into as many other languages as can be arranged. Although English is the scientific lingua franca, workers in other countries do not always read it easily and it helps greatly if the material can be read in a serviceable translation. For the same reason I took some trouble to oversee the publication of two books of translated foreign papers, mostly French and German, into English.

In recent years I have probably written and edited more material than at any other time. Some of this work consists in the writing up of research, some of it represents more general interests. Among these I would include the five volume *Handbook of Psychiatry*, the *Scientific Basis of Psychiatry* series, the volumes entitled *Psychiatrists on Psychiatry* and *Non-Specific Aspects of Treatment* and my *jeux d'esprit* on Sherlock Holmes and Sigmund Freud. The fruits of 'reflecting'!

GW *Did you have time to enter into formal involvements with committees and professional bodies?*

MS Certainly. Apart from sitting on the usual committees I was actively involved in advising on the mental health initiative taken by The Wellcome Trust. This has proved particularly important as money for research has dried up elsewhere. There was a spell on the Noise Advisory Council and the Council of the Section of Psychiatry of the Royal Society of Medicine, of which I was elected president. I have ongoing commitments to WHO and the EEC. And, of course, one is constantly involved in unofficial activities of an advisory nature, but I do not think there is much point in mentioning these. They come naturally as part of the job.

GW *Another special interest that you have hardly mentioned so far and on which you have been publishing more recently concerns historical themes in psychiatry.*

MS During the last 20 years professional historians have taken an expanding interest in the history of psychiatry. Several social historians have made a career out of the study of the social aspects of psychiatry. Many of them are gifted historians who know a great deal about the subject but they tend to be ignorant about mental illness itself. I have long felt that there is a place for a contribution to be made by medically qualified scholars who are familiar with the historical method and outlook.

I did this myself once on a small scale by working with a very eminent historian. It was an arduous but rewarding experience which taught me that it is necessary to place your medical material in its historical and social context and view it in relation to a whole host of non-medical factors.

Further, medical history can be of more than scholarly interest, especially in the less well-developed branches of medicine. If, for example, you take a topic like infectious diseases, which has moved from the pre-scientific into the scientific area with the coming of bacteriology, the miasma theory of disease is of largely academic interest. However, when dealing with a barely scientific discipline like psychiatry historical studies can be directly relevant to on-going issues.

GW   *Can you give an example?*

MS   A good example is provided by the current debate on the so-called recency hypothesis: did schizophrenia exist before the 18th century? This question has already attracted a great deal of interest among both historians and psychiatrists. It is not a purely academic topic in the sense of the miasma theory for it bears on the current discussion concerning the viral theory of schizophrenia. Psychiatrists in training would benefit from knowing more about the history of their subject. They would find that the broader aspects of the discipline can only be understood in their historical context. Many of these are illustrated in the three volumes of *The Anatomy of Madness* that I put together with Drs Bynum and Porter, both of them medical historians. Incidentally every issue of *Psychological Medicine* to date carries an historical article to help give the subject a boost.

GW   *Would psychoanalysis benefit from historical analysis?*

MS   Psychoanalysis is almost incomprehensible if it is not viewed in the context of the history of ideas. That is why some of the philosophical critiques are so cogent. Popper refuted its scientific pretensions outright. Wittgenstein[5] called it a 'powerful mythology' and remarked that 'this whole way of thinking wants combatting'. Gellner[6] refers to psychoanalysis as a 'complex belief system satisfying social needs in a scientistic idiom' and emphasises the need to appreciate that it is not only a doctrine but also an institution, a technique, an organisation, an ethic, a theory of knowledge, an idiom, a climate of opinion, a theory of culture, aesthetics and religion. An historical perspective is indispensable for an analysis (if I may use the word) along these lines.

GW   *You have criticised psychotherapy and psychoanalysis for other reasons.*

MS   I would not identify psychoanalysis with psychotherapy. What we now call psychotherapy, however it be defined, has been and remains part of the physician's placebological role as healer. In his authoritative monograph on psychotherapeutics, *Psychological Healing*, Pierre Janet[7] traces the evolution of the root activity from magical and religious practices to its various contemporary branches, of which psychoanalysis is one. Janet calls it a form of 'mental liquidation' and comments on its deficiencies from the standpoint of a psychopathologist. Over and above such considerations there is also the question of the place of psychoanalysis in medicine. Here I would refer to the situation in the United States where after World War II the subject was given its head in an unprecedented manner in most academic departments of psychiatry. Since then it has failed signally to live up to the expectations that were roused and its reputation has declined sharply. This is partly the reason for the swing towards biological psychiatry today. Whatever the future may hold for the psychoanalytical movement it will, I think, move increasingly away from medicine.

---

5. WITTGENSTEIN, L. (1989) Conversations on Freud. In: *Sigmund Freud: Assessments* (ed. L. Spurling). Volume 4. London: Routledge. Pp. 252–253.
6. GELLNER, E. (1985) *The Psychoanalytic Movement or the Coming of Unreason*. London: Paladin.
7. JANET, P. (1919) *Les Médications Psychologiques*. 3 Volumes. Paris: Alcan.

GW *Another question, indirectly related to this theme, stems from a remark you made at a symposium on the history of psychopharmacology – 'the dark before the dawn'. Drawing on your own observations made 30 years previously you conclude 'That was how the biological dawn appeared to one observer who is still waiting for the skies to lighten'. Would you expand on this?*

MS My contribution to that symposium was focused on one category of drugs, the so-called neuroleptics and their place in the management of schizophrenic illnesses. On the basis of my own experience I tried to indicate how far and why the situation was removed from the standard account of the matter. In a sense it represents a continuation of my interest in the evaluation of treatment, here viewed retrospectively in the light of the many factors that bear on the introduction, promotion and reputation of a treatment in psychiatry. An example of oral history.

GW *Do you have a last word on lithium?*

MS The lithium episode illustrates another aspect of the comment that I have just made. It arose as a result of the paper that I published with Dr Blackwell in 1968 just at the time when, unknown to us, the lithium bandwagon was about to roll. All we did was to discuss some of the flaws in a study published by the Danish workers, Baastrup and Schou, in the previous year, purporting to demonstrate that lithium could effectively prevent manic–depressive disease. We felt that the claims were premature and that more rigorous methods of evaluation should be applied. The heat generated by this controversy was in large measure artificial and served largely to publicise the topic. After 20 years the last word might go most appropriately to one of the Danish workers, Dr Baastrup,[8] taken from his paper on the subject delivered in 1987 at the 2nd British Lithium Congress:

> 'In 1967 Professor Schou and I published a joint paper entitled "Lithium as a prophylactic agent". We both considered the title a good one – what we intended to demonstrate was that continuous lithium treatment made it possible to change the course of a manic–depressive illness in such a way that the patient no longer experienced psychotic episodes. The use of that title was a grave mistake! And – having been brought up in a country where modesty is considered the prime virtue, we ought to have known better. We have been pretentious enough to claim that we could present a method for the prevention of mental illness.'

GW *This interview is to appear in an issue of the 'Psychiatric Bulletin' celebrating 150 years of professional psychiatry in Britain and perhaps we should conclude by saying something about the Royal College of Psychiatrists. Is it true that you have not involved yourself a great deal in College affairs?*

MS To say that I have not been asked would be a more accurate comment. I was quite actively engaged in the work of the Royal Medico-Psychological Association and was on a number of committees. Since the formation of the College, however, I have been more a well-wishing bystander than a participant. Many of my colleagues, I would add, have been in the same position.

---

8. BAASTRUP, P. C. (1988) Lithium reflections II. In: *Lithium: Inorganic Pharmacology and Psychiatric use* (ed. N. J. Birch). Oxford: IRL Press. Pp. 5–7.

GW　*Have you formed an opinion on how the College has developed in the past 20 years?*

MS　In many ways its development reflects its origins. Dr Howells[9] gave a very clear account of the tortuous way in which the College came into being and of the internal opposition to its formation. The extent of that opposition is manifest in the contributions of influential figures like Denis Hill, William Sargant, and Alexander Walk, to the debate on 'The Future of Organised Psychiatry in Great Britain and Ireland' held at the quarterly meeting of the RMPA in November 1963 and published as a special supplement of the *British Journal of Psychiatry*.[10] The people who were pushing for the College were principally the mental hospital doctors, who felt they would receive the short end of the stick under the aegis of the Royal College of Physicians. Numerically, of course, they constituted a substantial majority and when, rather unexpectedly, the College came into being, many of the original opponents of the College made U-turns in order not to be left out of the action. None the less, the two factions made uneasy bedfellows.

Since then a curious situation has arisen. On the one hand, as in other branches of medicine, the creation of a Royal College is clearly important. Many observers have remarked that this country is basically run by clubs, and Royal Colleges are special forms of clubs which have their own interests. In this case the College grew out of the RMPA which was essentially a club for mental hospital superintendents representing institutional psychiatry. Since 1970, however, the institutional base of psychiatry has been eroded by the run-down of the mental hospitals. The bulk of the psychiatric profession still retains links with the crumbling structure of the hospital organisation, but the pressure to develop some form of community psychiatry is driving them into uncharted waters. The resulting dilemmas were well summarised in a *Lancet* (1985) editorial entitled 'Psychiatry – a discipline that has lost its way', and when Professor Rawnsley (1984) devoted his presidential address to the theme of 'Psychiatry in Jeopardy', he drew attention to those difficulties from the somewhat inward-looking vantage-point of the College.

As a consequence of this trend it has become evident that whereas formerly the psychiatrists were undisputed masters in their own asylums, they now find representatives of several other disciplines snapping at their heels. I outlined this interprofessional rivalry in a paper – 'Who should treat mental disorders?' – that was based on material prepared for the College's Cambridge conference on psychiatric education in the early 1980s. It is evident that the general physician, the general practitioner, the clinical psychologist, the social worker, and the nurse, all lay claim to manage various forms of mental disorder and do not take the expertise of the psychiatrist for granted. The *Lancet*[11] editorial (for which I was in no way responsible) puts the matter bluntly:

> 'Much of the progress made by psychiatry in the past generation has taken place because psychiatrists themselves have led the way. It is sad that . . . their place as pioneers has been usurped by planners and politicians. It is time for the speciality to emerge from its torpor, cease its self-flagellation, and take on the mantle of leadership again.'

---

9. Howells, J. (1990) In conversation with John Howells (interview by H. Freeman). Part 1: *Psychiatric Bulletin*, **14**, 513–521. Part 2: *Psychiatric Bulletin*, **14**, 577–581.
10. British Journal of Psychiatry (1964) *The Future of Organised Psychiatry in Great Britain and Ireland. British Journal of Psychiatry* (special supplement, May).
11. The Lancet (1985) Psychiatry – a discipline that has lost its way. *The Lancet*, i, 731–732.

Here, I suggest, is both a challenge and an opportunity for the College. To meet the one and take up the other will call on all its resources, scientific as well as political. Many of us hoped for a strong research and academic dimension when the College was set up. This, I gather, is slowly evolving and should prove invaluable in the years ahead.

I should like to congratulate the College on this 150th Anniversary and extend my best wishes for its future well-being.

15 Tom Lynch

Interviewed by DAVID HEALY (1992)

Professor Thomas Lynch, DPM (Royal College of Surgeons, Ireland, 1951), FRCPI (Royal College of Physicians, Ireland, 1962), FRCPsych (1971). Professor Lynch was born in Dublin in 1922. From 1953 to 1961 he was staff psychiatrist, St Patrick's Hospital, Dublin, and consultant psychiatrist to Meath Hospital, Dublin. He was resident medical superintendent at St Otteran's Hospital, Waterford from 1961 to 1968. From 1968 to 1990 he was professor of psychiatry, Royal College of Surgeons in Ireland. He has been chairman and clinical director of the Eastern Health Board, chairman of the Irish Psychiatric Training Committee and chairman of the Irish Division of the Royal College of Psychiatrists.

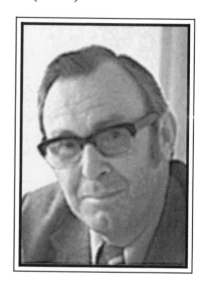

DH   Tell me something about your background.

TL   I was the first to do medicine in the family but I always wanted to be a doctor. My father came from a generation of National School teachers – his father and mother and grandparents. My mother's family had a grocery business in Tralee, but she was trained in teaching in England – which was unusual at the time.

They both became very involved in the Volunteer Movement for Irish Freedom. My father took part in the Rising in 1916. He was captain of the company in North King Street and he was eventually arrested and taken prisoner in the Four Courts. He was one of four sentenced to death and not executed (De Valera, Countess Markiewicz and Tom Ashe were the other three). He was subsequently transferred to prison in England – Strangeways – where he spent two years.

While in prison, he was elected to the first Dail as a TD (MP). He was not aware he was a candidate, but he was a good friend of Michael Collins, who was inclined to do this sort of thing – put one's name down and tell one afterwards. When he was released about 1918 in a general amnesty from prison, he took part in the Treaty Negotiations in London. He and Erskine Childers, father of the Erskine Childers who later became Minister for Health and President of Ireland, were two secretaries to the Treaty negotiations in Hans Square.

It all makes a good story. When we had the Spring Quarterly Meeting of the College in Galway in 1990, Tom Fahy organised a dinner of the Professors of Psychiatry Club. He wanted to get each of us Irish Professors to say a few words. Starting with me, he said, 'Of course you're not anything in Irish psychiatry, unless your father's been stood up in front of a British firing squad' – which was a typical Tom Fahy way to start things off.

DH   What about your upbringing?

TL   We were brought up in a middle-class family environment; my father was a Government Minister. When I was born, he was Minister for Education, and later on for Agriculture & Fisheries. To go to school, I had to brush up on English, because we all spoke Gaelic at home and all the staff at home were Irish-speaking girls.

My first memory of school (I was about 4) in Loreto, Stephen's Green, was of being collected and taken home in a tank, because at the time, the IRA were kidnapping Ministers' families. I learnt afterwards that it was the week after Kevin O'Higgins had been assassinated – one of the Government Ministers. I then attended National School for a couple of years, before being enrolled at St Mary's College, Rathmines, which is more renowned for its rugby. As I was reasonably good at tennis and rugby, I got on quite well there and I wasn't pushed for examinations.

DH   How or why did you decide on medicine?

TL   My father decided he would like me to study medicine in the College of Surgeons. I heard they had only a few dozen vacancies for students in 1941, so I realised it was important to get down to studying. I got a bare pass in the pre-clinical examinations in Chemistry and Physics, but managed a 2nd honours in Anatomy. I got first place in subsequent exams and the various scholarships that went with them, qualifying in the summer of 1946 with a First Class Honours Degree.

DH   What did you do then?

TL   I started in August on my Internship in the Richmond Hospital, now closed, and worked in Surgery with the late A. A. McConnell and later with the late Professor Leonard Abrahamson in Medicine. Towards the end of my intern year, I attended interviews with Norman Moore, when called in to examine patients for Professor Abrahamson. He asked me to come and join him in St Patrick's Hospital, but I said I was interested in medicine and not really in psychiatry. He reassured me that my responsibilities would involve the physical care of patients in St Patrick's. The arrangement was that I would study for my Membership in Medicine and during this time, I obtained it. My salary when I joined St Patrick's was £50 a year. When I got my Membership Part I, it went to £500 and when I got Part II, it went up to £1000, which was an enormous increase in the late 40s.

At St Patrick's I met M. O'Drury, Maurice Pillsworth, and Vincent Dolphin who are now regrettably all dead. With Norman Moore as Chairman, they ran very good case conferences every Monday, Wednesday, and Friday. I attended as many as possible, but without taking an active part. Con Drury from Exeter was also there. He was something of a philosopher; I was very friendly with him and although he was a most intelligent man, his main interest was cowboy films.

Within a short time, I adjusted to my new environment in a psychiatric hospital. It was not as traumatic as it initially seemed but the doors were locked on the wards. Norman Moore encouraged me to do my DPM while I was studying for my Membership, as the subjects in the Part I were much the same except for psychology, which I found dreadfully hard to tackle. However, I managed to scrape a pass in it; Part II was easy enough. Then Moore maintained that the Maudsley was the only place to go.

DH   Norman Moore – what was he like?

TL   He ran St Patrick's more like you'd run a boarding school. He was known as 'the Boss'. He ran every part of it paternalistically, but generally speaking, he was easy to work with. You started early – at 7.30 a.m. Myself and Joe Meehan used to start the list for ECT at about 8.15 a.m. We reviewed the night and day reports with Moore at about 9.00 a.m. Then to the grand round – on Monday the female side and on Tuesday the male side.

Every afternoon, Moore saw patients in his consulting rooms, from which he sent a constant flow of patients for admission. In the first year, there were only 300 or 400 admissions; this was easy to cope with, but it soon became a torrent. There was little time for reading. You could just about read a journal while falling asleep. But being off-duty meant that when 5 p.m. came, you were free; at 5.05 p.m., I was off down James's Street on my bike.

Norman was very articulate, intelligent, and influential; the case conferences were good. At least one of them a month would be taken up coping with administrative problems in the hospital rather than patients, and we learned how the hospital ran. It was a great help, in the sense that I learned about the funding of hospitals, which was useful when I went to Waterford and was responsible for everything down to the sheep that were savaged by the dogs.

St Patrick's Hospital also had a farm with 300 acres. I learnt something about farming; even helped to operate on a cow one night in an effort to remove a cyst.

We had a large influx of patients with all sorts of unusual problems to deal with in the case conferences. If you were in charge of the patient, you were expected to take a reasonable history and do a mental state and summary. Then the patient was interviewed. There was a very good standard of teaching in those days in Dublin; this helped me to cope when I went to the Maudsley. It was an awesome place, compared to St Patrick's which was hard-working and intense enough, but it wasn't frightening. Moore wasn't a frightening person, but he was authoritarian, and you understood where you stood and did your duty.

DH   St Patrick's is different to anywhere else in Irish psychiatry

TL   They always try to be ahead of the field. They would be innovative and take on everything new. At one stage, we were giving intravenous acetylcholine for various neuroses and also giving inhalations of carbon dioxide. It didn't catch on for any length of time, but we had given up insulin coma before they gave it up elsewhere. Once they discovered another less dangerous way of treating schizophrenic patients, they took that on board very fast and were quick to use the neuroleptics and antidepressants.

DH *Norman Moore and John Dunne seem to have been the two big figures of Irish psychiatry back then.*

TL   I think John Dunne probably in some way was envious of or resented Norman Moore's arrival on the scene, in the sense that Moore automatically took away the Trinity College students for teaching purposes. When I was doing psychiatry, teaching consisted of about ten lectures in Grangegorman Hospital at some stage between April and June. You attended there at about 4.30 p.m. and met all your colleagues from the three medical schools. We went into an enormous ward unit and sat around a dais; John Dunne stood on the podium and presented the cases. Even in my ignorance, I was often very embarrassed for the patient. I remember one who was quite theatrical being made to demonstrate that with the stethoscope, he could listen to Tokyo. It was comic stage stuff, rather than teaching. You got your attendance sheets signed, paid your fees, and the exam was a formality.

DH *Before Norman Moore how did St Patrick's operate?*

TL   There was a man called Thompson, who reigned three years. Before him was a Dr R. Leaper who was in charge of St Patrick's from 1906 to about 1942. He was credited with having changed the cells to rooms; he took out the straw and he put in beds and mattresses. He built a cinema and recreation centre for patients and was instrumental in purchasing St Edmondsbury as a convalescent hospital; that was never a locked facility. I remember Moore telling me that the first item on the agenda of the Board of St Patrick's when he arrived was the sale of St Edmondsbury, which he managed to stop.

Norman was keen on fishing and shooting, and St Edmondsbury was a lovely place with over 300 acres. He used to go shooting and fishing with us, in our single days.

The hospital had an old Austin 1929 car with a luggage grid in the back, which you could stand on. I was usually the lad without the gun and was selected to drive the car at night with the headlights on, while Maurice Pillsworth and Denis Doorley stood on the luggage carrier shooting rabbits. It was a different life at that period.

DH *You spent some time at the Maudsley*

TL   In 1952, I went to the Maudsley on leave of absence. I was attached to Felix Post. Also on the team were two other SHOs; one was Doreen Sherwood Jones, whose consultant was Harris.

Felix Post was one of the most pleasant consultants to work for; he wasn't at that stage fully involved in geriatrics. I remember I had brought over my Ford Prefect on a tourist visa. He had bought a new one, which I had to tutor him on driving and how to avoid stalling in traffic. One day, looking at his car engine, I remarked 'It's a beautiful engine; I'd love to swap it with the old one in my car'. They were similar cars, and later Eric Carr, who shared a flat with me, said that Felix Post was worried I might be able to do it, and he would never know!

My impression of the Maudsley was that it was a very strange hospital. Everybody was in absolute fear of Aubrey Lewis, who appeared to terrify all the registrars and social workers, and was even held in awe by the junior consultants. In my short stay, I was subjected to the usual Thursday morning conference with the non-PU registrars and I had to do one Monday morning conference and one journal club on a Saturday. I found him quite friendly. His only comment at the conference, in front of an audience of over 100, when I made a statement that this patient's choice of beverage was Guinness, was that it was presumably Thames rather than Liffey water, to which I replied that unfortunately, it was only Thames water he could get.

DH   When did you return to Ireland?

TL   I returned in 1953 to St Patrick's, where I was given the title then of staff psychiatrist and consultant to the Meath Hospital out-patient department.

On my return to St Patrick's, Denis Doorley was joined on the staff by Joe Meehan and the late A. J. Kilpatrick. Con Drury was in St Edmondsbury. Shortly after Thomas Bewley joined us for two years, with his sister Mary Bewley.

I left in October 1961 to go south to Watford as the resident medical superintendent of St Otteran's Hospital. It was an enormous change, but I always had ambitions to run a hospital myself.

DH   Tell me about the change

TL   My new colleagues were excellent! Paddy Meehan, who had been acting medical superintendent, Tom Toohy, and Jerry Fleming. They were somewhat older than I, but very friendly. One day, when we were doing a clinic in West Waterford at Lismore, I was informed by Paddy Meehan that we'd now have to go and buy some wood for the fish boxes for the patients' rehabilitation factor.

I was not only in charge of a hospital of just under 600 beds, but had an 800 acre farm with a piggery, cattle, and grain, and one of my duties every morning was to sign the chits for the bread, the milk, the pigs, and whatever else might be needed that day.

Fortunately, the chief clerk and secretary for the hospital saw my point when I said I couldn't be counting loaves of bread – it would be senseless and a waste of time. He agreed, and it stopped. Sheila O'Driscoll was a superb matron and her standard of nursing was excellent.

DH   How did St Otteran's compare to Grangegorman at the time?

TL   In parts, it was grim, but it was a small dolls-house of a hospital and easy to maintain. As I was working in a local health authority, you could contact the county manager and city manager very easily.

The one big achievement came when the opportunity arose to start a psychiatric unit in a general hospital, Ardkeen. It was possible in Waterford only because the district general hospital had been a sanatorium, with numerous units. These were changed into medical, surgical, obstetric, gynaecological, orthopaedic and eye units. There were spare chest units, half empty, and with the co-operation of the resident medical superintendent of Ardkeen Hospital, Dr Fintan Corrigan, and my own medical and nursing staff, we developed a psychiatric unit which opened in 1965. It was the first psychiatric unit developed in a general hospital in Southern Ireland.

DH   *Were you sure at the time that it was going to work?*

TL   Yes. At the time, Waterford Health Authority and the Department of Health funded me to attend two fortnight long residential courses at the King Edward Fund College for hospital administrators just off the Edgeware Road which were extremely interesting.

But it did take a long time to get the project off the ground. We had certain difficulties with our general hospital medical colleagues, but on the whole, they saw the logic of the concept. At the start, it was amusing – some of our own psychiatric nurses told us that general nurses were taking a different route to the dining-room, to avoid passing the psychiatric unit. But that ceased within a year, mainly as we were treating relatives of many of them on an out-patient basis, and they realised that we weren't ogres.

Within the space of a year and a half, we had integrated fully with the general hospital. We had reopened the rehabilitation, occupational therapy department, which had closed with the decline in the number of TB patients.

I was there six and a half years when a Chair of Psychiatry at the Royal College of Surgeons was advertised. It was conditional on having a consultant appointment for the Eastern Health Region, which I felt I probably would get. At the interview, the external assessor was Sir Martin Roth. I knew him vaguely from attending medical meetings, but I found it a trying and difficult interview.

We departed on holiday to Kerry the next day, only to find that we were being sought by the College by phone and telegraph. I had several phone calls to ring back to Dublin, to tell me that I had the Chair. I returned to Dublin in February 1968 to take over the post of clinical director of psychiatric services of the Eastern Health Board.

DH   *Do you think there's any scope for an Irish College of Psychiatrists*

TL   This has been mooted many times. It would be very expensive to have an Irish College. We have tried to look at the situation, since the Royal College of Psychiatrists' headquarters just happens to be in London. We are the Irish Division of the Royal College of Psychiatrists. Actually psychiatry, rugby, and hockey are the only truly joint ventures between North and South. We have never had any problem. In fact, I took over as Chairman of the Irish Division from John Fennelly, and was succeeded by Gordon McCallam of Belfast. At least one meeting in the year is held in Belfast.

At one stage, the Irish Division felt that if our Chairman had been from the North, it wouldn't be appropriate for him to negotiate with our Department of Health for conditions for either patients or staff in the South. So we decided, on the advice of Professor Ken Rawnsley who said there were some similar problems in Wales, to change our hats and just call ourselves the Irish Psychiatric Association when arguing in the Department of Health over conditions or such things. But in essence, we were the same body of men as the Irish Division of the Royal College.

Dermot Walshe was always keen to have an Irish College of Psychiatry, but that requires a lot of funding and I don't think it is practical. Norman Moore was very anxious that the Postgraduate Training Committee would be a faculty of the Royal College of Physicians of Ireland.

I was elected to the Irish Executive of the Royal College of Psychiatrists in the middle '70s, and was one of the first Irish examiners for the Membership.

In the winter of 1981, I was very pleased to be elected the Vice-President of the College.

The last committee of the Royal College I served on was the Court of Electors. I served for five years, and it gave me a link to the Royal College for over ten years. The man who succeeded me as Vice-President was Joseph Jancar. At one stage, I was senior Vice-President, Joseph Jancar was junior Vice-President, and Tom Bewley was the Dean – all three using an Irish passport.

About this time, I became involved with the American Psychiatric Association and managed to persuade the APA to have a mini-meeting in Dublin after their main meeting in Toronto. I remember Sir Desmond Pond asking if we would consider having it in the Isle of Man as a neutral venue! But I had already contacted all the relevant bodies in Ireland to get funding to entertain the Americans. The Royal College did join us in Dublin, and we had 300 to 400 delegates here for a three-day meeting at the end of May 1982. As a result, I was elected an honorary corresponding fellow of the APA.

DH *The Royal College of Surgeons has an unusual role in the Irish medical scene, doesn't it?*

TL There are several Royal Colleges in Ireland; they have individual Charters which they cherish greatly. The RCSI was granted its Charter by George III in 1784, and the Royal College of Physicians was chartered 100 years before that. The two colleges work as a Conjoint Board. The Royal College of Surgeons is an undergraduate school, as it once was in England and in Scotland. They have recently created a Chair in General Practice. When I was first appointed in 1968, it has a small medical faculty and you could get things done quickly. But of course, it has expanded enormously and meetings now last much longer. Everybody is seeking teaching space in the curriculum.

The College itself has been generous, in the sense that one man could not possibly cater for the needs of undergraduates, and cover all that has to be covered in psychiatry, so they have funded four senior lecturers. They also permit the co-option of our senior registrars as tutors in psychiatry and fund lecturers to given specialised talks to students.

DH *In Ireland there's a mix of private and public service. The UK is moving towards Trust hospitals and is becoming quite concerned as to what's going to happen to psychiatric services. Do you think there's anything that the Irish experience can offer as a pointer to the future?*

TL The system in Ireland works very well but it is complex. There is a mix of state-owned hospitals, state-run institutions, and privately run hospitals in the sense of those run by religious orders, or those by lay boards such as St Patrick's Hospital and Stewart's Institute for the Mental Handicap. Also, the voluntary hospitals, which are semi-private – voluntary in the sense that they were self-funded, though the state now has to underwrite these costs, but they are independent and they can appoint their own consultants.

All usually work together very well, but there is a point that is exercising the minds of the present members of the Psychiatric Training Committee about senior registrars. Currently, if a trainee on the Eastern Health Board Programme starts in one of its hospitals, he or she stays there. It is rather difficult for them to move, say, from St Brendan's to St Patrick's or St Vincent's, and then on to St John of God. It can be done, but only by leaving the Health Board's employment and obtaining a post in the other facility.

The Health Board probably offers the most extensive training, in the sense that they have available not just big psychiatric training centres and general hospital units such as we have in Blanchardstown Hospital; but also facilities for child psychiatry, forensic psychiatry, and mental handicap services.

DH   You were in St Patrick's when the modern psychotropic drugs came out first – at the time there was a feeling of a revolution

TL   I remember Norman Moore was one of the first to use these new 'wonder' drugs. The only therapy had been ECT for the psychotic depressed patients and insulin coma for the schizophrenic patients. I ran the insulin unit for nine months. We had 18 to 20 patients every morning for insulin coma, and also an enormous number of patients for ECT every day of the week; of course, it was straight ECT. I was there when scoline first came into use.

The first neuroleptic to arrive was chlorpromazine, reserpine and shortly after that, serpasil came on the market, but unfortunately, we had many patients who became very depressed while medicated with serpasil.

At the time, there was a constant stream of drug representatives with 16 mm films depicting the beneficial effects of these drugs on monkey behaviour – they stopped clawing and biting you. About the same time, marsilid appeared on the market as an anti-depressant. Imipramine came on stream a year or two later; later again, amitriptyline and subsequently a plethora of similar drugs. The first benzodiazepines arrived shortly afterwards.

DH   Did insulin coma work?

TL   I think it helped schizophrenic patients because they were treated as a specialised group, 15 to 25 at a time, on a 50/50 ratio, male/female.

What was really happening was that these were a group of fairly acute schizophrenic patients, who were young and were kept activated. There were special rehabilitation and re-socialisation programmes for them. Activation alone was probably as good as any insulin course. When insulin was discontinued, tranquillisers were substituted to minimise the more acute symptoms, and make them more amenable to psychotherapy and other treatments.

Regarding neuroleptics, my first dramatic experience was with an out-patient in County Waterford, a young boy who was prescribed a small dose of chlorpromazine. He had paranoid symptoms and while he was on the drug, was symptom-free, but when he omitted to take it, he would relapse within weeks. This was very dramatic, so much so that I became convinced that it wasn't just purely damping down the psychotic symptoms, until they naturally abated of their own accord.

The depot neuroleptics appeared in the late 1960s. It was clear that they were effective, and in some patients dramatically so.

DH   At the time you were prescribing neuroleptics, what kind of doses were you actually prescribing – what seems to me to have happened is that what was prescribed would now be called low dose, and then somewhere in the mid to late 70s the megadose regimes came in, which were no more efficacious, so that we are on the way back now to the kind of regimes that were first prescribed.

TL   I think that's probably true. Also, one was prescribing low dose regimes of several drugs, rather than sticking to one in a higher dosage. There's no doubt polypharmacy was practised.

DH   *Do you think medication made a big change?*

TL   I'm quite certain that it wasn't just that patients were coincidentally getting better for other reasons. Certainly, there were other improvements – the patients' conditions were improving, and the public were getting interested in patient care. I suppose you could say that medication made these other changes possible. The drugs certainly did subdue many of the unwelcome symptoms of disturbed patients. They make it more possible to communicate and develop rapport. Use of the neuroleptic drugs could have a very dramatic therapeutic effect, even in quite small doses.

Many of us have the experience of patients, well-controlled on depot neuroleptics, indeed so well controlled that they decided to stretch the intervals between their injections. Remaining well, they eventually decided – 'I can do without' and in a matter of three or four months, they are back in hospital, having relapsed.

DH   *St Patrick's, even though they had locked wards, would have been a much less horrific place then Grangegorman.*

TL   It did not have to cope with the great numbers of elderly mentally handicapped patients, whom you have in public mental hospitals. When you have to cater for the severely mentally handicapped patients you cannot keep the wards in pristine condition. Hospitals like St Patrick's and St John of God's do cater mainly for social class I–III. Such people, because of greater facilities available to them at home, would be better motivated and have a better chance of recovery. Having said that, they did admit and treat acutely psychotic patients to St Patrick's.

Grangegorman (St Brendan's) on the other hand, was always considered the end of the line. When St Patrick's or St John of God's couldn't cope, patients were sent there. Actually St Ita's used to be the very end of the line for the public patients.

DH   *In England, 'private' as regards medicine is a somewhat dirty word; it's not the same in Ireland – can you explain it?*

TL   I used to have the opinion that it was a socialist view that brought this about, but I don't believe so now. Many times at the Court of Elector meetings, some members expressed a contemptuous attitude to the private sector. I remember protesting at one meeting that if it wasn't for the private hospitals, their President, Dr Thomas Bewley, and myself would not have been trained in psychiatry.

In Ireland, there is a different attitude to the private sector. St Patrick's Hospital was founded in 1745 for the poor of Dublin – Jonathan Swift's will specified this and the hospital always provided accommodation for people from the deprived areas of the City; it runs out-patient clinics for the surrounding sector subsidised by the hospital.

DH   The fact that places like St John of God's are being run by religious orders and aren't profit-making makes some difference?

TL   St John of God's have funded wonderful improvements in the hospital, as have St Patrick's – elegant foyers, offices, and accommodation that certainly in no way resemble the old-style hospital. It's difficult to find such money for a public mental hospital – politicians and the public in general scrutinise where our tax money is spent. It's a pity that more emphasis isn't spent on upgrading the public mental hospitals. St Patrick's Hospital and St John of God's Hospital are a credit to Ireland; indeed, the Royal College of Psychiatrists hold the membership exams there.

DH   That's alright for the service within the hospital, but what about trying to run a service in the community.

TL   You mean the private hospitals do not run a community service. This is extremely difficult; the service in the community really has to be funded by the State. There can be no profit in it, and to keep themselves going they have to be solvent; there could be no capitation fee to cover the number of patients they treat. For example, the number of psychiatric patients seen in the out-patient department in Blanchardstown General Hospital on a Friday morning is usually about 50. Granted there are four psychiatrists there and four can readily manage that number. But those 50 do not have to pay anything. They will also get their prescription drugs free.

It needs a health authority to give this back-up, as well as to provide hostels, day centres, workshops and other facilities required for rehabilitation.

Community services need state funding if they are going to succeed. The state has provided some funding, but unfortunately community services are not cheap. Many consultant psychiatrists suspected that the motive for closing hospitals was to save money, but most administrators now realise that community care facilities are not a cheap option.

DH   Can you tell me something about your role in the Mental Health Association?

TL   I am a founder of the Mental Health Association of Ireland, and currently hold the post of Honorary Secretary. It was founded 25 years ago and is a limited liability company. Its aims were to set up rehabilitation facilities for psychiatric patients and to educate the public. The aims remain the same, with the emphasis on the latter. It is a big organisation now, with more than 50 local branches throughout the country. Our Chief Executive Officer, Mary O'Mahony, is a very live wire, although the Board tends to be getting old now and most of us have reached retiring age.

MIND in England has gone a different road, but we did not follow their lead. They became political and were often used as a stepping ground for higher things in politics. One of the reasons for my staying on the Board has been to ensure it keeps its original aims, to try and increase knowledge and stimulate public interest in psychiatry. Of course, there are still prejudices and stigma; you do not counter centuries of prejudice over a matter of a few decades.

DH *You've been a clinical director on the Eastern Health Board. Has the example of Irish clinical directorates any lessons to offer the British?*

TL A clinical director in theory meant that one could look after one's own clinical material, be responsible for that, and allow lay people to manage administration. But as clinical directors, a number of my colleagues have become so involved in administrative work that they can spend little time in clinical work. I continue to run my own out-patient clinics, day centres, and workshops, and I continue to see patients on the wards. But it's more and more difficult, because administration problems are lumped upon you, and you pick up too many committees.

At one stage in my career, I developed an interest in rehabilitation, so I was appointed to the National Rehabilitation Board, to the Central Remedial Clinic, and to the Rehabilitation Institute. In addition, I found myself a member of the National Drugs Advisory Board. Added to that, there were the Royal College of Surgeons and the Royal College of Psychiatrists committees. When I was senior Vice-President of the Royal College of Psychiatrists, I was run off my feet.

DH *What else do you think we need to do in the next ten years in Irish psychiatry?*

TL Here in Ireland, further development of the training programme is a first priority. There are not less than 20 to 25 vacant consultant posts being filled by locums throughout the country. Creating more senior registrar posts and, of course, getting them funded would help solve this. Psychiatry has become a much more acceptable speciality. The standard of medical personnel intake nowadays is very good, many aspirants having double membership.

This is a problem. Only the academic lecturers and professors have higher medical degrees. Many people in psychiatry think that is an old-fashioned view. I think it shows a very good broad education, not just in the psychiatric field, but in general medicine also.

What is needed now is an expansion of the service by increasing the number of consultant posts in mental handicap and in child psychiatry. At the moment, with cut-backs, psychotherapy is almost off any menu. We have, however, managed to get the Health Board and Department of Health to accept that future senior registrar posts in psychiatry should be so structured that candidates get some experience in psychotherapy.

DH *What do you think psychiatry in the United Kingdom has to learn from the Irish?*

TL We are very alike in our views regarding psychiatry, though the Irish are probably less intense in their approach. I wonder if that is a good thing to recommend to the UK. The majority of our colleagues in Britain have similar interests and hobbies. I think that they have much better organised research facilities.

DH *Have the Irish better clinical and rehabilitation facilities?*

TL I think so. I have experience of clinical work in England, and work in the community. I do not think the facilities in the community are as well organised. Workshops, day hospitals, day centres, and hostel places are very well provided throughout Ireland.

Our nursing staff are better trained in Ireland. I also think that the concept of psychiatric nurses in the community is more advanced in Ireland. We have some excellent community services, developed by these nursing staff. In the

UK there is a dichotomy between community and hospital. The only separation that exists here is between the community physicians and community directors, i.e. the medical personnel in charge of community physical health as distinct from mental health. They developed from the old style medical officer of health and are only remotely linked to the hospital service.

16   Ismond Rosen

Interviewed by HUGH FREEMAN (1992)

**Dr Ismond Rosen, MB, BCh (U. Witwatersrand),
(1946), DPM (1951), MD (1954), FRCPsych
(Foundation) (1972).** Dr Rosen was born in
Johannesburg in 1924. He was a student at the Ecole
des Beaux Arts and the Academie Julien, Paris. He
was at the Maudsley and Bethlem Royal Hospitals from
1952–58 and the Portman Clinic, 1958–59. He was
research psychoanalyst, the Hampstead Clinic 1967,
and consultant psychiatrist, Paddington Centre of
Psychotherapy from 1958. He has been an exhibiting
artist from 1947 and had exhibitions at the Whibley
Gallery and and the Camden Arts Centre, and the
Royal Academy, London. He is a Fellow of the Royal
Society of Medicine, Royal College of Psychiatrists,
Portrait Sculpture Society and a member of the
International Psychoanalytical Association and the
British Psychoanalytic Society.

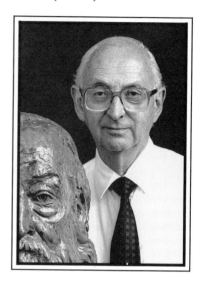

HF   Were there any important influences from your early life in the development of your career?

IR   I had significant relationships and influences with both my parents; they
were caring and courageous people, who valued emotional closeness.

The circumstances surrounding my birth were very dramatic. I was born
prematurely and unexpectedly. My father ran out into the street for help, saw a
nurse in uniform, picked her up bodily and carried her to my mother's bedside,
where an aunt had already cut the cord. My mother was hospitalised for three
months and required an operation for a retained placenta and septicaemia.

It could be said that both my mother and I were fighting for survival at that time.
Only recently have I realised that she must have focused on her new-born babe
as the spur to her own survival. This early maternal deprivation, together with
the compensatory intense closeness and over-protection, contributed a sensitivity
in me to the quality of togetherness in relationships, which may also have gained
expression in judging aesthetic proportions in art. I have observed patients with
a history of severe early deprivation who seemed to have compensated for such
deficiency with enhanced intellectual capacities, as if they were trying to restore
an emotional gap with some area of perfection under their own control.

I grew up in a large hotel, run by my parents in the centre of Johannesburg.
My mother was a gifted listener, and complete strangers would pour out their
problems and life histories to her. My father had been part of the mass
immigration in the 1880s from Russia into the United States. On arrival in
New York, at the age of 6, he sold newspapers; had his own business, with
assistants at 14, and gave up a flourishing photographic studio at the age of 19,

when he emigrated to South Africa. He photographed Cecil Rhodes and the officers of the Argyll & Sutherland Highlanders in the field during the Boer War, then led a very romantic life, farming, losing everything, and beginning again. My parents expected success from their offspring.

Their warmth and family dedication were applied equally to the atmosphere of the hotel. This was my developmental background – a service institution where I came into everyday contact with members of the public, to whom I was expected to show a sense of responsibility and tact, though they included artists and players from touring companies and drunks who were potentially violent. All very good practice for dealing later with difficult psychiatric patients.

A typical chore, when my parents were away on holiday, was to cash up in the bar around midnight and write up the books, wake at 4 o'clock in the morning to go to the fruit market, return for breakfast, and then be on time at the medical school for 8 o'clock! There was no particular remuneration for this; it was just one of the routines.

HF   Could you say a little more about life in the hotel?

IR   Another advantage was the experience gained working in every kind of hotel environment – in the office, kitchen, dining-room and bar.

My first clinical experience as a psychotherapist occurred when I was a second-year medical student, aged 17. I was quite friendly with a young barman, whose wife had given birth to a stillborn child. A few days later, he asked whether I would see his wife, who was mute and refusing food. I found her in bed, with her parents sitting in silent despair. With no previous experience to guide me, I intuited that I had to be alone with her, and summoned up the courage to ask her parents and her husband to leave. After what seemed an eternity of silence, the very young girl and I became acquainted, as words came to me and she gradually became able to reply. We talked about her feelings regarding the stillbirth, and she came right out of the depression.

The barman was much gratified, and as we walked back to the hotel, I recall telling him that this was the sort of work I would like to do in life. My previous experience was of helping boys with their problems at boarding school, where, as a prefect, I called them in for 'peptalks', which in retrospect, were short-term psychotherapeutic interviews.

HF   How was your time as a medical student?

IR   I became a medical student a few months after my sixteenth birthday, in 1941. There was some sense of guilt at not having joined the army, but I was under age and had to help with the hotel.

As students, we worked and played hard; there were some who subsequently became distinguished academics internationally, but who never shone as students. Our intake at Wits medical school was the last one without formal selection procedures, yet our year's record of professional achievements was head and shoulders above that of subsequent ones.

HF   Why was that, do you think?

IR   It could have been a higher quality of motivation, but of course, that's very difficult to measure. As students, though, we were fortunate to have fine teachers, among whom were magnificent models for identification.

One who taught us much about personal behaviour was Raymond Dart, the Dean and Professor of Anatomy, who was also a famous physical anthropologist. He thought in historical and developmental perspectives, using his studies of ape-men and aggression as the earliest human behaviour. An example of his thinking occurred early in the second year. Two hundred students dissecting in the anatomy hall were chattering away, clattering their wooden stools on the concrete floor with deafening effect, when Dart quietly entered, took up a position in the centre and hurled a stool to the floor, creating an instant, if frightening silence. With all attention now riveted on him, he raised the same stool above his head and set it swiftly on the ground without a sound. This was anatomy in action! Dissection took place in hallowed tones thereafter.

He used to invite his great rival, Robert Broome, the palaeontologist to lecture to us – 'He will probably only talk about the beauty of the Karoo', Dart would say, 'but he is a real personality'.

I became involved in the rivalry between these two great men after qualifying, when I modelled the soft tissue reconstruction for Australopithecus ('southern man-ape') Prometheus. Dart, its discoverer, called it this because fossilised ash had been found in the breccia. He showed how animal bony remains at the site had been used as weapons and instruments for stripping flesh, which he believed was the first evidence of human aggression and violence, though later researchers regard the bony markings as due to other scavengers. Photographs of my soft-tissue reconstructions appear in Dart's book *Adventures with the Missing Link*.

HF   Could we talk about how you first got involved with psychiatry?

IR   During our fourth student year, we had formal teaching in it at Weskoppies, the country's main mental hospital, in Pretoria. A few students would spend some days there, wandering about on their own, familiarising themselves with the patients.

The chronic patients were kept in back wards connected by an interminable corridor, built according to a Victorian design, while the acute patients inhabited buildings like large country houses, each with its grounds encircled by tennis court fences. Entering one such day room, we found a solitary patient standing on his head on a settee. We waited for about ten minutes, until he eventually came down, and I wondered what to say to him. He appeared to me to be Jewish, which prompted me to ask 'Are you the Messiah?', to which he immediately replied, 'Who else?'. I was chuffed at the encounter, feeling I had made some special contact. I found the patients fascinating to meet and understand. Of course, we were all rather scared before we went. Afterwards, the most frightening aspect was the isolated beauty of the place, where contact with the outside world and life's endeavours had ceased to exist.

At that time, there was an enormous amount of public hostility and stigma attached to the mental hospitals, which I felt required altering, but I was heading for a career as a plastic surgeon, based on my interest in portrait sculpture. Since the end of my first year in medicine, I had regularly done minor surgery at Casualty, stitching up the wounds which resulted from the endemic violence. In my fifth year, though, I went on to do the first three years of the dental degree. It was only after I qualified that I decided against taking up plastic surgery because I had a partial red-green colour blindness, and opted for psychiatry instead.

Personal limitations play as important a part in determining career choice as talent or preferences.

HF Can I ask you how your artistic work began?

IR   I saw one of the young Africans who worked in our house making small clay figures of oxen, when I must have been about six. I found it quite easy to make things, and produced my first sculpture, which happened to be a skull, when I was about eight; I used to carry it round in my pocket as a sort of talisman. In high school, we had Walter Battiss, the foremost artist in South Africa, as a master, but it had been decided by the family that I would do Latin rather than art.

So from then on, there was always a conflict – medicine or art – I wouldn't give up one for the other, and the conflict went on until I realised that the two weren't in conflict at all. I had to do both.

HF If you produced your first sculpture at the age of eight, that seems quite remarkable. How did you know what to do?

IR   I don't know. I sort of just did it. My father had never had a formal schooling, but he believed that if you needed to do something, you just went ahead and did it. This was very important for me later with things like therapeutic experience, because when I actually started to work with psychiatric patients, one could get very little guidance from any of the consultants. They were mostly organic psychiatrists and had very little experience of talking to patients psychotherapeutically, so when I started in a psychiatric hospital, I discussed things with my immediate colleagues. We all helped each other, and that was a wonderful experience of learning without a competitive spirit, but rather with one of mutual enlightenment.

Contemporary registrars with me who attained high academic status were Professors Dick Cheetham, Fred Frankel, Lynn Gillis and Lionel Hersov. We unknowingly emulated the experiences Freud went through – in that we taught ourselves to hypnotise. At that time, there were still quite a few hysterics around, and we found that with hypnosis, you could get a severe hysteric who was completely unable to walk, to start walking.

It took further experience, though, to learn that severe hysteria is a much more serious condition than appears in the presenting symptoms, and several of these people from whom we had removed their hysterical defences subsequently became much more ill. For instance, one had a heart attack. In that way, we learned that there were unfathomable depths and layered defences in human personality. It then became clear that what might initially have been something of a gift or a sensitivity to unconscious mechanisms was insufficient; one needed formal training.

HF How did you actually start psychiatric work? Did you become a medical officer in a mental hospital?

IR   I did my house jobs – medicine and surgery and some casualty work – and then was appointed medical director of the John Gray Community Health Centre. This was in the poorest white section of Johannesburg, funded by the money collected during the university rag. The director was Helen Joseph, who gained fame afterwards as an anti-apartheid campaigner. So it had a certain prestige and research capacity and one of the specialists attached was Dr Wolf Sachs, who was the only practising psychoanalyst in Johannesburg at that time. I was one of the few male staff, with a lot of females, most of whom were psychologists or social workers. That year was one of an initial coming to terms with dynamic problems, both in the family and in the community.

HF   What was the next stage of your psychiatric odyssey?

IR   I was appointed as one of the first registrars at Tara Hospital, a fine house in beautiful grounds which was administered by the provincial authorities. This was quite new for psychiatry, as all the other psychiatric services were in large mental hospitals under central government aegis. Tara was a neuropsychiatric service, so that we registrars were trained in neurology, and in treatments for neuroses, personality disorders, and early cases of schizophrenia, such as ECT, insulin, and psychotherapy.

Maxwell Jones came out from England, which fired our enthusiasm, so that we started groups of every description – small therapeutic ones, those where patients were responsible for administering their activities, and a large weekly group where one of the registrars met all 100 patients.

One of the ideas I formulated then was 'group handling for nurses', the sisters being trained to conduct these with the nurses: one would act the role of the patient and another that of the nurse, in some difficult or aggressive situation. We imagined the same thing must be going on everywhere else, and that everybody knew about it, so no-one thought of writing it up. It was all done again much later in England by people like Bertram Mandelbrote, who was a registrar at the Maudsley when I arrived, but there was no knowledge there that we had already done it.

HF   Did you have experience of working in a large mental hospital?

IR   One of the aspects of our South African DPM training, which was for three years, was spending six months at Weskoppies Hospital. I was given 800 patients from the chronic wards to look after, yet we weren't overworked. One visited the wards every day and did the notes and examination of patients, according to statutory needs. Within a short time, I found I was running the malarial ward, the dispensary, the insulin ward, and giving ECT and then I went on to take charge of more active units, including the forensic ward. The hospital was an active treatment centre, the consultants were friendly, and we all worked happily together. One of the pleasures at that time, being in my early twenties, was residing in my own house in the hospital grounds. Black patients tended the garden, where they secretly grew their own marijuana. I did a lot of sculpture portraits, both of the patients and staff.

At Tara, I had to deal with a patient who was one of the main broadcasters over the radio in the morning. At a time when there was no television, he would wake the whole country up with his sunny personality. Unfortunately, his voice was reduced to a croak because of an hysterical aphonia. He had suffered this twice before and had been given a last opportunity for treatment, with the understanding that if he didn't improve rapidly, he was going to lose his job. Through hypnosis, I tried to reveal the basis of his problems as quickly as possible, which fortunately was achieved. Waking up every morning, I would switch on the radio to see how the treatment was progressing. What I discovered with this patient, like Freud previously, were the limitations of hypnosis. In this case, the cure was based on the working through of the sexualised use of his voice, in an oedipal conflict.

In 1948, we were doing sodium amytal interviews at Tara with people suffering battle stress from World War II. I applied this experience to one of the chronic catatonic schizophrenics who hadn't spoken for nine years and who would stand immobile in the exercise yard, where he would be moved by other patients so as not to be burned by the sun. Yet, within a few interviews, this man emerged as an apparently normal human being, who talked and assumed a completely different physical demeanour from when he was catatonic. He remained normal for a few days, and then slipped back. I didn't have the knowledge to keep him out of catatonia, and there was a very painful episode after my seniors decided that he be given ECT. We took him up for treatment and he literally fought like a wild tiger; the ECT regressed him right back into catatonia.

HF You seem to have had a very wide experience in psychiatry.

IR   I feel that I was privileged in being able to be part of some of the major developments over the last five decades. We had many cases then of GPI, which were treated with malarial therapy, though it was being superseded by penicillin, which was only just beginning to be available. Insulin coma was a particularly awful treatment to have to give. It was highly dangerous and the nursing staff and I used to celebrate every morning with a particular feast – avocado sandwiches – when all the patients had come out of coma. There were times when you literally had to fight because a patient in deep coma had bitten off the metallic end of the airway with clenched teeth. The danger of death then was from suffocation, so one had to force open the locked jaw, extract the airway, put a new one in, and of course bring the patient out of the coma. When I was at the Maudsley later, on the insulin service again, Brian Ackner was in charge. He did the double-blind study on insulin coma which gave the *coup de grâce* to the whole thing. So, I was part of that as well.

There were experiences too in public duties. After I had gone back to Tara, I was asked by our superintendent to attend the inauguration of a mental health society in Pretoria. I was to get a lift with the Johannesburg Medical Officer of Health. Though I wasn't qualified yet as a psychiatrist, he insisted on me going, saying that I wouldn't have much to do except be present in case some little old ladies wanted to ask a few questions.

Travelling with the MOH, we were laughing most of the way, until I asked him if he had the programme. This proclaimed the inauguration of the Pretoria Mental Health Society at the City Hall, under the aegis of the Mayor. The wife of the Minister of Interior and various speakers were named. 'Main Speaker' had a space opposite. I asked 'Who is the main speaker?', at which the MOH said, 'You are!'.

The laughter became a little hysterical on my part and a few minutes later, we drew up at the imposing City Hall, with the Mayor in his robes waiting to greet us. I was shown into a large assembly room, filled with men in dark blue suits who were looking very severe. I spoke about the work I had done in individual and group therapy, including work with the delinquents, and about the need for services for young people attempting suicide.

What I then realised was that this was a politically determined meeting, at which the University of Pretoria was aiming to take over the mental health services, and that no one from the Government service or from Tara Hospital had been invited, apart from myself.

One of the things about growing up in a country like South Africa was that, as a young man, one had opportunities like this. We quickly became very responsible and experienced clinicians with the confidence to deal with people.

HF   How was it that you decided to come to England?

IR   In South Africa at that time, most people wanted to have a European experience. I wanted to further my artistic work, make the decision whether I should go into art or stay in medicine, and also get more experience in psychiatry. So as soon as I completed my DPM requirements, I left home.

I arrived in England in October 1951, rang up the Maudsley, and arranged to see the Dean. I found David Davies very kind and he arranged for me to see Professor Lewis. Of course, we had all heard of Aubrey as a most formidable figure, but he was also quite charming to me at first, though rather formal.

In those days, I was a rather 'nice young man', fairly shy but wanting to get places, and the interview wasn't at all easy. He asked me what I had done and then what I'd read. In South Africa, we followed the Scottish model and our textbook was Henderson & Gillespie. I told him I had read that and a few other books, which I thought was really quite an accomplishment, but of course he said, 'What else have you read?'. I mentioned a book on personality, and when he asked me who the author was, I couldn't for the life of me remember! That made me feel an absolute idiot, though previously I'd been rather proud of having read it.

He asked me what I intended doing, and I told him I wanted to go off for about a year, study art, and give myself a chance at that, but would be very happy if I could get a job at the Maudsley in a year's time. He said he wouldn't be interested in giving me one in a year's time, but would think of giving me one in six months. I agreed to that, spent a few weeks in London, and on the day I was to leave for the Continent, got a letter from him confirming the offer.

HF   How was your French experience?

IR   I arrived in Paris with some artist friends and went to the art school I had chosen, the Academie Julien, but that evening, I got the most awful news – that my mother had died suddenly. The shock was compounded by the fact that my friends had gone off. Then the school closed, as it was December, and I was all alone in Paris, unable to speak French.

This was supposed to be the opportunity to discover if I had any creativity, but mourning was hardly the occasion for that. However, when the school re-opened, I did some stone carving at the Ecole des Beaux Arts, as well as life drawing, and then travelled south – being at the first post-war Mardi Gras in Nice – and right through Italy, reading Freud in Florence in the morning winter sunshine, and on to Rome.

There, I had a dream which seemed to resolve my conscience, because it said quite clearly – choose medicine. At that point, in late March, I decided to return to London and resume my psychiatric studies at the beginning of April.

HF   So you followed Freud, who also I think had dream experiences relating to Rome?

IR   Yes, these things seem to be significant in one's career. Starting at the Maudsley, though, was a very curious experience, because the atmosphere was so unlike what I'd been used to at Tara, with its warmth and feeling of working together.

There was a most cold and distant relationship between everybody. I can remember sitting at a table with two senior registrars, neither of whom talked to me at all. A friendly American sat down, waved his hand at them, and said 'Hi-ya fellows'. They both looked up at him, said nothing, looked down again, and went on conversing between themselves. The idea at the time seemed to be that nothing that you could say when you arrived was worth listening to. You were really an infant, needed to be regressed, and after this treatment for a couple of months, you would start to learn what they wanted to teach you.

I was on the Professorial Unit, which had two institutions through which Aubrey Lewis operated clinically; one was the Admission & Discharge conference and the other was the Monday morning conference. I am very grateful to him for one thing – he was one of the great teachers, if you could only learn from him – and what he taught me was how to think. I didn't know how before that, but I responded to this systematic questioning – the Socratic form, plus the Cartesian view that there is nothing I can be sure of except my doubt.

Later, as a senior registrar, one of one's important tasks was to prepare junior colleagues for the Monday conference. We developed the skill to think of every question that one could possibly ask about the particular patient, and this was where the thinking process came in.

However, I was due to assist Denis Hill with the DPM clinical examinations one day, when I got a call in the morning that my father was severely ill and that I should fly back to South Africa, which I did immediately. When I arrived, he was said to be dying of cancer of the lung. I didn't think my medical experience was all that wonderful, but there was one thing I could do, and that was to be like Aubrey Lewis and systematically go through and question everything that had happened to him. What we eventually found was that he only had a calcified mass, which was an end-on view of one of his vessels in the lung. This had been misdiagnosed by the radiologist, and they had then given him deep therapy and burned his chest. In fact, what they took for cachexia was really a depression that he had developed with the prognosis, but in two or three weeks while I was there, he was completely cured. He would have died, I'm sure, otherwise.

So that in clinical work, asking questions, and taking the history in detail, and going through it again, seems to be the most important thing you can do.

HF   What were your other experiences of Aubrey Lewis?

IR   In 1952, at the end of the year, the registrars put on their first pantomime. It was 'Dick Whittington' and was about a professor from Adelaide who sold his soul to the Devil for the Chair of Psychiatry in London! This was dynamite. I had been chosen to play the professor, which I did as compassionately as possible, but there was Aubrey sitting in the front row. He looked on with a smile, but deeply pained underneath, as I could see. This was given as two performances, on the Friday and Saturday nights.

On the Monday, as I was Lewis's assistant in the out-patient department, I had to present two cases to him, and the whole staff waited to hear what he was going to say to me. As you can imagine, I was terrified. Aubrey came in, we saw the two cases, one after the other, and did the letters. He never said a single word about the pantomime, which I thought was quite extraordinary. I don't know whether he didn't know what to say or felt it was the best thing just to say nothing.

However, when I came to leave for a job at the Portman Clinic, and started in private practice, I 'phoned the Maudsley on the first day, to see if there were any messages for me. I was told there were two people trying to get hold of me. The first was the Professor, who asked if I was going to apply for the Chair in Psychiatry in Johannesburg. I asked him why he was asking me this, and he replied that someone else had asked him to be the referee for them, and he felt that if I was going to apply, he would rather be the referee for me. I was enormously pleased, but said that as I had to find time for both my analysis and my art, I had given up the idea of an academic career. The other person looking for me was David Stafford-Clark, who was referring a new patient – so both calls were very welcome.

HF   What was the feeling toward psychoanalysis at the Maudsley then?

IR   When I joined, it was highly ambivalent. I remember Aubrey asking me if I'd thought whether I was going to do analytic training. This was really a difficult question to answer, because I had already applied and had been accepted! He said 'Of course, you realise that you aren't going to do your work as well as possible, and it will interfere with you getting a Chair', and various things like that.

But on the other hand, I had his support when I was doing psychotherapy with an extremely difficult patient – and of course, the Maudsley got some impossible patients to deal with. He asked me when I was going to present this case, and said he would particularly like to come and listen – as he did. Another time, he asked me if I wanted to be a senior lecturer in psychotherapy, but I said it wasn't something I was interested in doing then.

The Maudsley experience was one where eventually one made many friends, at a depth of intensity that doesn't occur in other training experiences, and of course, so much original work was being done.

I also worked with Erwin Stengel, a most eminent psychiatrist with an enormous clinical facility and a way of helping research and the writing of theses which Aubrey never had. He encouraged us, and in many cases, our theses were based on his own interests. He had a wonderful sense of humour, but with a very political twist to it. He used to give a clinical demonstration once a week; one particularly difficult man occupied over half an hour, making manifest each of his vignettes of clinical deviation. At the end of this, Stengel said, 'Of course, you do come to the Maudsley for other purposes as well, don't you? Perhaps you could tell us about them.' The patient said 'Well, I come up here to the psychology department, I'm one of Professor Eysenck's normals'. Of course, there was enormous conflict between Eysenck and the analysts particularly. He seemed hell-bent on trying to destroy psychoanalysis, perhaps because he was trying to clear the way for behaviour therapy.

HF   Did you have experience of psychotherapy with schizophrenics at the Maudsley?

IR   Yes. I found that I could tolerate a good deal of anxiety from the patients, which perhaps many clinicians couldn't. Following the work of John Rosen, I spent up to five hours a day continuously with some severely regressed patients. I took one man into a side-ward, where there was a piano, and as we were talking, he lifted up the lid and tried the keys, but they were silent – it was a practice piano. He had been a most brilliant scholar, who knew several languages and everything about music, but practically nothing about the real world. He was in such emotional pain that we gave him one or two ECTs and later, he completely recovered; perhaps as a result of the psychotherapy he had, he could make the jump back to normality. At that point, he said to me, 'The one point in the treatment when I realised that you really understood me was when you took me into that side-room with the practice piano, which was silent. You realised I was silent in quite the same way.' These chance matters can have a considerable bearing with such patients.

HF   Have you any particular recollections of the introduction of the neuroleptics into psychiatry?

IR   I was indeed present when neuroleptics were introduced at the Maudsley and also when Linford Rees was doing the first double-blind studies.

With the introduction of chlorpromazine, we certainly could see how helpful it was for psychoses, and when double-blind trials were being done on the same set of out-patients with successive different neuroleptics, improvements occurred serially from each one, which seemed a bit remarkable. But some would relapse back and we didn't know at that time how long people would have to stay on such drugs, and that some would have to stay on them almost indefinitely.

The Maudsley was always wary of sedatives or anxiolytics as 'wonder drugs'; routine serum bromides were still required when I joined the staff. Continuous baths were also preferred to drug sedation for mania, until more specific remedies became available.

My later experience was of being involved with psychotherapy patients who required anti-depressant treatment. There was a school of thought that people should not be given any drugs at all, because it would interfere with the therapeutic process, but I was never of that opinion. I believed that the needs of the patient were always the first criterion, and if there was suffering, something had to be done to relieve it. In this way, some patients could make progress that they would not have been able to make in psychodynamic therapy if pharmacological treatment hadn't been available.

Curiously enough, a group of analytically trained psychiatrists at the Camden Clinic, of which I was one, published the first out-patient controlled trial of Tofranil.

HF   Shall we talk now about how your involvement in psychoanalysis began?

IR   As I mentioned earlier, in South Africa I had met Wolf Sachs, who gave me some supervision. Just before leaving, I gave a lecture on group therapy in a prestigious Philosophy of Science series, which I then thought was my major interest. The reader in Philosophy, Dr Yourgrau, very kindly gave me a letter of introduction to Anna Freud, so that I made an appointment to see her after I arrived. I remember feeling that I should be with her as little time as possible, because she was so important.

When I returned to England in April 1952, I saw her again and applied formally for training at the Institute of Psychoanalysis. I was duly accepted after being seen by Winnicot and Mrs Hoffer, both of whom were masters at interviewing. After an interval in my formal training, I qualified in 1958.

The one thing that I recall was the enormous amount of work one had to put in. During the last year of training, one was required not only to be in personal analysis five times a week, but to analyse two people daily, as well as attend seminars most evenings. So the schedule ran something like this: I saw my first patient at the Institute at 8 o'clock. At 9.15 I had my personal analysis for 50 minutes in Chelsea, and then went to the Maudsley as rapidly as possible to start the day's work until 5 p.m. which, being senior registrar on a Professional Unit, was a taxing occupation. At 5 p.m. I would see my second analytical patient at the Maudsley, then have dinner rapidly, attend life drawing classes until 8 p.m. at the Regent Street Polytechnic, and then pop round the corner to the Institute of Psychoanalysis, where the seminar would run up to 9.45 p.m.

This was quite an exhausting schedule over a year, and there wasn't much time for socialising or even for reading, which one was supposed to be doing. But somehow one managed.

HF *Sounds like the life for a bachelor.*

IR   Yes. It was, but what happened in my case was that I intended to marry after finishing the full training and, fortunately, that worked out very well.

HF *Shall we talk about the culture of psychoanalytical training?*

IR   What was most acute at this time was the rivalry between the various groups at the Institute, particularly between the Kleinians and the Freudians, with the 'middle-group' or independents led by thinkers of their own.

The original standard-bearers of these scientific theories were then present and very active. If you were presenting a patient to Melanie Klein, for instance, she would run riot over you. Then, if you took up what she was saying, as I did on one occasion, and presented another case in that manner to Anna Freud in the following week, you got into hot water all over again. It seemed to me that people coming from the Continent had a loyalty not only to individuals but also to a philosophical system of ideas, which was somewhat at odds with British pragmatism and with the eclectic approach with which I was familiar in South Africa.

There were logical reasons for both points of view, once you accepted their premises, but at times one could be put in an invidious position through these conflicts.

HF *Can we talk next about when you left the Maudsley?*

IR   If one had trained there, this was the springboard to the major step in one's career. I was looking for a psychodynamic institution in which to work, and so was very pleased to take a job at the Portman Clinic, which specialised in problems of sexual deviation and delinquency. There were notable consultants such as Harry Rubenstein, Edward Glover, William Paterson-Brown, and later Adam Limentani. I had already had experience in the delinquency field, working with Peter Scott, who had wanted me to stay in that specialty, but I felt it was too narrow.

When I did my MD thesis on 30 cases of schizophrenics with obsessions, I found that if you wanted to do research, it was important to have as many suitable patients as possible. So I tried to restrict my Portman patients as much as possible to one particular type. Many patients had been sent by the courts because of exhibitionism, so I decided to use both individual and group psychotherapy for them.

This turned out to be a very good idea, because 1960 was World Mental Health Year and I organised a national congress on sexual deviation at the Royal Society of Medicine. It was a great success and I was able to present the results of my studies there. This was followed up with a book, with other British contributors, which was published by Oxford University Press in 1964 under the title, *The Pathology & Treatment of Sexual Deviation*, and it became quite a standard work in the field.

HF   I did a review of it at the time.

IR   I remember that. Fifteen years later, though, with leading world authorities, we produced what OUP described as the Second Edition, but which was really a brand new book called Sexual Deviation.

My idea was that all the various approaches towards deviant sexuality would be brought together. But the analysts said there wasn't enough psychoanalysis in it, and the psychiatrists said it was full of psychoanalytic lingo, so that they couldn't recommend it. I think it was you who said 'What are you worried about, when everybody's reading it and buying it?'.

I was very pleased when it was quite clear that it was being used as the basic text by very serious places of study all over the world. Now that another 15 years has almost passed, the question is whether to produce the next edition, because work doesn't proceed very rapidly in this field.

HF   How did you find the process of editing books?

IR   I had been spending a lot of time producing a major art exhibition, and hadn't given enough time to the book, for its second edition. When I did get busy with it, it seemed to take an inordinate length of time; many contributors wouldn't send in their material, though as usual, those of the highest standard were the speediest.

One day, I received a telephone call from Phillis Greenacre, the doyenne of American analysts, who asked me what was happening with the book. She had already sent her chapter in, and now someone else had written to her, asking for a contribution on that topic – which was fetishism – for another volume. I had a fright with this, because I knew that if she withdrew her chapter, there would be no book and everyone else's work would literally go down the drain. So I promised her we would do things as soon as possible, and the book finally appeared.

On a later visit to New York, where she entertained us to dinner, I reminded her of this. She said 'You know, I did it on purpose, just to buck you up.' So distinguished analysts are not always people who just listen and never act.

HF   In recent years, childhood sex abuse has become a very important topic. How did it figure in your work at the Portman Clinic?

IR   From psychoanalytic work with adults who were abused in childhood, one knows that all such children should have access to psychotherapy.

Psychotherapy with such adults is very time-consuming and particularly testing of the counter-transference.

The Portman Clinic emphasised that the abusers also require just as much treatment. Indeed, the whole family does, but where are the trained people who will have the skills to deal with these problems? The fact that many offenders who are sent to prison don't receive any treatment whatsoever is disturbing, because there is evidence that in selected cases, one can achieve life-saving results. Magistrates and others involved haven't sufficient knowledge that offenders who go into prison may re-offend, and that this is part of the acting-out before such behaviour can be dealt with in a therapeutic relationship.

A great deal of education is still required in the field of sexual deviation. We do know that sexual behaviour is the final result of a complicated pathway in development, which has biological as well as psychological and social determinants, so that we shouldn't fool ourselves with any simplistic approaches.

We also have to face the fact that the scene has been affected by the politicising of homosexual attitudes. One of the points I have tried to make in TV broadcasts such as Channel 4's *Comment* and the *After Dark* programme is that young people with homosexual behaviour should not be made to feel that they have a fixed homosexual identity, but should have the opportunity of psychotherapy to be given a 'second chance' to mature in relationships and sexual preference.

Of course, we have to be tolerant of all people, but still recognise as psychiatrists and as scientists that we have a right and a duty to understand the psychopathology of people with every type of sexual behaviour, including the normal, and to help where we can.

HF   Did your first consultantship involve both the Portman Clinic and other places?

IR   I received an appointment to the Camden Clinic shortly after I joined the Portman, preferring to keep my interests as broad as possible. The Clinic was a small house on Camden Road which originated under the name of The British Hospital for Functional Nervous Disorders. It was the first psychiatric out-patient clinic in England, and was set up by private subscription. We were happy doing general psychiatry as well as psychotherapy, but some years later, were amalgamated with the West End Hospital for Nervous Disorders and the Paddington Hospital as the Paddington Clinic & Day Hospital, in Harrow Road.

We had a very prestigious start, but were subsequently run down in number of consultants, and in 1974, the option came up whether or not we would join St Mary's. As the only consultant left, I became chairman and had to deal with a most hostile group of professionals. We decided, however, that we would try to make a go of remaining an independent clinic, and were able to appoint some experienced consultants. However, the staff in the Day Hospital had what they regarded as their own particular brand of treatment, which finally culminated in a legal tribunal examining the work of the consultant concerned. I spent five days in the witness box, having my whole administration put under the microscope.

HF   Does that cause célèbre have any general lessons for the question of consultants' responsibilities?

IR   I think that a consultant, although responsible for his own work and acting according to his own judgement, should nevertheless still be responsive towards the attitudes of his colleagues. There is a very fine boundary between clinical freedom and abuses requiring collective responsibility for patient care.

Where a specialist psychotherapeutic function had been adopted, some psychologists, social workers, and nurses at the Paddington Centre were loath to accept a medical consultant's responsibility for their work. They felt they had sufficient training to be fully responsible for their psychotherapeutic way. This applied particularly to social workers, but the administration refused to grasp this nettle, because they did not want to make a judgement between the medical and social work staffs. This remains an unresolved issue.

HF   From your experience of the Paddington Centre, what do you feel about the relationship between psychiatrist and administrators?

IR   Having avoided absorption by St Mary's Hospital in 1972, the Paddington Centre came under heavy fire by the district administration as an easy target by which to save money. After three experiences of almost being closed down, we became more adept in showing ourselves to visiting assessors, so that fear at having to reveal our clinical work gave rise to a more confident outlook. The administrators then became personally involved in understanding psychotherapy and turned into staunch supporters.

I think we were among the first NHS clinics to practise modern techniques of survival. When under threat by the administration, it was important, firstly, to target and reveal the anonymous individuals in the administration who were responsible for decision-making.

The second aim was to arouse professional and public opinion, whose weight was brought to bear on the administration. Because of our excellent relationships with local bodies and services, they gave active support and enlisted other institutions such as the House of Commons. In a situation where the administration wasn't really interested in whether one service or another should continue but where they had to save money, they were often swayed by the weight of such opinion.

The effect of the losses and the pressure to survive wasn't wholly negative though. We had to show statistics on the number of patients that we were treating, and having a high ratio of consultants to junior staff, we discovered that we could give supervisory training in psychotherapy to honorary therapists, who would then treat the patients and so help many more than the staff could alone.

Sir Keith Joseph, as Minister of Health, complied with my request that the Paddington Centre for Psychotherapy be recognised as a psychoanalytic clinic within the NHS.

HF   You have had a lot of involvement over the years in the fields of public education and the media.

IR   This began rather early in my career. In South Africa, we were encouraged to look at the wide implications of psychiatry, particularly through the activities of the National Association for Mental Health, as well as having more direct contact with the public. Before I left, I had organised the first series of radio broadcasts on psychiatry, which did something to reduce its stigma at that time.

While at the Maudsley, I became a founder member of the Public Information Committee of the NAMH, and appeared as the psychiatrist in one of the earliest television series, *Fantasies of the Night*, on understanding dream interpretation.

Later, I was privileged to take part in some of the prestigious productions such as *Life-line* with people like David Stafford-Clark, and created TV programmes for BBC2 *Horizon* on sex education, violence, and particularly with the production of a documentary of one of Freud's cases called the Rat Man.

This had an interesting origin, commencing with a letter from Anna Freud stating that she has been approached by the BBC about a documentary on the Rat Man and would I please deal with them, which I took to mean I should refuse on her behalf. Some unconscious ambivalence was expressed in a simultaneous letter to the BBC, referring them to me as being very experienced and able to give them every assistance.

Bruce Norman, the BBC producer, came to see me and, within a fortnight, we had a shooting script prepared from the very complicated material. One had not only to make the analytic process intelligible, but also invent Freud's dialogue with the patient.

The BBC then realised they didn't have Miss Freud's official permission. I declined to act as intermediary, so that when the BBC approached Miss Freud directly, she replied with, 'Didn't Dr Rosen tell you that I never give permission for such things and that the answer is no?' The BBC were aghast because they had already sunk £10,000 into preparing the sets.

Eventually, she gave permission for the production, with the condition that a disclaimer appeared at the end of the film, stating that it had nothing to do with her or her family! Her attitude was based on Freud's notion that the complexities of psychoanalysis would be over-simplified, and therefore corrupted, by the mass media. The film, in which Edward Fox (of *Day of the Jackal*) played the patient, went on to win many awards. It is an excellent teaching aid for the understanding of this case, in which Freud unravelled the psychopathology of obsessional neurosis from a psychoanalytic point of view.

Later in the year, I presented the film in New York to a meeting of the American Psychoanalytic Association, where it was very well received.

HF   Why do you think almost all analysts in this country live in North London?

IR   I must preface my reply with the experience I had when I first arrived in England. Out of choice, I wanted to live in Chelsea – probably because of the romantic associations of the district – but then rented a room in north London because I was told all the analysts lived there. When I eventually went into analysis, I had to travel daily to Chelsea, where my analyst lived! I don't think we really know why they all live in north London. It's a very beautiful area and was where Freud settled initially. But perhaps the main reason is that it's fairly close to the Institute, so that analysts would naturally tend to live nearby.

HF   Of course, all this time, there had been another side to your life, which was your artistic activities.

IR   I decided I would always continue them as best I could. As a student, I had already done two medical busts – one of Lister and one of John Hunter (which is now in the Royal Society of Medicine).

When I came to London and was appointed to the Maudsley, having come directly from Rome where I had been studying Michelangelo's Moses,

I thought it most appropriate to do a head of Henry Maudsley. Professor Lewis supported this, and I think he may have paid the £50 which it cost to cast it in bronze out of his own pocket. This is a very large head with its flowing beard; it's one and a half times life-size.

I had the opportunity to do the work at the Royal College of Art, because one of their prize-winning young painters had developed a schizophrenic illness, was admitted to the Maudsley, was put under my care, and made a very good recovery. As a result, I became friendly with one of the professors of painting, and hence the *entrée* to the College.

One Saturday afternoon, when the College was closed during the summer holidays, I was busy casting the Maudsley head. I was pouring plaster into the negative mould to form the positive cast. The mould was delicately balanced on a chair, and as I was turning it and swirling the plaster around inside, it somehow managed to slip off and crash onto the floor – which I thought was the end of the Maudsley head.

I was going to the theatre that evening and was in rather a hurry, so the only thing I could think of was to take some string, tie the two remaining halves of the negative mould together, place the shattered pieces together as best I could, and pour in the rest of the plaster, leaving it to set and hoping for the best.

In fact, it turned out perfectly, except for a small bit missing at the cranium, which I was easily able to remodel.

The following year, the head was honoured with the most prominent place in the Sculpture Hall of the Royal Academy Summer Exhibition.

HF   How do you combine an artistic career with a clinical career?

IR   I think one gets urges, ideas that one wishes to make into reality – whether it be a sculpture, a drawing, a painting, or a scientific paper. It's the strength of wish which really forces one into action. You never find the time for creative activity, you have to make it. Of course, you have to work harder.

When I was a houseman, we used to work from 8 in the morning until 6 in the evening, as well as completely through the night on two evenings a week, including working through the next day. I would come home from the hospital, have my supper and work on my sculpture from 8 o'clock until midnight. I always had a lot of energy and feelings of dedication and pleasure in what I was doing.

My most difficult time was in 1973–74, when I was concurrently chairman of the Paddington Centre, running a busy private practice, and spending every spare moment preparing over 100 new works – stainless steel sculptures, paintings, lithographs and etchings – for a major exhibiton at the Camden Arts Centre. During the year, I did the catalogue with its essay on creativity and a lecture at the Tate Gallery on the Psychology of Richard Dadd. Of course, I was very tired at the end of it and took quite some time to recover. Even if I had only ten minutes to spare, I could go up and do some work on a sculpture or drawing, and each activity would somehow freshen me for the other.

When you are working under that sort of schedule, all sorts of remarkable coincidences occur. This is an area I am researching at the moment, but which we don't take a lot of cognisance of as psychiatrists. I think that in research, whenever one has coincidental experiences they should be recorded, much as one would record experimental observations, and at the same time, one should try to record one's inner feelings about them. I believe that if you recorded these, you would find that the experience of coincidences would go on day after day, sometimes for weeks, particularly if one had a 'creative phase'.

Professor Lewis was apparently said to feel that the head of Maudsley was like his super-ego outside his office, and was very pleased when it got moved to the Institute of Psychiatry! I also did the bust of Henry Rey for his retirement from the Maudsley; he and I had shared rooms in Harley Street for years.

There's also the head of Dame Betty Paterson in the Paterson wing of St Mary's, named after her as Chairman of the North West Thames Regional Health Authority – a most gracious lady, an expert administrator, and very reminiscent of the Queen Mother. She arrived for the first sitting at my studio with her chauffeur bearing her television set. She didn't think she could just 'sit' and in any case, she wanted to watch the snooker! In fact, though, we dispensed with the television set and initiated a most wonderful series of discussions.

There are many modes in which art, psychotherapy, psychoanalysis, and psychiatry function in common. A good portrait isn't merely a likeness produced by looking at the person; something mysterious happens when your hands create an image in a different medium. A whole communicative process occurs, ranging from the perception of the person to the final aesthetic proportion and expression. The meaningful portrait is the resultant image of the relationship that is set up between sitter and artist.

HF   What about people who are dead, like Henry Maudsley?

IR   He was really prettied up for his portrait. I had pictures of him, and the wonderful inspiration of Michelangelo's Moses helped to give some embodiment to the spirit and idea of the man, as well as to the idea of the Maudsley Hospital. It was a challenge to make mature interpretations of both Maudsley, and Stengel, some 40 years later, which Lundbeck Pharmaceuticals presented to the College for its 150th anniversary.

I have been fortunate in the quality of sitters I have been commissioned to portray; for example, the bust for the retirement of Professor Dorothy Stuart Russell from the chair of morbid anatomy at the London Hospital Medical College. I felt I was in the presence of a remarkable personality and that it was important to capture her evident femininity, which she had preserved in what was originally an all-male preserve, as the first woman consultant to be appointed to the hospital. She took me to the window of her office, from which we could see a sign – 'Mission to the Jews'. She explained that having had to work so hard to overcome the traditional prejudices against females in medicine, she felt a sense of identification with the Jews.

HF   Do you feel there is an artistic side to psychotherapy?

IR   I certainly do. Good psychotherapy is essentially a logical and aesthetic pursuit of understanding and togetherness, much like an artist in realising an inner vision. It's part of an 'aesthetic' approach when one takes a good history, revealing an image of the balance of forces within that individual.

I liken this process to the uncovering in a good anatomical dissection, where, like a good sculpture, the planes are in correct perspective. One can be either very sensitive or not to how the facts relate, particularly to those areas which are silent and require further elucidation. At the end of a diagnostic interview, one can have an 'artistic' appreciation of the make-up of the personality and of the problems and relationships of this person.

When it comes to therapy, the balancing becomes more complex, because correct timing of therapeutic interferences has to be taken into account. These may be in the nature of imparting understanding, reassurance, or explanations linking unconscious material with transference relationships. Therapeutic interpretations are most potent where one demonstrates to the patient patterns of behaviour which have occurred in childhood, in the present reality and in the transference relationship, and their relevance is clearly communicated and understood, leading to intellectual and then to emotional insight. That to me is an artistic process, and it imparts the same pleasure to therapist, patient, or artist.

HF   What about the relationship of dynamic aspects of the mind to the organic structure of the brain?

IR   I have a very good case illustration on this point. When I was appointed to the Camden Clinic, I inherited a lot of patients who had been attending for a long time. One particular man, who was into his middle 70s, was a depressive and suffering from what appeared to be arteriosclerotic difficulties, in that he was very forgetful, but just able to find his way home.

We became friendly and he started to tell me about factors in his early life. He related how, as a boy, he had come from school and when he met his father, he mimicked another boy at school who had a stammer. His father objected to him imitating the stammer, though, and told him to stop it; the boy took fright and couldn't stop stammering, at which his father struck him to the ground and he had stammered ever since. In fact, he stammered while telling me the story.

A few sessions of working through the affective aspects of this traumatic experience resulted in his stammer disappearing. He remarked how sad it was that he hadn't had this sort of help early on. He used to play the piano in a bar, had a good singing voice, and would have loved to sing there, but he couldn't because of his stammer. In this elderly patient with organic brain damage, the repressed affects were still dynamically available in the unconscious, and his life-long symptoms could be relieved by simple, compassionate psychotherapy of the kind every trained psychiatrist should be happy to do.

HF   How do you see yourself working in the future?

IR   I am engaged in projects which integrate my various activities and experiences. The most significant of these will be an exhibition to be held at St Paul's Cathedral in London, of 'The Holocaust Chapel and Sculptures', where three full-size bronze figures depict Christ as a Jew in the Holocaust, as a symbol of Nazi atrocity, and as representing the need for universal religious tolerance.

17 Robert Cawley

Interviewed by HUGH FREEMAN (1993)

Professor Robert Cawley, BSc Hons (1947) PhD (1949), MB ChB 1955, DPM (Conjoint Board) (1958), FRCPsych (1971), FRCP (1975) Hon FRCPsych (1990). Robert Hugh Cawley was born in 1924 in Birmingham. He was senior registrar at the Bethlem Royal and Maudsley Hospitals. Professor Cawley was Senior Lecturer and First Assistant at the University of Birmingham Department of Psychiatry from 1962–67 and then became consultant psychiatrist at the Bethlem Royal and Maudsley Hospitals from 1967–89 and at King's College Hospital from 1975–89. He was Professor of Psychological Medicine in the University of London at King's College Hospital Medical School and the Institute of Psychiatry, 1975–89 – Emeritus since 1989. Professor Cawley was an examiner in several universities, and was Chief Examiner for the Royal College of Psychiatrists from 1981–87.

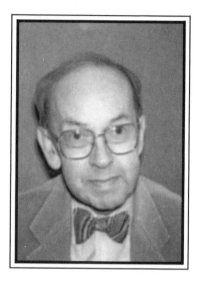

HF   You have described yourself as a late developer – as a psychiatrist and indeed as a doctor. Could you tell us something about your earlier life?

RC   I was born in Acocks Green, an unpretentious suburb of Birmingham, and lived there until I was 16, when the family home was blasted to pieces by one of Marshal Göring's landmines. I was fortunate in obtaining a scholarship to Solihull – a minor public school – which was remarkably good in many ways and rather appalling in others. I owe a lot to the place. Perhaps the only teacher who made any lasting impact on me was Margaret Noyes, one of two women appointed to meet the exigencies of Hitler's War, who did much to repair the depredations left by those earlier responsible for educating me and my luckless colleagues in music and the visual arts. Thanks to her, I was able to establish a love of music, which has been one of the outstanding pleasures of my life.

At the age of 16, when I took the School Certificate (now called GCSEs), I was interested in arts subjects – English Literature and Modern Languages. I had a lofty attitude to science, which was for the boors. But already, I was having long episodes of illness, which caused me to slip back three years in my school career. I spent long periods in hospital, with severe anaemia, which nearly killed me and was eventually cured by splenectomy. The doctors and medical students were all very friendly and in fact provided engaging seminars on my condition. I learned about reticulocytes and normoblasts, mast cells and differential counts, and picked up some rudimentary immunology. I became fascinated by the subject and also developed an enormous respect for medicine as a career, deciding to aim in that direction. But in my enfeebled state after the illness, I had some difficulty in changing tack and turning to physics, chemistry, biology and mathematics. I eventually obtained these higher certificates ('A' levels), but by that time, I was nearly 20. At the eleventh hour, I was rejected as a medical student because the authorities considered I wouldn't have the stamina. So I turned to zoology, which became my first love, academically speaking, and my first degree.

HF   Is there anything else about your early life or pre-university period that you would like to recall, or which you feel may have influenced you in your later career?

RC   Our family structure was a bit unusual, and perhaps illustrates my parents' approach to family planning. I had one brother and one sister, respectively 16 and 15 years older than myself. My arrival must have been a shock for all concerned. They were very decent about it, and I had quite an agreeable childhood. My father was a headmaster and my mother had qualified as a teacher at the turn of the century; two of her sisters and numerous other relatives did the same. My sister became a teacher, but my brother escaped, though even he married one. So I was brought up in a milieu where teaching was an unremitting topic of conversation, day in, day out. The strange and fearsome political and social events and alignments of the 1930s were also kept under review, and so was gardening – my father had a nice garden. It was a pleasant, sheltered, and essentially humdrum childhood, but by the age of 14, the health problems I have mentioned began to dominate my adolescence. In one of my several attacks of haemolytic anaemia, my haemoglobin went down to 18%, causing an episode of right hemiparesis and dysphasia, which gave me my first neurology lesson. It also alarmed me, and everybody else, more than somewhat. I recovered from that fairly quickly, with the help of blood transfusions. In those days (1940–41), there were no blood banks to speak of in civilian hospitals. So it became the duty of the unfortunate registrar, who shared my blood group, to become the donor. I remember him well, an extremely nice man named Christopher St Johnstone, who later became a consultant physician at the Queen Elizabeth in Birmingham – and sadly died prematurely – not from bloodlessness, thank goodness. His chief was Sir Leonard Gregory Parsons, FRS, an illustrious paediatrician and general physician. So my development was interrupted, but I met some fascinating people and the world seemed a generous and indulgent place, even though I was very aggravated by these recurrent illnesses.

HF   Could you tell us something about your time as a zoologist?

RC   I wasn't a very good one. Never having collected butterflies and moths or gone out fishing, I wasn't particularly competent as a natural historian. But I became interested in genetics and ecology, and in marine biology, spending some time in marine biological stations – at Millport in the Firth of Clyde, at Port Erin in the Isle of Man, and at the very famous one in Plymouth. In my final year, Lancelot Hogben, the head of department, returned from the War service. He was a remarkable man – displaying vast knowledge and enormous energy, sparkling originality and passion, debunking the conventional wisdom, all with a background of infectious enthusiasm laced with flashes of impatience and interludes of moroseness. With him, there were no dull days, but often some pretty testing ones. Recently engaged in developing medical statistics in the War Office, he was planning to exploit its powers and expose its follies more generally in medicine and biology. A most gifted teacher, he was very clear about the social and political implications of science, being for example a vociferous opponent of the then popular eugenics movement. Through him, I became more interested in human genetics and medical statistics, and in experimental biology. Later, I moved into his new department, and completed a PhD in Medical Statistics. At that stage, I found that though careers in biology or statistics had their attractions, I was still intrigued by medicine, and kept looking in that direction. Lancelot alleged that I was out of my mind, stormed at me, and tried very hard to dissuade me by offers of some fascinating jobs – in the end, though, he graciously accepted my refusal to take his advice, and our friendship lasted till the day he died.

HF   Is there anything about your first university career, your life as a BSc student, that you would like to recall?

RC   It was a curious time. I went to the University of Birmingham in 1944, at the age of 20, and of course most able-bodied men and a lot of women as well were doing their War service, so it was a very attenuated group of students and staff. I had had an instructive medical board for National Service, being required to stand naked in front of several ancient, whisky-sodden doctors, who staggered round me, and said they didn't think much of me. Therefore, I was graded Four – unfit for any form of National Service, which was all rather humiliating when most of my contemporaries were heading for accelerated maturation in the armed forces. But at least I started my university career then, instead of much later. It was, I suppose, like the university in pre-War years; we felt ourselves to be privileged and made the most of it. I did a bit of work as a reporter and later editor of the university newspaper and subsequently of a literary magazine. I can't remember that I worked very hard, but on graduating, I was fortunate enough to be awarded a University Research Scholarship, which enabled me to stay on without having to pay any postgraduate fees, which I didn't have the money for. So I did my PhD work on that scholarship, and later my own research grant, for 2½ years. It was then that I really learned the meaning of work and also something about research under Hogben.

HF   Were there other people who influenced you during your studies of biology?

RC   The acting head of department was Minnie Johnson, herself a gifted teacher. Her methods were informed by a great interest in social psychology and group dynamics, though that was all a bit lost on me at the time. She was an articulate person who could take a warm interest without being intrusive. Forbes Robertson, who has only recently retired from being the Head of Genetics at Aberdeen, was a very bright, amusing Scot, who gave a superb course in genetics. There was Michael Abercombie, married to Minnie Johnson, a man of great erudition, with enormous scientific flair and curiosity, who later became Director of the Strangeways Laboratory at Cambridge and a leading biologist of his generation. John Waterhouse, a Cambridge mathematician, was a most agreeable man and an excellent expositor of statistics as applied to biological and genetical work. To him in particular, and to the others, I owe a great deal. Later, I was also influenced by a man a bit younger than myself, Raymond Wrighton. He had achieved the heights in his mathematical studies at Cambridge, and worked in R. A. Fisher's department where he obtained the rather rarefied Diploma in Mathematical Statistics. He tried to teach me how to mistrust authority, but I lacked the mental power to follow him closely.

HF *I'd like to ask you now about your time as a medical student, which I think was also at Birmingham.*

RC   It was. First I had to persuade the school to admit me, and secondly I had to find the money. Neither of these were easy, and I was impeded by Charlie Smout, the Sub-Dean, who looked and behaved rather like a complacent churchman, authoritarian and ever on the look-out for sin and idleness. He considered I had already had my innings: with a first degree and a PhD, it was unfair that I should occupy a place in the medical school when some bright boy from King Edward's school down the road might be taking it. And, he said, working your way through medical school is out of the question. So your wishes can't be fulfilled for two separate, valid, and unalterable reasons, he concluded with relish. I was not the first, or last person to have trouble with his suburban outlook, but two people came to my rescue. The first was Sir Leonard Parsons, the Dean, who had known me since I was his patient, years earlier. I had an interesting encounter with the two men, in which Charlie's pugnacity was elegantly reformed. The second was Thomas McKeown, the Professor of Social Medicine, who offered a part-time research fellowship in his department, which would provide me with enough to live on. I have felt eternally grateful to those two men.

Having started, I found anatomy extraordinarily difficult – I couldn't remember things and I sometimes questioned the authority underlying some of the assertions we were expected to swallow. I managed to struggle through, but it was a humbling experience, because I wasn't nearly as good as the bright boys who had come straight from school, with their state scholarships. Once anatomy was over, I enjoyed reading medicine, though I didn't distinguish myself: I was occupied with other things which I thought I could do fairly well, such as medical statistics, research, and teaching. I graduated six months late, at the end of 1955, at which time I was 31.

HF *Presumably your extra years and the experiences you already had as a scientist must have given you a rather different outlook on the medical course, compared with the students around you. You said you questioned the anatomy teaching, which must be a very rare event. What other differences do you think there were in your approach to medicine from those of your colleagues?*

RC   It's not that I was so arrogant as to question the anatomical structures, but I felt upset by the naive biological assumptions about form and function. I had been trained to doubt. I enjoyed all the clinical work, but found some of the underpinning of clinical knowledge – much of the pathology, biochemistry, and microbiology – disjointed and uninspiring. As a result, my clinical work obviously suffered, but the general approach, the clinical reasoning which I was taught, I found congenial. The Professor of Medicine particularly interested me: Sir Melville Arnott had a most rigorous approach to clinical medicine, as well as a huge store of knowledge.

K

HF   What about your exposure to psychiatry during your time as a medical student?

RC   We weren't formally taught anything to speak of. There were a few visits to the local mental hospital with the Medical Superintendent, J. J. O'Reilly; his demonstrations carried conviction, but I don't think anything very much was conveyed, though he and his colleagues certainly did their best in limited time. There was also Myre Sim, in the teaching hospital; he tried to teach me something. In my year, there were precisely 100 students and at least 12 of us became psychiatrists, including Alwyn Lishman and Michael Rutter, later my colleagues at the Maudsley. I think this must have been the play of chance, because there was nothing to link the teaching we had with a wish to practise psychiatry, nor any common thread binding the 12 of us.

HF   Any other personalities you would like to recall from your student or early medical career?

RC   Tom McKeown's department had some talented people – Reg Record, Ron Lowe, and Brian MacMahon – each of whom later reached the top of the tree academically. They were extremely friendly and encouraging and taught me a great deal, not only about medicine. In Arnott's department, there were two excellent senior lecturers, Trevor Cooke and Ken Donald, as well as George Whitfield, who was a superb teacher; I was fortunate, when I graduated, to become one of two house physicians in the Medical Professorial Unit, and then a house surgeon in neurosurgery with Professor Brodie Hughes. He was a cultured and sceptical man and neurosurgery was, of course, a fascinating topic, having some relationship to what I hoped to do in the future.

HF   At the end of your pre-registration year, what did you decide to do next?

RC   In earlier years, while I was doing my PhD, I met another doctoral student, a medical graduate named Vera Norris. She was appointed to the Maudsley as a lecturer in medical statistics, about the time I became a medical student, and made a very considerable impact there. She wrote the first *Maudsley Monograph* and did a lot of work in collaboration with the medical staff. We were good friends and she was enthusiastic about the Maudsley; what she said attracted me greatly. When the time came for her to leave, to accompany her husband to Scotland, Aubrey Lewis, having heard that I had been reared in the same stable, was quite keen to meet me. This happened when I graduated, before my house jobs; it was the first of my fascinating encounters with him, and he invited me to take Vera Norris's job right away. He thought that having obtained a medical degree, I would be wasting my substance if I trained as a clinician and was rather keen that I should get on with developing medical statistics in relation to psychiatry as soon as possible. I resisted with some difficulty because, of course, I was very flattered by his offer. However, I wanted to become at least a registered medical practitioner, even if I decided not to train as a psychiatrist. Incidentally, Vera Norris died with a tragic illness, two or three years later, while still a young woman.

HF   Having resisted that flattering invitation and completed your year as a houseman, what did you do then?

RC   After two or three months completing some research, I went to the Maudsley as a senior house officer. I found it immensely rewarding, and became convinced that clinical psychiatry was the career for me. So I went through the training, and the consultants I was working with taught and inspired me – Felix Post, Kräupl Taylor, Michael Shepherd, and Edward Hare. In due course, I became a senior registrar. I had been encouraged by Aubrey Lewis to take the Conjoint DPM, which I could get more quickly, so that I could accept a lectureship. It was agreed between us that it should be a clinical lectureship, rather than one in medical statistics, and after I had completed my DPM, the plans were activated. I had been very careful to say that I wished for an honorary senior registrar post but, for reasons which were pretty complex, it turned out that Lewis wasn't able to manage that. So he told me that I would be a clinical assistant in out-patients, and I told him I would have to withdraw my acceptance of the job. We then had some rather frank meetings and correspondence, in which he told me I would be throwing away my career if I rejected the post I was being offered, but I said I wanted to be a clinician and therefore had to do what was necessary. Soon after, I was appointed as an NHS senior registrar and a little later achieved what I wanted – being appointed a clinical lecturer and honorary senior registrar.

HF   So it sounds as though Sir Aubrey's prognostication on that occasion was not very accurate – was it really important to stand up to him, and perhaps possess a strong personality of one's own on that sort of occasion?

RC   Well of course, people used to find Aubrey a rather awesome person, but I had been brought up in the school of Lancelot Hogben, who could be far more scorching than him. With Lancelot, the legend was that if you could last a year, nothing would destroy you. I never found Aubrey anything but charming and genial, although we did have the occasional brush. He thought on two occasions that I was making a great mistake with my career, but he later conceded that he had been wrong. There have been a great many panegyrics of course about him, but none I think has given the right emphasis to his sense of humour. As long as one wasn't intimidated by him, he was a delightful person, with an immense sense of fun; he could throw back his head and laugh and demonstrate a belief that one should be flippant only about serious topics. When in that vein, he was an entertaining, warm and friendly man.

HF   I must confess that I saw little evidence of any of these particular qualities that you're describing in my encounters with him. Can you say a little more about the personalities you were in contact with at the Maudsley or who taught you then?

RC   Felix Post, my first consultant, struck me from the beginning as a man with an impressively logical approach to clinical problems. It was a general psychiatric unit – he later specialised in old-age psychiatry, of course. To a beginner, his logic was compelling and he set high standards of clinical reasoning. He never failed to recognise the distinction between facts and suppositions, observations and conjectures. He emphasised the value of a detailed, objective examination of a person's mental state. So he taught me the basic stuff, and I have found myself going back to things that I learnt from him on many occasions. Then I worked for Kräupl Taylor, who some unfriendly people said was a psychotherapist who didn't believe in psychotherapy. That was a harsh judgement, not correct by any means. He was a superbly intelligent, able man, demanding of rigorous standards in his registrars. Case presentations never took less than an hour, and often at the end, he would indicate his disappointment that you had really said nothing of value. He was critical, fierce in some ways, but immensely engaging and again very logical. He assumed that you knew your psychopathology and was very fretful if he found you didn't. He argued that psychoanalytic technique was far more important than the content of its theory, so that you might use the techniques associated with transference and interpretation to the advantage of the patient, though you didn't have to accept the theory behind them. From that developed what was known as his challenge therapy – prokaletic psychotherapy – in which, on the basis of having established a good transference relationship with the patient – not an easy task – you were then able to challenge or encourage him or her, and offer interpretations of the subsequent response. The doctor's approval or disappointment had a strong meaning and effect, especially for someone with a personality disorder. It certainly helps the patient to reflect about his/her own feelings and assumptions, and this is potentially very important. Kräupl Taylor described it in detail in a paper in the *British Journal of Psychiatry (1968)*, but unfortunately, it is hardly ever referred to now.

HF   I can confirm what you said about Felix Post, because my own first placement was with him, but so far as Kräupl Taylor is concerned, do you think anything is left now of that rigorous intellectual tradition that he maintained?

RC   That question is very important and difficult to answer optimistically. A lot of that searching, critical, insightful approach to psychopathogenesis is a thing of yesterday. We now find a great emphasis, perhaps correctly, on descriptive psychopathology and phenomenology, which have recently come into their own, whereas psychoanalytic or dynamic psychopathology is very difficult to understand, unless your standpoint is that of a psychoanalyst. It's understandable only within its own terms. Beyond that, I would find it very difficult to think of any strand which measures up to the highly intellectual and at the same time ingenious approach that Kräupl Taylor practised.

HF   Does anybody now practise psychotherapy with the challenge as part of the technique?

RC   From time to time I make use of it myself, though not quite in the same rather stringent terms that Kräupl Taylor demanded. Any challenges I have employed in trying to help patients have been rather less overt than this. KT would emphasise that you had to establish a good working relationship with a patient before you start challenging him or her. However, this was too much to ask for some of my colleagues, and I do remember one trainee, now eminent, uttering a premature challenge to a woman with problems of emotional control, 'Now you're angry and I think you're going to throw that bottle of ink at me', whereupon his prediction was fulfilled and he acquired a new suit, courtesy of the House Governor (according to the theory, the patient should have denied being angry). Another story was that in the ultimate challenge situation, KT failed altogether. When a man pulled a gun on him in out-patients, instead of issuing the challenge, he rushed for the door and shouted for Sister Lawley! My belief is that it's a very difficult strand in psychotherapy, which calls for careful training. I don't know of anybody who works that way now.

HF   What about some of the others in your list?

RC   I learnt much from Michael Shepherd, and agree with others that he has an outstanding intellect. Edward Hare was a clinician with strong interest in the uses of epidemiology – he was one of this country's pioneers. His influence was great, though he had an idiosyncratic approach to clinical teaching, which at the very least taught one to examine one's own utterances critically. I never worked personally for Eliot Slater, but he was a very influential man at the Maudsley. At his case conference, he seemed to have a rather lofty attitude, but with a firm basis of experience and his feet very much on the ground. At the same time, he was a tremendous humanist and a man I admired greatly. A very different kind of psychiatrist was Denis Leigh, for whom I was senior registrar for a while. He was hard-headed and blunt, yet compassionate and highly successful in the market place. Douglas Bennett, who arrived at the Maudsley just as I was about to leave, was the first person who made me aware of the scope and future of community psychiatry.

HF   Would you like to summarise the essence of the Maudsley at that time in a few words?

RC   It was a University hospital in the best sense. The things one learnt were as much from one's peer group as from seniors. Some of the senior registrars were six or seven years ahead professionally, so there was a whole range of people with greater or less experience, talking and arguing in the common room. The set-up was superb as a place for learning a difficult subject; one could both obtain enormous help and support and have a very enjoyable and stimulating life. I looked forward to the days all through that period.

HF   I know that many people (including myself at times) experienced the downside of the institution. However, shall we go on to your next phase, at Birmingham?

RC   The downside became very apparent to me at a later stage in my career. Meantime, I was appointed as Senior Lecturer in Birmingham in 1962, six months after Bill Trethowan came to the Foundation Chair. He'd come from Sydney, where he had led an influential department, so he was an experienced professor, who earlier had known the Maudsley very well. I had mixed feelings, though, about leaving: one left behind one's own coterie and support system. I left the excitement of London for the relatively drab existence of Birmingham at that time, yet it was good to have more responsibility and to see an academic department shaping. It was hard work because in those days regional training schemes were non-existent and Bill was one of the pioneers in establishing organised training for senior registrars. I used to make parochial visits to all the mental hospitals in the Birmingham region, like a bishop's chaplain, and learnt quite a lot about what was going on in them. Earlier, I had been round many mental hospitals in my work for the MRC; so I came to have a pretty extensive view of mental hospital practice. I saw a lot of the better and the worse things about them. Many of the medical superintendents and other consultants in the hospitals were most interesting people, with great humanity. I can remember being impressed, though also sometimes baffled by many aspects of mental hospital practice that I witnessed.

HF   Could you give a few impressions of the mental hospital in the Birmingham region that you saw at that time, in the early 1960s?

RC   There was the Central Hospital at Warwick, at which the medical superintendent for a long time had been Edward Stern. It was known as 'Stern's Place' and a wit had said that the hospital was run by the Stern Gang. It was a large hospital in the most superb countryside of South Warwickshire, but obviously insanitary; years later, they had one of the most notable outbreaks of typhoid in recent times. Teddy Stern was highly authoritarian – the king of the whole creation. I think everybody there – staff and patients – saw themselves as in fealty to him in some way. One of his lieutenants, Clifford Tetlow, did quite a lot towards the evolution of the College from the RMPA, but I think the other consultants had their heads down so much that they weren't able to see what was going on around them. Stern was quite a scholar and wrote a few good historical papers; he reminded me a bit of Sir George Pickering, then Regius Professor of Medicine at Oxford. I think they were the same type of person, that one doesn't see in medicine so much now – tremendously authoritarian and having reached an exalted position, stubborn, with a benign mien, and unduly influential. They weren't people one would cross swords with. On the other hand, there was a hospital at Lichfield called Burntwood where Clegg, the medical superintendent, believed in including his consultants in all important decisions.

I think your question is really asking, though, what it availed for the patients. It was difficult to understand. At that time, extremes of psychopathology were the striking features of a walk through a mental hospital. There was a lot of established catatonia but also other very strange behaviours and emotional outbursts. I remember those phenomena as characteristic of much that I saw, though they're now much rarer, fortunately. As a visitor, it would have been unusual to have a coherent conversation with a patient, yet whenever I did try to do so, I was always a bit surprised by the amount of sanity which existed in even the most dishevelled or bizarre person. I don't think the lessons from that era have been fully learnt. For example, community care with inadequate provision must be pretty pathogenic, and there may still be a place for total care in a residential setting for a small number of mentally ill people. But have the rational principles for effective community care and modern treatment in institutions really been worked out? So often, they seem to be based on *a priori* assumptions rather than experience.

HF   Let me ask you what else has influenced you in becoming the kind of psychiatrist you are.

RC   From psychiatrists, there has always been opportunity to learn how *not* to do things as well as what to take as exemplary. I have learned a lot about techniques and styles from observing, not only my seniors, but also my contemporaries and juniors. There have been, of course, tremendous advances in the scientific disciplines and knowledge underlying psychiatry – the psychosocial and biomedical sciences – as well as impressive advances in clinical psychiatry itself. So it has become a clinical/academic subject of distinction, though the best people academically aren't always the best psychiatrists clinically. I don't wish to imply that high academic achievement necessarily rules out high clinical competence, but the association is by no means complete.

Often, I have met junior trainees and predicted to myself that this or that person is going to be a first-class psychiatrist, but I'm not sure what gives me this feeling of confidence. Knowledge of the scientific basis of psychiatry is absolutely essential, but by no means sufficient for high clinical competence.

HF *I think there is at least one special patient you might want to mention*

RC   There is one I can mention by name, because she has mentioned me by name in some of her writings, and that is Janet Frame, now a distinguished New Zealand writer and poet. Her autobiography, in three volumes, has been condensed into a very good film called *An Angel at my Table*. She was certainly a most amazing person to have as a patient. She had spent years in mental hospitals in New Zealand, and had seen the worst side of psychiatry. Consistently (and mistakenly) diagnosed as having chronic schizophrenia she had received more than 200 applications of ECT unmodified. But she survived this and remained a superbly intelligent, articulate, imaginative person, an original thinker, whose scope and confidence increased over the years. She has achieved many prizes, fellowships and honours. I was her registrar during a long admission to the Maudsley and I subsequently continued to see her and correspond with her, but I'm glad to say she needed no further psychiatric treatment. She was really quite ill but certainly did not have schizophrenia. She showed a most interesting interplay of original thought and imaginative awareness of her very rich inner experiences. She was a most instructive and rewarding patient, who publicly made generous (though not uncritical) attributions to myself and others, and to the Maudsley. She is in no way to blame for the fact that in the film, I was played by a New Zealand actor, whose name I can't remember but who seemed to take the view that I must have been a classy existential psychiatrist of the 1960s, with a shaggy beard and a rug over my shoulders, eating chocolates and drinking tea whilst talking to my patient. Fortunately I appear for no more than two minutes. I like recognition, but not of that sort.

HF *In the mid-1960s, you wrote a chapter with Thomas McKeown, on the balanced hospital community and psychiatry, for a book I was editing with Jim Farndale. It seemed at the time that this was a very important idea for the future development of hospitals, but somehow nothing much ever came of it.*

RC   This was Tom McKeown's idea. His vision was, as you say, called the 'balanced hospital community', and he applied it to the Queen Elizabeth Hospital site in Birmingham, where there was a lot of room for development, contiguous with a university campus. Tom's idea was that all hospital specialities should be represented on this site, through substantial building programmes, and that their structure and function should reflect the age-structure and the kinds of illness, acute and chronic, in the community. With that notion, there was another one – that hospital is only one phase of treatment for any disorder, and that the community services should be developed at the same time as the building of new hospitals. In this way, the whole campus would become a centre of operations for hospital and community work. He was always a bit vague about where general practice came into it, but this was in the days before the Royal College of General Practitioners. At that time, general practice was not a well organised specialty, and I think he failed to recognise that it would inevitably play a leading part in any comprehensive medical developments.

I was asked, while I was a lecturer at the Maudsley, if I would produce a project on the psychiatric component of the balanced hospital community. This entailed planning for services which included in-patient, day hospital, and out-patient care, as well as reaching out into the community, and which had to be multiprofessional and integrated as fully as possible with the other aspects of both hospital medicine and community services. I wrote several of the memoranda for that project, and I think it was at that time that you invited me to write a chapter for your book. But the idea didn't come to anything. If you go to the QE now, you will see an enormous development, with the new specialist hospitals and units and a post-graduate centre, and it's certainly an impressive group of buildings, but I think it has failed to exploit community links, or hospital care for the less severe acute illnesses, or the problems of chronic disabilities. Perhaps this was because there wasn't the necessary staffing and leadership from the community, and because the GPs remained very much outside the hospital centre. There were loopholes in the plan, although McKeown was a man of great originality and flair – a pioneer. But he wasn't close enough to the practice of any kind of clinical medicine to be able to deal with some of the very difficult aspects. What community services can do and what they can't do nowadays is, of course, a very live topic and a difficult problem to work out.

HF *In his later writings, McKeown played down the contribution that technical progress in medicine had made to the improvement of health, as opposed to the advantages that come from high standards of living. As someone who has been very much at the receiving end of technical medicine, would you accept his view? Was his balance of opinion right on the developments of medicine?*

RC   As one who owes his survival to high technologies, I have to say no! But I would certainly accept his point that a higher standard of living and improved public health measures did a great deal to eliminate infectious disease, reduce certain deficiency disorders, and therefore to prolong life. The arguments he produced are absolutely valid, but he didn't foresee any of what we now regard as the medical problems associated with a higher standard of living or with longer duration of life, or the consequences of high-technology medicine, or the effects of cultural shifts. Ischaemic heart disease, for instance, has become more prevalent because people are living longer, and perhaps also because some are living a sort of life which makes them particularly prone to that kind of disorder. This is one of many new public health problems of the present day. Longer survival and altered social mores are causes of different patterns of morbidity in the population. Disease does not disappear when conventional public health measures become standard, and when modern treatments become gradually available. This was believed when the NHS was introduced in 1948, but it now seems absurd. I think Tom got some of it right, but he missed some of the rather big tricks in the game.

HF *One of the main principles he expounded about hospital was that the structure should be flexible because needs would change and change quite quickly. Yet if one looks at the hospital buildings of the last 20 years, it seems that what has been done has, in fact, been quite the opposite. They are highly technical structures which are very difficult to change.*

RC   That is absolutely right. He wasn't able to foresee the technological revolution, if that's the right word, in medicine and nursing – the developments which require very expensive accommodation and staff and sometimes, as in intensive care units, expensive machinery. The idea of hospital architecture changing to represent functional change doesn't seem to have much said about it nowadays. You could mention mental hospital wards being converted into day hospitals, even the introduction of day surgery, but otherwise it's difficult to see how the structure should be reflected in the design or in planning for the future. Tom was associated with Llewelyn Davis, the architect; the whole of his department of architecture at University College at that time seemed to be dedicated to adapting structure to function. They used some of the biological models of growth such as could be found in D'Arcy Thompson's book *Growth & Form*, where you could use coordinate transformations to demonstrate how living things change in shape – their relative dimensions – as they get larger. It was a very interesting attempt at biological analogy, but I doubt whether it really has any pay-off in the foreseeable future.

HF   Let's go now to 1967, when you left Birmingham. What did you do next?

RC   I went back to the Maudsley as a consultant, and did a lot of clinical work during the following eight years. I had a unit in general psychiatry at the Maudsley and one at Bethlem, and also half of the psychogeriatric unit at Bethlem, which I shared with Felix Post, before Raymond Levy was appointed. I also became heavily involved in a certain amount of administration, and eventually became Chairman of the Medical Committee, a member of the Board of Governors, and so on. In those days, it was all transacted in a most gentlemanly fashion. It was before the managerial revolution, and I suppose still the sort of job it had been in the earlier days of Carlos Blacker, Brian Ackner, Denis Leigh, and Felix Post. I had a very satisfying eight years as a full-time consultant. When I returned to the Maudsley, Denis Hill had just been appointed to succeed Aubrey Lewis and he (Hill) was keen to involve some of the more junior consultants in teaching in his department. He appointed Alwyn Lishman and myself as First Assistants, with defined teaching responsibilities. That was all very satisfactory, but in the early 1970s, there was a move to establish a Chair of Psychiatry at King's College Hospital across the road. The institute was very interested in seeing this Chair established, but the process went through several stages, one of which revealed that King's didn't have enough money to do it, but said they might be able to pay for half of the total expenses of a small department. So in late 1974, it was settled that there would be a joint Chair and that two senior lecturers, a lecturer, and secretarial staff should be a joint responsibility. It was suggested that I might apply for the Chair. Of course, I had observed academic departments growing up elsewhere, and had really set my face against a return to the academic world, feeling that my line was to be a practising psychiatrist and post-graduate teacher. But rather to my surprise, when this joint Chair came up, I found myself interested by the unique opportunities it seemed to offer. So I applied and was appointed. I started in October, 1975 and then it was that I really began to know the meaning of trouble.

HF   In what way?

RC   The department at King's had been a small one in a general teaching hospital. It was called the Department of Psychological Medicine, and when I took office, the senior consultant explained that it was altogether superior to the Maudsley which was only a *mental hospital*. This was a department patients attended if they didn't want to go to a mental hospital, so that we saw more interesting cases – sensible people not lunatics – and practised a better standard of psychiatry. No mention was made of the fact that it was not at all representative in its clientele. This harked back to 1967, when the Maudsley had first taken responsibility for a district service. Before that, all the long-term patients who might otherwise have been admitted to King's or the Maudsley had gone to Cane Hill in Coulsdon, Surrey. The Maudsley's new district commitment meant that it would take responsibility for the acute management of patients living in the old London Borough of Camberwell, with a population of about 130,000. The other part of the Health District was in the Borough of Lambeth, with about 100,000 people. In 1967, that remained part of the responsibility of Cane Hill, but already it was recognised that King's too would shortly become responsible for its own district.

So I moved into a situation where a self-satisfied little hospital department regarded itself as very superior to the Maudsley, and relied on the out-of-town mental hospital for providing the bulk of the psychiatric services. The psychiatric beds at King's had dwindled to a token number – four – on the neurological unit. However, a consultant from Cane Hill, John Hutchinson, had just been appointed to King's, as a first step towards King's taking on a district commitment. I was also told on my first day by the senior consultant that I would get the support of everyone in the department, but must recognise that nobody would go anywhere on the coat-tails (sic) of the Maudsley. A stony silence answered my protest that I had been appointed to forge academic links between the two places and was in the business of trying to integrate, rather than compete. So I was not popular at King's, and on crossing the road back to the Maudsley, I found I was not at all popular there either. Wherever I turned, I was a quisling. My friends weren't particularly inclined to support what I was trying to do and were suspicious of my motives. Neither King's nor the Maudsley wanted any kind of integration (Denis Hill, Jim Birley and Tony Isaacs were exceptions at the Maudsley, along with Nicky Paine the House Governor; Steven Greer was the only exception at King's). The arguments were that integration for teaching and research must inevitably lead to joint development of services, so that for King's, the much-valued identity of the department would be lost. For the Maudsley, it would lead to a larger district commitment at the expense of funds, staff, and accommodation for the 'special' services for which it was rightly famed.

When I started at King's, I decided to adopt three major objectives, which would take perhaps three years to complete. Firstly, there should be a joint training scheme; there were about 70 registrars and senior registrars at the Maudsley and 12 at King's. Creating a joint rotational training scheme would bring King's, with its general hospital psychiatry component, into the Maudsley circuit. This I thought should take about a year; in the end, the prejudices (on both sides of the road), together with the institutional barriers (the Maudsley was a Special Health Authority and King's was at the time part of an Area Health Authority, under the aegis of the SE Thames Region), caused it to take nine years.

The second objective was to have medical students coming over to the Maudsley on a regular basis; I thought that might take a couple of years, but it took ten years of pleading, memoranda, committees, and clandestine meetings.

My third objective was to have a joint service, rather than two separately administered ones. This I thought might take a little longer than the others – say three years. In fact, it had not been achieved when I retired in 1989, after 14 years, despite help from a number of sources, including the Health Advisory Service. So my plans can hardly be said to have got off to a flying start.

I'd hoped, of course, that the Camberwell Register, which had been developed by John Wing's MRC Unit, could be expanded to include the East Lambeth population about to be served by King's, but my preliminary proposals for that arrangement were most unwelcome. My friends were not interested in any of my proposals. You mentioned the downside of the Maudsley, and for me this was it. I was very surprised and disappointed. In the course of time, I had a lot of moral support from King's and made a lot of friends there, but there was no new money for these developments. Yet they had to take place before the joint Department could function as it should, providing a comprehensive service for its own District and a basis for teaching and research in general hospital psychiatry, as part of the Maudsley/King's post-graduate training programme. It was certainly the unhappiest phase of my career. I still enjoyed clinical work, did a lot of post-graduate teaching at both the Maudsley and King's, and reorganised the undergraduate teaching. There were ways in which the Department was successful, but in what one might have thought the essential prerequisites, it was still grievously underdeveloped when I retired.

Of course an unsurmountable problem was the Maudsley's near-total preoccupation with its 'excellence'. The lesson is that the pursuit of 'excellence' is on all fours with elitism and isolationism – both enemies of progress. It has nothing to do with meeting the challenges and opportunities of the day. Therefore, the concern with 'excellence', as opposed to impeccable practice, awareness of context, and imaginative planning, can never succeed. The place had moved far from the Maudsley of Aubrey Lewis. As a result, in recent years the Maudsley has been forced to incorporate King's psychiatry, on very unfavourable terms.

HF   *We need to come now to one of your biggest areas of interest, which is your involvement in research. Of the many research areas you've been associated with, you said the first was human growth and development.*

RC   That was when I was a zoology student in my final year. Lancelot Hogben had designed a study and gathered a lot of data about human growth and development during the years from 10 to 16. The project was called Studies on Puberty, and my first assignment was to help with sorting and analysis of data for the first paper, which was on the qualitative changes during puberty. This was quite a complicated bit of analysis, my first venture into serious research, and as a reward for much labour, I was mentioned in a footnote.

That was the way things were done at that time: I was very proud of this acknowledgement.

The second study was on the quantitative aspects of puberty – the growth spurt, along different dimensions of the body. The analysis of these anthropometric data was the main content of my PhD thesis – my very own project. What was hitherto not well recognised was that there is differential growth at puberty, not at the same rate along different dimenisons of the body. For example, arm length and leg length don't increase at the same rate as height, while neck girth, shoulder girth and pelvic width don't change at the same rate, and so on. Not only was there variation between individuals, and different axes of the body, there were also striking contrasts between males and females. One was able to combine that with the previously published qualitative data and produce a sort of calendar of sexual maturation and its variations. The measurement principle I used was a development of a theory which Julian Huxley had made use of in animals – the 'allometric equation' – which is a way of relating growth along one dimension of growth along another. We were still in the era of desk calculators and Hollerith sorting machines, long before computers. So dozens of hours had to be spent, and careful thought had to be applied *before* setting out a detailed regression analysis rather than, as nowadays, afterwards. If you made what Bacon called a radical error in the first concoction, woe betide you, because you were liable to find you'd wasted three weeks' effort.

HF   The next one, I think, was pedigree analysis.

RC   That didn't occupy a very great deal of my time, but in those days, human genetics was at a relatively primitive stage. In that kind of genetics, a lot of the work is in the assignment of probabilities of particular family constellations, and thus making predictions regarding genetic mechanisms. It also provided the basis for an early form of genetic counselling.

HF   What about the work you did for the MRC?

RC   In about 1973, I was invited to be a member of the Project Grants Committee of the Medical Research Council's Neurosciences (Neurobiology & Mental Health) Board. An awful lot of the work was in basic sciences, but such projects as the MRC funded in clinical psychiatry also went through it. After about three years, I became Chairman and a member of the Board – the parent Committee. In due course, I became its Chairman, and a member of the Council itself. Those were interesting times, because they provided me with some rather high-powered seminars on a lot of subjects in neurobiology and basic medical sciences. It gave me an opportunity to affect developments in a very small way, and it opened my eyes to the range of basic sciences which might have a bearing on psychiatry. There was always a very large pile of documents to study before these meetings. I doubt whether this work really paid off in terms of the advancement of psychiatry at King's or the Maudsley, but that wasn't the object. I spent in all about eight to ten years with those activities with the MRC before I finally came to the end of my stint with the Council in 1981.

HF   It sounds like a good time to have left.

RC   That's absolutely right. The day had already arrived when many grant applications were highly rated and yet not funded, so that applicants naturally became very discouraged. The decisions and chances of success have become immensely more difficult in the last ten years.

HF   One study that might be a bit more controversial was the MRC randomised controlled trial of treatments of depressive illness.

RC   That was an earlier venture. The MRC had established the practice of multi-centre randomised controlled trials with streptomycin in tuberculosis, and in 1959, the hope was expressed by its Psychiatry Committee that the same method could be carried out on some of the newer treatments in psychiatry. The obvious candidates for this sort of process were the antidepressant drugs, since one needed to have an acute, time-limited condition. I was brought into this trial as an assistant, and it became my function to co-ordinate it and to carry out a good deal of the statistical analysis, during 1961–64. I usually spent a day a week in or around London attending to this.

   The first problem was to recruit patients for the trial. They had to be in-patients in psychiatric hospitals or units, suffering from clear-cut depressive illness according to closely-defined criteria. There were meetings of large numbers of consultants, the first of which I remember was held in the Westminster Public Baths, and the attempt was made to secure their co-operation. The next stage was for visits to the mental hospitals, nearly all by myself, in order to go over the detailed procedures and listen to the objections of some of the prospective participating consultants. In that way, I was able to visit pretty well every psychiatric unit in all the four London Regions and also in some of the hospitals in East Anglia, Cambridge, and Oxford. In due course, we collected enough patients for the trial, went through the procedures, obtained the data, analysed these, and presented the results to the Secretary of the Committee, Michael Shepherd. They were also presented to the main Committee, the Chairman of which was Sir George Pickering, who understood psychiatry as might a general physician. The paper was published in the *BMJ* in 1965. There were no names at the head of the paper but several, including my own, in a footnote. The results were that for moderate to severe depressive illness, the most effective of the treatments on trial was ECT, imipramine following a close second and thirdly, placebo and phenelzine, differing very little for that particular kind of illness in that setting. Naturally, there were many people who didn't find this result very palatable, and William Sargant was quite tireless in his attempts to discredit our methods. Nevertheless, the trial was accepted as at least the first plank in the modest edifice of multi-centre controlled studies of treatment in psychiatry in this country.

HF   Your conclusion about phenelzine was not that held by most clinicians who had used it. Do you think there might have been some problem about the dosage or the selection of patients?

RC   The selection of patients is a big limitation in any clinical trial, and this was no exception. We had to select patients with moderate-to-severe depressive illness, requiring admission to hospital, and for whom ECT could be a form of treatment. So they were pretty ill people, and yet of course, they had to be people who might start with no treatment other than a placebo. It was a restricted group, by no means representative of all depressive disorders. If we had been able to construct a stratified trial with more people and a wider range of illnesses, we might have seen some differentials according to the severity and type of disorder, and phenelzine might well have proved to be more effective than it was in our particular series of patients.

HF   I think your next project was an attempt at a randomised controlled trial for the assessment of psychotherapy?

RC   That was in 1969–70 and I think the first, last and only research collaboration between the Maudsley and the Tavistock. The question was – can you assess the efficacy of dynamic psychotherapy by a controlled trial? The answer, in a word, was no. Our feasibility study was worthwhile in demonstrating this. There were a number of reasons why the method proved to be inapplicable, one of which was the problem of choosing a suitable control treatment. People included in the trial had to be deemed by psychotherapists as likely to benefit from dynamic psychotherapy, but they had also to be seen as at risk of receiving a control treatment which included only supportive treatment. This put rather a strain on the psychotherapists who, for regrettable reasons, start off with the firm conviction that their treatment is effective and therefore necessary for some people. That selection factor meant that it was possible only to include a very small and atypical series of patients in the study. It wouldn't have done at all for the very expensive business of a randomised controlled trial with long-term follow-up. One other limitation was in the large number of criteria of change and improvement which would have been necessary, including not only those of descriptive psychopathology – the symptoms and social adjustment – but also dynamic variables. These were agreed upon only after very difficult arguments among the research group, and they were less easy to establish in a reliable fashion than were the more descriptive criteria. So our pilot study was successful, but the answer was negative.

HF   There were also some projects on psychiatry in general hospitals.

RC   That was when I went to King's. The first that I myself was involved in was with Geoffrey Lloyd, looking at psychiatric sequelae of myocardial infarction; he was at that time working in my department, and wrote several papers on the topic. In other projects, my main role was as an initiator or adviser, and subsequently as a person mentioned in footnotes. I've been mentioned in quite a lot of footnotes in my time. Unlike many professors, I believe that authorship of papers should be restricted to those who have done really substantial parts of the work.

HF   We should now come on to one of your most important areas of research – in connection with education and examinations. You were, of course, Chief Examiner for the College.

RC   I became Chief Examiner and Chairman of the Examinations Sub-Committee in 1981. That was when James Gibbons retired from that office, and it was already being promulgated that changes should be made to the examination. In fact, what was required was a root-and-branch revision of the whole thing, so as Chairman of the Examinations Sub-Committee, I became

Chairman of the Working Party for reviewing the examinations, and our work took nearly five years. We had a very good group of about eight people (including a representative of the Collegiate Trainees Committee), all of whom worked very hard on reviewing the previous examination, and possible modifications for the new one. We produced our report, which then had to go through the Court of Electors and the Council. It was accepted, and the new examination was phased in from 1986, over a five-year period to 1991. I think the examination is due for further review, which I hope may not have to be as radical as the last one. We continued to have the clinical as the central part of the examination, though steps were taken to improve the reliability and uniformity of standards. As far as multiple-choice questions were concerned, we agree that these were the best way of testing certain kinds of factual knowledge. So the MCQ was considerably revised, the MCQ bank was diversified and cleaned up, and certain rules were devised for setting MCQs and testing their performance. This provided opportunities to test reliability and validity. We set great store on the reliability of all other parts of the examination by introducing quite elaborate schemes for the training of examiners and monitoring the results.

The biggest change was in the distribution of the examination between the first and the second parts, because hitherto, the first part had been devoted to basic sciences and only after passing that did the average student get on to serious reading on clinical psychiatry. That was the wrong way round – too reminiscent of the traditional procedure in the undergraduate curriculum – and we introduced a clinical in the first part of the examination, together with an MCQ on clinical topics. The second part includes the basic sciences, as well as the more advanced assessment of clinical knowledge and skills. One other big change we made was in the essay paper. Previously, this had included questions inviting a display of factual knowledge, and it had been very difficult to obtain a reliable way of marking these, because there was so much muddle between factual knowledge and opinion, between reasoning and presentation, and so on, in the answers. So it was agreed that factual knowledge should be tested by the MCQ or the newly introduced Short Answer Questions (SAQ), while the essay would address a broader topic, the candidate being required to answer one question out of a choice of six. This would display the standard of their presentation, argument, and reasoning. Another change was in the oral examination in Part II. Previously, this had been a random collection of thoughts which came into the examiners' heads, which the candidate would be questioned about. We introduced the ruling that the viva would focus on very specific problems of managing patients, and that examiners would prepare themselves for this by having their own card index of about a couple of hundred case vignettes. We talked for a long time about having a second clinical, not based, as the main clinical had always been, mostly on hospital in-patients, but to include patients seen in general practice, out-patients, or in wards in a general hospital, with a wider range of psychiatric disorders. However, with 300–400 candidates twice a year, it would not have been possible to organise second clinicals in all the centres or to recruit suitable patients for them. So the oral on patient management problems was the nearest we could get to the second clinical examination in Part II.

HF As Chief Examiner, I would imagine you have had some experience of other higher examinations. How do you think this College compares with the others?

RC I feel very optimistic. The conjoint DPM changed very little from its traditional pattern. Several University departments have introduced master's degrees, usually with emphasis on research methods and a project – but these are supplementary to the MRCPsych, not substitutes. The Australasian College of Psychiatrists has a very good high-level examination (MRANZCP), including case books and advanced knowledge and experience, which differs from the MRCPsych in being an exit qualification. After passing it, the candidate looks for a consultant post. After passing the MRCPsych, a further three or four years higher (senior registrar) training is required. However, I am glad to know that steps are to be taken to harmonise the two. Among other specialities, the MRCP (UK) hasn't very substantially departed from its old form, but of course, it can be said to serve its purpose as an examination in general medicine. An examination in psychiatry should be very different, and I think we have got away from any stereotype we might have taken over from the MRCP. A nearer one for comparison might be the MRCGP, which is obviously immensely difficult to arrange, because of the diversity of general practitioners' work and the types of decisions they have to make. They have worked very hard on their examinations, and now they have a very well constructed one. I would be confident in saying that the MRCPsych is the most appropriate examination feasible for its subject in today's climate.

I mentioned that on the review Working Party, we had a member of the Collegiate Trainees Committee, who was responsible for finding out what the trainees thought about various issues. One thing which surprised me very much was that the trainees didn't want to have local examinations or rely on local assessments by consultants with whom they had worked. They wanted a central one, rather than to be assessed by their own tutors and teachers. I think that was an important principle, because it can so easily be argued that the exam should be based on local practice and cumulative performance, with either no test or only a simple one. Nevertheless, if such an arrangement might be introduced some time in the future, it is likely that standards would vary considerably from one locality to another.

HF As an individual, you have perhaps experienced being something of a surgical battlefield and you have had long periods of illness, from your adolescence onwards. Do you think this has influenced your general outlook in the way you practise medicine?

RC It must have done. I've mentioned the long period in hospital in my adolescence. In later years, I had a connected series of misfortunes. I had a partial gastrectomy of the Polya type when I was 33. Ten years later, I had to have my gall bladder removed and that became complicated by the scarring round the blind loop of the duodenum, left by the gastrectomy. Although my surgeon could not have been more eminent in his field, he told me it had been a long and difficult operation and he believed he had left a stone behind. But I remained very well until, ten years later, he was proved correct when I had an obstructed pancreatic duct and acute pancreatitis, pancreatic abscess, pseudocyst, subphrenic abscess, and empyema – a whole lot of nasty things which kept me in hospital for more than six months. Some people write books during their illnesses, but I was never able to concentrate my mind for that. However, I've had plenty of opportunity to observe doctors, nurses, and patients, and I suppose I learnt a lot from my experience, though so far, I haven't experienced the psychiatric battlefield. I have probably become rather sensitive about what is good and bad practice in doctoring and nursing, but I don't know how my ideas can be generalised or how they might have affected my own practice. One learns something about oneself from being a patient, but perhaps not a great deal about how to practise medicine.

HF   One of the subjects you've thought about is team work in psychiatry. Where do you feel that has got to at present?

RC   I think psychiatric practice has reached the point at which it is recognised that at its best, it's a multiprofessional affair, so that the psychiatrist works best in association with a team of people. These include the psychiatric nurse, who is now much more than a handmaiden, the social worker, the clinical psychologist, occupational therapist, and specialists in rehabilitation. A psychiatric service of the best kind would be one in which all those people work together in assessment, management, and prognosis – identifying a patient's needs and doing as much as they can in meeting those needs. This means that they make decisions jointly, as well as practise in harmony with each other. I think that trend is one that many psychiatrists would agree with, as a most desirable move away from the hegemony of the psychiatrist in the management of mental illness. However, the trend has been rather tripped up by the fact that the other professions are now developing not only technically, and in their training and career structure, but also a need to go it alone and to be in competition with each other. The result is that social workers, for example, sometimes only very reluctantly work with psychiatrists; psychiatric nurses, if they are community nurses, may prefer to work with general practitioners rather than psychiatrists; clinical psychologists often compete rather than collaborate with psychiatrists, and the whole aspiration for team-work has tended to be thwarted. I feel sad that the opportunities for team-work have diminished because of this fragmentation.

HF   What can be done about it?

RC   I would like to see some policy discussions at the highest level. Perhaps the College should talk about this with the other professions, in order to establish something like a code of multidisciplinary practice, emphasising the duties rather than the 'rights' of each profession. It would be a code for multi-professional division of labour and collaboration in the interests of the patient or client, and, although one could foresee difficulties in agreeing details, it shouldn't be a hopeless task. Otherwise, we are going to continue to have a position where there's a lot of repetitiveness and fragmentation, rather than integrated effort. And that means a lot of wasted time, energy, and resources. It may also mean that a lot of the really important clinical decisions will be made by managers rather than practitioners, of whatever kind.

HF   You are preparing a lecture, I believe, on 'Is psychiatry more than a science?' Is it?

RC   It was a title I chose myself, and I have some misgivings about it. Psychiatry is very clearly based on the biomedical and psychosocial sciences.

There's no doubt about psychiatry's scientific basis and about the huge advances that have been made in recent years, so it can certainly be dignified by being called an advancing clinical scientific discipline. However, I do believe there's significantly more to psychiatric practice than science. What that extra is, though, I find difficult to characterise. But it seems to me important that somebody should be thinking about this.

HF   Can you take it any further at this stage?

RC   It's often said, of course, that medicine itself is an art as well as a science; that is rather obviously true. I believe, though, that in psychiatry, the non-science component – the X factor – is bigger than and different from what it is in the rest of medicine. Some people would claim that this X factor can be understood only by recourse to psychoanalysis. I strongly dispute that. I suspect it can be defined as something more primary, more basic to human experience than psychoanalysis, which is a relatively late invention. There are those who would say that the X factor – if it is admissible to concretise it for the purpose of this argument – is that aspect of psychiatry which belongs to the humanities. I can see the point of that argument, but I think it should be taken further. For the sake of our understanding of mental illness and its management, I hope somebody will be able to crystallise it one day, and I believe it will remain outside the purview of science.

HF   In passing, you mentioned psychoanalysis in relation to psychiatry. It has been said that psychoanalysis is not so much a doctrine or body of theory, but more a climate of opinion – something which is now an integral part of our culture. Would you accept that view?

RC   Certainly. Whatever role psychoanalysis may have as a treatment in itself or in the general run of psychiatric problems, it's fundamentally a way of looking at human experience – a viewpoint which has become assimilated into our culture. Perhaps its importance to psychiatric disorder is small, compared with its significance in cultural and social anthropological studies and in the imaginative literature of successive periods of human history. Aside from that, though, it is sad that within psychiatry, even nowadays, there is so much antagonism between those whose practice is based on psychoanalysis (exemplified by the Tavistock Clinic) and those who forswear it, believing it to be extinct (exemplified by those who base their practice on neuroscience alone). The dogmatism, on both sides, horrifies me. Perhaps the majority of psychiatrists are sensible people who occupy the middle ground and sometimes admit to uncertainty. I fervently hope this is the case.

18 Jozé Jancar

Interviewed by HUGH FREEMAN (1992)

Dr Jozé Jancar, MB, Bch, BAO (NUI) 1952, DPM (NUI) 1955, FRCPsych (Foundation) 1971, Hon FRCPsych 1988. Dr Jancar was born in Slovenia in 1920. He was a student at Ljubljana, Graz, Galway, Dublin and Bristol Universities. He was taken to a concentration camp in 1942 during the Italian occupation of his country and after the war he and his wife went to Austria. They came to England in 1948 and he became a nurse of the mentally handicapped at Hortham. In 1961 he became a consultant psychiatrist at Stoke Park Hospital. He won the Burden Research Gold Medal and Prize for research in mental handicap in 1971. From 1979–1983 he was Chairman of the Mental Deficiency Section of the College and was Vice-President of the College from 1981–1983. He is the author of *Stoke Park Studies – Mental Subnormality* (1961) and co-author of *Clinical Pathology in Mental Retardation* (1968).

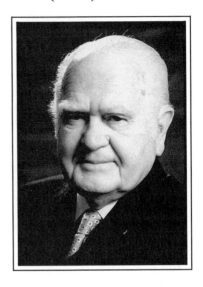

HF Your early life, I think, was very different from most of the people who have been interviewed previously for the Bulletin. Could you tell me something about it?

JJ   As you know, I was born in Slovenia. I had a very happy childhood and young adult life until 1941. I attended a grammar school, called the Real Gymnasium in Ljubljana. I travelled by train to the city every morning from my home in a village nearby. I earned my keep by helping other pupils who were not doing so well at school. I became head boy and received quite a few prizes, but the most exciting thing was when I was invited by King Peter, with the other 40 best pupils in Yugoslavia, to stay with him for a week in Belgrade, at his White Court.

HF Could you tell us a little more about your experience of going to the Palace in Belgrade, because this must be a very unusual experience for a psychiatrist?

JJ   When we were told that we were going, the grammar school where I attended made sure that we were smartly dressed; they gave us each a new suit and new shoes. Then, the Court sent a royal railway carriage to Ljubljana and five of us, with a Professor, went in this, attached to the Belgrade train. When we came to Zagreb, the Croatian contingent came on. As you know, Yugoslavia was then divided into eight provinces, and from each, the five best pupils had been selected. When we arrived at the special station in Belgrade for the royal train, we were taken to a hall, where each of us was fitted out with a Crombie overcoat. Each of us was then allocated to a boy from Belgrade, who was our own age and also one of the best pupils. It was an honour for him to receive one of us in his home. I was taken to the home of my host, whose father owned an insecticide factory.

The next day, we went to the Court, where we met the King for the first time, and there I also met, for the first time, an English nanny. We each received a silver and gold medallion of Peter II. We visited the grave of King Peter's father in Oplenac, went to the theatre one day, to the Mint, and to the Airport to see the first German Junkers passenger plane. However, every night, we went to the Court to visit the King, where we were received and had a meal with the Marshall of the Court. The final day was the day of 'Materice', which is a Serbian custom where the mother of the family has to give something to each member: it is like a Mother's Day in reverse. At the Palace, there was an international assembly of ambassadors to the Court, and it was a really beautiful evening, with Court music and presents from the Queen Mother. The Press had been with us all along, and Fox Movietone News were filming it all. Everybody had a few drinks, including me, and then, suddenly, the Marshall of the Court came along to our Professor. He said one of the Slovenes had to thank the King, as well as one of the Croats and one of the Serbs. Our Professor came over to me with a bunch of carnations, which is a Slovene flower and told me I had to give them to the King, and give the vote of thanks. I said I wasn't prepared for it, but he said I had to do it. The next day, I read my speech in the newspaper '*Politika*' and it seemed to be quite good, but I don't remember having given it! Next morning, we were saying goodbye to everybody, went to the train, and came home. It was a fantastic experience.

During the summer, I travelled a lot, learning about people and life; I cycled along the Dalmation Coast and in late summer I used to climb, as well as participating in athletics and winter sports. Unfortunately, when I matriculated and started medicine in Ljubljana, the War began in the spring of 1941, and we were occupied by the Italians. They let us study for about two years, and then the university was closed. We students were helping in various hospital departments; I was working in the Eye Department with the famous Professor Jevše, who had an international reputation; he was very encouraging to young people. Unfortunately, I was taken to a concentration camp in Gonars in 1942, and when Italy collapsed in 1943, the Germans occupied us. Once again, we were working with the Underground, helping in hospitals and treating people who had been involved in fighting against the Nazis, the Communists, and the Fascists.

HF   How do you think your wartime experiences affected you later in life?

JJ   They taught me a lot about psychiatry, particularly in the concentration camp, when men's masks dropped, and you see each man as he really is. There were both University professors and road sweepers who were most helpful and real people; while others, without their masks, weren't really the people we had been seeing before. I spent a week in the death cell at Ljubljana. When I was arrested, they said that if any Italian was shot outside, they would take people from our cell to shoot them.

HF   You were hostages?

JJ   Yes; it seems unbelievable, but we became stoically indifferent. They would come at 4 a.m. and call out names; these people would be taken out, and we just put names on the wall and went to sleep. Everybody who walked out neither cried nor swore – just defiantly walked out.

When we were being taken to the camp, they chained us together and put us in cattle trucks. We sang on our way to a concentration camp because we were out of the death cells. At St George's Station, near Gonars, we were thirsty and you know how the railway engines used to be fed with water; we put our hands out to catch some of this water, but the soldiers beat us back – wouldn't allow it. When we were walking towards the camp, people spat at us, and called us 'Banditi'. Yet, two years ago, I went to visit Gonars and I met the people there; they were so nice! We went to see the memorial to the people who died in camp and it is very well kept. I said to myself, how can man be so incited, for religion, for politics, or for nationality to do such cruel things? This was a great school of experience for me – one which I don't want anybody to repeat or go through, but I learnt a lot from it.

HF   *I believe that when you got out of the concentration camp at Gonars it was through the intervention of the Vatican. Is that right?*

JJ   That is correct. Our Bishop from Ljubljana intervened through the Vatican to release the Slovene students, and pressure was brought on the Duce – Mussolini – and we got free.

HF   *What happened next?*

JJ   At the end of the War, I went to Austria as an anticommunist refugee, where we were in camps, hoping that one day, we would be able to restart our studies. Unfortunately, the three Austrian Universities were in the wrong places: Innsbruck was under the French and Vienna and Graz under the Russians, so we had no hope of going to any of these.

HF   *How did you manage to continue your studies?*

JJ   We had a great friend, John Corellis, who was working for UNRRA, and with his help, I was able to go illegally across the Dolomites to Padua, in August, 1945, but if I had been caught, I would have had to deny that we knew each other, or we would both have been in serious trouble. There, I met a Jesuit priest, whom I knew from Ljubljana, and I asked him if he would arrange an interview with the Rector of the University. I brought with me all I had salvaged, which was my University documents. He was a very charming man, and asked me what kind of curriculum we had had. When I told him that we had been occupied by the Italians, he said this curriculum was according to Italian law, and he smiled and said, 'Right, I will accept you, and your wife and sister', but I added that there were about 80 others. He replied, 'All right, anyone who can produce a document from Ljubljana University will be accepted, providing they find their own money and accommodation'. However, when I came back, the Russians had left Graz. It was much easier for us to study there because, Slovenia being such a small nation, we couldn't produce our own medical textbooks, and so we used German ones. It was terribly difficult to find anywhere to stay there, because there were thousands and thousands of refugees. I met Captain Ryder, who was chief of that sector for UNRRA, and he was very sympathetic. We went round and round Graz, to see if there was any place that could accommodate students, and found the 'Keppler Schule', an empty grammar school, and we moved into it just before Christmas. There were some difficulties in acceptance of some students because their documents were missing, and denazification was taking place. Luckily, I had documents stating that I was in the Gonars concentration camp, which helped, and that I was representing the Slovene students in Graz. Also, the Dean was of Slovene origin, and when we were on our own, he started to talk to me in our language, which was a great relief to me, and he was then very helpful. Soon after, we were moved into ex-German barracks, and were able to start studying, but life was hard. The first Christmas, we had only about 600 calories per day – a bit of soup with cabbage in it. Then a young lady came along – Iris Murdoch, a student herself. She was deputy director in the refugee camp, and we became very friendly; she is the godmother to my daughter and we are regularly in touch.

When I was in the final year, we had to do three weeks' residency in the neuropsychiatric department. The regular Professor had left through denazification, and they had recalled Professor De Gasperi, who was nearly 90 years of age. He was a contemporary of Adler, Jung, and Freud, but didn't belong to any of these three schools; he was independent. He said to us, 'Psychiatry has a great future, providing you remain a doctor first, then a neuropsychiatrist. You have to examine each patient carefully because he has both a mind and a body, and you have to know which is affecting which'. He was a really excellent lecturer, and I got so involved there and then, I decided to do psychiatry.

HF   When did you come to England?

JJ   In 1948. We landed in West Wrating, near Cambridge and again, Iris Murdoch was there, as an undergraduate, and she was very anxious that I should restart my medical studies. She took me to London to meet the Duchess of Atholl. I was very impressed to meet a Duchess for the first time; she spoke very good German, as well as French. Of course, I didn't have any English then. She said, 'If you go away for a year somewhere to learn English, then we will be able to get a place for you either at Oxford or Cambridge'. But I had come to England as a European Voluntary Worker, and there were only two places to go – either mines or agriculture. I had to get out of those, though, if I was going to be able to continue medicine. One day an ex-Indian Army Sergeant Major came along, looking for someone to act as a male nurse in the YMCA Camp at Gloucester. I went there, but there was really nothing to do, because they were all healthy people. They spoke every language from Europe except English, so I didn't learn any English, and I was getting quite frustrated.

I went into Gloucester one day, looking for a Catholic Church, hoping that somebody would know some language other than English. There was in fact a young priest who spoke Italian, and I asked him if I could get a job as a nurse in Gloucester. He said, 'No, it is impossible', but he added, 'I know a doctor near Bristol who is in charge of mentally handicapped people; would you like to work with them?' I said of course I would, because I wanted to do psychiatry. One day he collected me, and we went to see Dr Lyons at Hortham Hospital near Bristol, where he was the medical superintendent. This was the longest interview I have had in my career; it took nearly three hours. What he wanted to know was all about the War and what had been happening in Europe; his wife knew a bit of German and the priest translated into Italian.

Then he said, 'I'll take you, providing that you don't wear the clothes you're wearing now' – because I went in my best suit – 'that you are kind to the patients, and that you learn the English measures of medicine'. These were the three conditions, and I was appointed to the highest possible grade, which was nursing assistant Grade I.

When we finished the interview, I asked him if he could also give a job to my wife. He asked, 'Does she speak better English than you?'. I said she did, she had learnt English in Graz, when she was a medical student. He accepted us. When I had been there for over a year, he called me into the office one day and said, 'Now, you are finished here', and I was worried because I thought I had got the sack. 'No', he said 'you are going to be all right. You have learnt enough about mental handicap, but you will need a lot of terminology in English and Latin, so you must go to a general hospital'. I went to BRI where I worked for over a year. I was rotated through every department, on both day and night duty, so that I had really great experience. I came to think that every medical student should have at least six months working as a nurse. When I became a doctor, I was able to ask nurses what I knew they could do and also criticise what I knew they were doing wrong. Meanwhile I wrote for admission to all Universities in England and Ireland. Bristol were willing to accept me, but I would have had to wait two years, because there were so many ex-servicemen, who had priority. However, I got very friendly with Professor Darling, who was in charge of the Dental Department, where I was nursing his patients. He said to me, 'Would you like to do dentistry?', and I said I would; I had given up hope of doing medicine. He arranged an interview with the Professor from Newcastle. He accepted three years of my medical studies, with some extra time to qualify as a dentist.

Just then, a letter arrived from Professor Shea, who was Dean at Galway, and he offered me a place there. This was in January, and he said could I come as soon as possible, so that I wouldn't miss the term. Of course, I had to get a visa, and somebody had to give a guarantee for me. My wife and I were able to save some money, and with the help of friends, I managed to scrape together enough for the journey, and off I went to Ireland. There, the Rector asked me if I had means to support myself; I said yes, and I started, but it was very hard work. I remember reading Boyd for the first time, until about 3 o'clock in the morning; I had only got through about 20 pages. I realised how much English I lacked and I went to Professor Kennedy and asked if I could do my exams in October, but he said I should do them in June. He told me he had studied in Heidelberg, and agreed that what I didn't know in English, I could do in German. We had to do philosophy and psychology, for which we had a Franciscan priest as Professor. I went to see him and told him about my diffi-culties with English. He said, 'Are you a Latin scholar?'. When I said, 'Yes', he told me that what I didn't know in English, I could put in Latin, and this would be acceptable. This was another encouragement, but then came a crisis.

I remember so vividly that it was St Patrick's Day when I walked along Galway Bay wondering what to do next. My landlady was asking me for money, and I owed her two weeks' rent already. I thought the best thing would be for me to go to the Police and ask them to deport me. I didn't know anybody to borrow money from, and there seemed to be nothing else I could do. The next day, Iris Murdoch sent me £100, and this saw me through. At that time, all Galway students had to go for their final year to Dublin. This was really important to broaden our knowledge. There are three medical schools there and one examining body, each with their own professors and hospitals. We Galway people could travel round them, and we found out from the Dublin students which were the best in the various specialities. We made our own timetables, and the standards were very high, the schools were competing and the senior professors had all had experience in Europe, England or America. One course in particular I enjoyed very much was obstetrics and gynaecology, and I became very friendly with the Master. When I was leaving, he called me in and asked what my plans were when I qualified. I said, 'I am going into psychiatry' and he said, 'You are wasting your time'. He offered to appoint me as Assistant Master, which at that time was a big job. I thanked him, but let him know later on that I would stick to psychiatry.

At that time, there were quite a few hospitals in Dublin at which you could train for the DPM. I had my wife and daughter in Bristol, and I had to find a secure job, somewhere. I went to Grangegorman and other hospitals, but all the junior posts were booked. There were a lot of graduates from Dublin, and I had come from Galway. They advised me to try Ballinasloe, where I obtained a job. It was a 2,000-bed hospital and McCarthy was the superintendent; incidentally, he was also a co-editor of the *Journal of Mental Science*. He had worked in Canada with Banting and was a very brilliant man. When I had been there for about a fortnight, he had a heart attack and died. His deputy was Jack Delaney, who was a great character, and a good psychiatrist.

A lot of people are saying today that mentally handicapped people should be having the same service as people with psychiatric disorders, but I saw the tragedy of this at Ballinasloe; severely mentally handicapped patients were placed with chronic schizophrenics, and the mildly subnormal with acute cases. They were badly treated by the patients, and nurses didn't know how to deal with them. I think this is the biggest mistake people can make if they are trying to develop 'generic' services; I witnessed that it doesn't work.

HF   They had no special services for the mentally handicapped?

JJ   In 1950 they were poorly developed. However, I have visited and lectured in West of Ireland more recently, and they have developed very good services now.

After some time in Ballinasloe, I felt I was so tired of books that I wouldn't attempt any other qualifications; it had been such hard work, struggling to get my degree. However, a new medical superintendent was appointed, Dr Shea – the brother of the Dean who had accepted me. He said, 'Look, you have to get your DPM, or there is no future for you. You will always be junior'. So I started again, but the requirement for the DPM then was that either you passed the lot, or if you failed any part, you failed it all. It was very hard, and there was no time off and no tutorials; I had to take my exams in my study leave.

HF   What happened after the DPM?

JJ   I thought I was lacking in medical experience, and I went straight to the Mercers Hospital in Dublin where I had been a student, and asked if I could have a place there. They offered me a post as a senior house physician, and I spent a very happy year there. After a few months, they called me to the Board Room, and I was quite worried as to whether I had done anything wrong. There was a colonel, ex-British army, who was the Chairman, and he said to me that they were watching my progress, and would I be happy to accept the post of Registrar, being in charge of the hospital? Nobody was actually running it then. There were students and junior doctors, and the senior staff were coming and going, but there was no organisation.

As Registrar I organised both the students and the housemen, so that every consultant had a student and a junior doctor. Unexpectedly I had a call from Dr Lyons in Bristol, who asked me to come and see him. I went, and he said, 'If you want to succeed, you must come back to England and prove that you are capable of doing the job'. So on 15 May 1956, I came for an interview at Stoke Park, and met a tall doctor called Alan Heaton-Ward, who was the medical superintendent. There were five people with the DPM for one JHMO position. After we had been interviewed, I was told I had got the job. Just before I left Ballinasloe, Dr Shea produced a book, and said, 'Read this, and you will see where you are going; how lucky you are. It is a very famous hospital'. It was the first *Stoke Park Studies* by Professor Berry, so I was very apprehensive when I arrived to start my career at Stoke Park and in Bristol.

HF   What were your first impressions of England?

JJ   When I came to Cambridge, I found the English countryside very flat. Of course I had come from Slovenia, which is a mountainous country and the part I came from had nice valleys and fields. Also, they were talking in a language which I couldn't understand at all, though I knew German, French and Italian – as well as my own Slovene tongue. In England I saw this cool, calm, Nordic type of a man or woman, who wouldn't give much away, but when he or she knew you, a real friendship would develop.

HF   What were your impressions of Ireland at first?

JJ   Mixed feelings – I met people in England who had very little good to say about Ireland, and I met people there who had very little good to say about England. I began to see that both sides had some justifications but what impressed me was that there was a new generation of people in Ireland who did not want to talk about the troubles in the 1920s. They wanted to build a new Ireland. When I was at Mercers, which was a Protestant Hospital, there were many Catholic people in it; I am a Catholic myself, and they knew that, but nobody held that against me. At the same time, the Lord Mayor was a Jew. This tolerance is something we are all striving for. I was also impressed with the medical teachers in Ireland.

HF   Shall we talk now about your early work in Stoke Park in the 1950s and 1960s?

JJ   I was very fortunate. Alan Heaton-Ward was really a very good colleague to me: he gave me freedom to develop my work. There was a very congenial atmosphere in the hospital. The medical superintendent, Matron, and Hospital Secretary were like a family. They knew every patient and every problem with the staff, and they were respected. I worked hard because I knew I had to prove myself, and we also used to work most Saturdays and weekends. I was also very fortunate that Professor Berry, who was 90, was still in Bristol, as were Ronald Norman and Fraser Roberts. Dr Norman was an authority on neuropathology, and Fraser was an outstanding geneticist. They were both very kind to me and very encouraging. The other person who interested me very much was Grey Walter, like Golla, he was a very difficult man to get near to, but he was very helpful to me. I could go to him with any neurophysiological problem of the cases that I had. I was therefore very lucky to be in this milieu. From the psychiatric point of view, one of the greatest researchers at that time, was Professor Golla, at the Burden Institute.

Because of this grounding, I was able to move then towards other departments at Frenchay General Hospital for help. They became interested in the field of mental handicap; as I was asking things which they didn't know, they had to search for them, and become involved. There was Frank Lewis at Southmead Hospital who started to study the chromosomes of our patients and became internationally renowned. I was, if you like, a catalyst to them, and we developed a service which I thought was second-to-none. My patients had priority before normal people for outside consultants. I think that it is a tragedy that anti-doctor, anti-psychiatric and anti-hospital people have become so influential in this field. I was also very lucky to have two great tutors in Penrose, who was the greatest man in the country in mental handicap, and Dent, who came to see me often.

HF   Could you say something about those two, Penrose and Dent?

JJ   At first, there was a little tension between Stoke Park and people from other centres, particularly Penrose. Here was the first multidisciplinary centre in the world for the subject, and he was a single-handed man. But when he realised what we were trying to do, he became very helpful. I had a huge correspondence with him about rare cases. He was a man for all seasons – calculus, or genetics, or even psychiatry; his Maudsley Lecture was an example of this, and the message was that mental handicap is the basis for future research in psychiatry. Dent was a biochemist, and was very anxious to find out more about this aspect of mental handicap. He examined hundreds of specimens from our patients.

HF   How were you involved in the development of services?

JJ   In the 1970s, when there were various enquiries up and down the country about bad buildings and overcrowding in mental handicap hospitals, Heaton-Ward and myself were telling Ministers that we could not provide a good service if we didn't have money and facilities. However, the question of community care was creeping in already, and we had great difficulty in persuading the Department to give us permission to pull down old buildings and create small units. We persevered and eventually succeeded; we totally rebuilt both Purdown and Stoke Park Hospitals. What we achieved were specialised units for spastics, for the blind, for psychotics, and for the elderly; the last one was the first purpose-built unit for the elderly handicapped, which is an important issue at the moment. We also provided a unit for disturbed patients and an assessment unit. At case conferences in the community, we noticed that certain patients needed further assessment, so we admitted them to this special unit where all the professionals involved, both from within the hospital and outside, could be called in to make their contribution.

We also opened two clinics in Bristol and one in Gloucester where parents and other relatives could come with patients, and we were able to help and advise them. I feel whatever the future holds, we should never forget that in our service, the hospital is part of the community. Community care is great, providing that you give people the same quality of service as we gave.

HF   Tell me about your work for the College.

JJ   Those were very interesting times. I was groomed for Chairmanship of the Mental Handicap Section by two old friends, Alec Shapiro and Alan Heaton-Ward, who were Secretary and Chairman. They planned for Valerie Cowie and myself to follow in their footsteps, and we did. What was exciting in the RMPA time was the battle to improve the Section for Mental Handicap – what was then called 'mental deficiency' – and support for this did not come either from the Department or from the RMPA itself. It was difficult, but we had help with good leadership, particularly from Alec Shapiro, though he was too strong-willed for some people.

HF   He once described me as a 'self-appointed pseudo-expert', in a letter to The Lancet, because I had expressed some views on mental handicap, but we afterwards became very friendly.

JJ   Yes, he could be difficult, but he had a vision and he was the one who, with Harvey Stephens, an American, created the International Association for the Scientific Study of Mental Deficiency, which now has an international congress every three or four years. Its preliminary meeting was in London in 1961, and then the organisation was formed in Copenhagen four years later. It now awards a special Stephens & Shapiro Prize.

My Chairmanship of the Section was at a very difficult period – one of the hardest times at the College. I was at the same time Vice-President. The President, Ken Rawnsley, was very ill, Gerald Timbury, the Registrar, had a stroke, and Natalie Cobbing, the College Secretary, was failing in her health. There was the 1983 Mental Health Act and also the battle over Russian expulsion from the World Psychiatric Association, which was really spearheaded from the College. I used to go to see Ken Rawnsley in hospital, and he was very supportive. The junior Vice-President, Michael Gelder, and other senior members of the College were also very helpful.

The hardest was the battle over the Mental Health Act at that time; the anti-psychiatry and anti-hospital lobby was very much in the forefront. If it hadn't been for the College, we would have had a very poor Mental Health Act. Bob Bluglass was chairing the special sub-Committee; he was a tremendous help to the President, and did a lot of work behind the scenes, lobbying various MPs and Lords. The Department was also very helpful, in spite of being very severely pressurised, and I should mention two of their people here, Pamela Mason, their senior medical officer and, particularly for mental handicap, Rodney Wilkins. They came regularly to the College with new proposals and ideas and were constantly changing different parts of the Bill.

The first White Paper on amendment of the 1959 Act was quite reasonable, and mental handicap was recognised in it, but then suddenly, the feeling was strongly anti-medical and anti-hospital. The College then tried to restore something like the old Board of Control, and succeeded in this, although under a different name –

the Mental Health Act Commission. But it was only through raising the issue of people who had suffered brain damage from head injuries that we were able to salvage something for mental handicap in the 1983 Act.

HF   It was unfortunate that so much time and effort went into that legislation, when some fairly modest amendments to the 1959 Act would have been much better. On another subject, what about your involvement in research?

JJ   I have never been a full-time researcher. I was a doctor first, a psychiatrist second, and a specialist in mental handicap third, yet I always felt that we need to record whatever we observe. Through systematic recording, all of us who are working in the field will accumulate information which will help future generations. In the last 20 years, I have been particularly interested in the problem of ageing. With the late Dr Carter, I analysed the changes in age of the mentally handicapped during the last 50 years. It was remarkable how many were living longer and nearing the longevity of the normal population. We need to know what kind of facilities we have and what type of disorders will be found, compared with those of normal people. This is a very exciting area and, luckily, we have a lot of material from the past which can be used for comparison. We were the first to publish data on cancer in the mentally handicapped, with information on what particular types are more prevalent in different groups. When I was in Australia at the last ISSMD meeting recently, we had a symposium on ageing and people from many countries presented papers on the subject. I am anxious that young psychiatrists coming into the field should be encouraged to join in this research effort.

HF   What about your activities outside psychiatry?

JJ   I believe it is very important to join with the other specialities in medicine, and I was very proud when I was elected President of the Bristol Medico-Chirurogical Society, as it is one of the oldest medical societies in this country.

HF   What date was it founded?

JJ   In 1874. My presidential address was on the history of mental handicap in Bristol and Bath. In Bath, there are records of a hostel going back to the 14th century, kept by the monks.

I think it is very important that psychiatrists should not be isolated. They should be working with their medical colleagues. Often, the people do look upon psychiatrists as being something different, but when they realise that you are also a doctor and are interested in various aspects of medicine, they accept you. I have never felt a stranger amongst my colleagues and, similarly, when the new Medical History Association of Bristol was formed, I was invited to be one of the founder members.

HF   How was your time on the Mental Health Act Commission? We were both present at its first meeting, at Sunningdale, in 1983.

JJ   As you know, the campaigns leading up to the 1983 Act were reflected in the Commission – some members of the Commission were anti-medical, anti-psychiatric, and anti-hospital. However, I was very fortunate that in my team, there were people who were highly professional and experienced. We covered Wales, the West of England, and parts of Broadmoor, and I had a very happy four years with them. I believe we did some good for the patients, that we were Commissioners not 'Commissars', and that the staff also benefited. Very often, when we went back we were welcomed, which I thought was very encouraging. I am also pleased that we were able to take care of mental handicap patients. Thanks to Gillian Shepherd, who was our first Regional Chairman, and Shirley Turner, who was the second Chairman, we were able to form a special team. We made quite a good impact in making sure that patients in mental handicap hospitals, not just the ones who were legally detained, were provided with the services needed. But on the whole, the Commission has become too cumbersome, and I believe the Scottish arrangement is much better. They appointed permanent staff, with very senior people, like the old Board of Control, and this was what the College really wanted.

HF   Can you tell me about your involvement with the BMA?

JJ   On the whole, the BMA had very little time for psychiatry, they were so much involved in politics of their own. When I joined the Mental Health Group Committee, it was Professor Linford Rees who had invited me there, and also proposed me as vice-Chairman. I realised that they were anxious to learn about our problems. I was keen that we should help all the doctors from various groups who were dealing with mental illness, for whatever reason, and we should bring them all together, under the umbrella of the BMA. Before I retired as the Chairman, we succeeded in gaining a permanent member on the Council. The College should continue to strive to have a good liaison with the BMA. One notices with pleasure that two past presidents of the College became presidents of the BMA.

HF   Could you say something about your writing?

JJ   The book, *Clinical Pathology in Mental Retardation*, resulted from a combination of interests between two people – a pathologist and a psychiatrist. Bob Eastham and I often discussed common problems, and neither of us had a relevant book which would be able to help us in what we needed to know. So we started to work together and to our surprise – this was in the 1960s – so much seemed to be happening in this field; the more we researched, the more we found. The book came to fruition, and was very well received; it was translated into Italian.

HF   Has any new book appeared on the subject?

JJ   There are now books on pure pathology and new ones on mental handicap, but no such combination as the one we created.

HF   What about other publications?

JJ   The College is very fortunate that Dr Blake Marsh left money for the lecture named after him. Many eminent people from the field of mental handicap have been the lecturers. When I was invited by the College to lecture, I felt very honoured, but also worried what to produce. It had to be something original. I started to look at various skin disorders associated with mental handicap. I was very interested in how skin disorders could reflect on the development of the brain and mind, as well as in how certain pathogenetics reflect them and are diagnostic of the nature of disorders. The lecture was published in your Journal, and it is still often quoted now as a topic which had not been researched enough. The same is true of skin disorders in general psychiatry too.

HF What do you feel about present developments in mental handicap services?

JJ   We must never forget that there is nothing new under the sun, so we must look back to see who tried things before, where they tried them, and how they worked. One must never dismiss new ideas as being irrelevant, but must judge how much advantage or disadvantage there will be for the patients, for the staff, and for the society. If you look back over the last 50 years, you see so many people wanting to claim they have all the answers. Multi-professionalism is very important and, whatever we are trying to do, we should share the same vision and the same experience.

A good example is the question of community care. In the 1900s, the first President of the MPA who worked in mental handicap talked about the same problem. Our work at Stoke Park in the 1950s aimed to provide as good a service outside as in hospitals. The Victorians built hospitals for those people who were on the streets and in workhouses. Of course, there were some bad hospitals, but we mustn't condemn them all and say, 'All was bad yesterday and all is good today'. We always tried to copy the Americans and Scandinavians, but we don't copy them now, when they are telling us what trouble they are in with non-institutional care. Many people don't realise how much families of mentally handicapped people suffer.

At the moment, there are about six different labels for mental handicap floating around the country, confusing parents, professionals and others. I have been through the use of several different labels in my career, but I have never seen one to make any real difference to the patients and their families. The Department of Health has had to give in to yet another change. Even some chairs – and incidentally, we now have six chairs for mental handicap in this country – are being relabelled to make them more fashionable.

HF What do you feel now about your native country?

JJ   I was born in a beautiful part of the world. We had our 'Peasant Revolution' in the 18th century, when we became independent from feudal obligations to the aristocracy. We kept our history, language, and nationality intact throughout all occupations – by the Austrian monarchy and before. The people are industrious, and now they have eventually reached something we were always striving for – independence. When we were in Yugoslavia, we wanted to have a genuinely federal state. However, we Slovenes have no ethnic problems, with a river dividing us from Croatia and the Alps from Austria and from Italy. Culturally, we have one of the highest proportions of literate people and the highest rate of publication of books for a little nation of about two million. We have very good education, with excellent grammar schools and university departments. Our Professors have been educated in the capital cities of Europe. Slovenia had suffered heavy losses in 1991 during the attacks by the Yugoslav army, but the people have survived, are working hard, and a new Slovenia is emerging.

Finally, I would like to say that I have been here since 1948, and everybody knows that I am Slovene, a political refugee, a foreigner, but I have never been treated as such. I obey the law of the land, I respect the nation, and people here respect me. I have never had any problems, either at work or elsewhere, from that point of view. I am grateful for what this country has given me and also for what I have learnt here. I also hope that I have given something back.

19   Hugh Freeman

Interviewed by GREG WILKINSON (1993)

Professor Hugh Freeman, BM BCh (1954), MA, DPM (1957), MSc (1980), DM (1988), FRCPsych (1971), FFPHM (1989). Professor Freeman was born in Salford in 1929. He won an open scholarship to St John's College, Oxford, and afterwards was a clinical student at Manchester Royal Infirmary. He was a Captain in the Royal Army Medical Corps and was a Registrar at Bethlem Royal and Maudsley Hospitals. He was Consultant Psychiatrist from 1961–88, and has been Honorary Consultant Psychiatrist, Salford Health Authority, University of Manchester School of Medicine, since 1988. He has travelled widely, mainly on behalf of the WHO. Books he has edited include *Community Psychiatry* and *150 Years of British Psychiatry* with German Berrios. He was an assistant editor of the *British Journal of Psychiatry* from 1978–83 and became Editor in 1983.

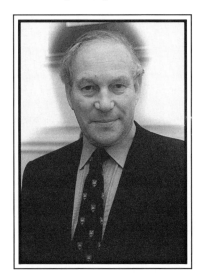

GW   I would like to begin by asking you to set your professional contribution in some general context. What do you see as being your main achievements?

HF   My main interest, over many years, was the development of a service for a community. That community was Salford in Lancashire, which is where I was born and, as many people know, has often appeared in paintings by L. S. Lowry, and in plays and films. It was an archetypal Industrial Revolution place, and when I started work there in 1961, still had a largely unchanged 19th-century environment. It was dirty, usually covered in a pall of smoke, and people were mostly living in very overcrowded conditions, but it had a tremendous sense of community, and that was something that largely disappeared in the course of redevelopment in the '60s and '70s. This experience was what primarily turned my attention, some time later, to the relationship of mental health to the environment. But in the '60s, most of my efforts went into integrating the very poor psychiatric resources we had there into a service that would respond to the needs of that population in the best way possible.

GW   Most people will think of your contribution in the editing field.

HF   I should explain that I'm a rather reluctant scientist. I was an arts person at school, and went to Oxford with a history scholarship, but because of family influences, I changed to medicine. The arts subjects, though, particularly history and English, have always been my principal love, and so it was that side of medicine that I tried to include in my work.

I went up to Oxford in 1947, and two of my contemporaries as medical students were Michael Gelder and John Cooper. Our life there was nearer to the world of *Charley's Aunt* than to that of today's egalitarian universities. It was a privilege to live among the incomparable buildings and gardens of St John's College, and Oxford itself wasn't yet ruined by traffic and redevelopment. After the restrictions of wartime provincial life, I found it a cornucopia of new and exciting experiences.

After that, I was a clinical student at Manchester Royal Infirmary, which brought me back to reality with a jolt. There were some outstanding teachers there, including Robert Platt and Douglas Black, but also some very inadequate ones. Psychiatry was taught by Bill Trethowan, who was one of the best lecturers I encountered in the whole of my studies.

GW   So there were strong social and community influences on your development. What took you into psychiatry?

HF   There were three main things. When I was at Oxford, I did a degree in psychology, and one of my tutors was Oliver Zangwill, whose special interest was neuropsychology. Secondly, as a house surgeon, I worked in the department of neurosurgery at Manchester Royal Infirmary, which brought me into contact with Sir Geoffrey Jefferson. He had been one of the original neurosurgeons in this country, after being trained by Harvey Cushing in America in the 1920s. In 1955, he'd been retired for several years, but was still extremely active; one of the most impressive things about him was his unflappability if anything was going wrong in theatre. The techniques in use then were fairly primitive by today's standards, and anything like brain scanning was still in the realm of science fiction. I knew I would never be a neurosurgeon, but it increased my interest in the central nervous system.

But the main influence was my late uncle, Jack Kahn, who was one of the great pioneers of child psychiatry in this country, though I don't think he's been as well recognised as he should have been.

GW   What was his influence?

HF   He was a GP for 20 years in Yorkshire, before he even started psychiatry, and therefore he had an understanding of the realities of illness in the community, in a way that I think many doctors probably don't have, if they become specialists straight after qualification. He had also been in local government – Chairman of the Health Committee in Huddersfield – so that he knew how to deal with local authorities. He set up a remarkable community-based child psychiatry service in the East End, in Newham, which I believe hasn't survived all the upheavals of recent years. I was very much influenced by the kind of model that he created, and also by his writings. Two of his books – *Unwillingly to School* and *Development of Personality* – have been widely read for many years, and we will publish a new edition of the first one next year. We also republished his *Job's Illness* – a psychodynamic interpretation of that part of the Bible – which impressed biblical scholars as well as psychiatrists and psychoanalysts.

GW   I'm struck by the obvious feeling that you had for that Salford community, and then for a community model of psychiatric service in the East End of London. These conjure up uncomfortable images in my mind. What does that tell us about you: that your interest was in doing something positive, in these very difficult conditions for psychiatry?

HF   You have to remember that I was a child of the 1930s, at the time of the Great Depression, and also of the rise of the dictators in Europe. So from the beginning, I was very much aware both of the terrible poverty that surrounded us, and also of the political dimension of things – that medicine couldn't be practised in a social vacuum.

My very humdrum, lower middle-class childhood, though, was interrupted by an extended visit in 1935–6, with my mother, to relatives in South Africa. At that time, apart from people in the armed forces or colonial service, only the rich travelled abroad normally, so that this was a very unusual experience. Our journey then took us three weeks by sea; when I went back again for the first time, last year, it took 11 hours.

GW   Is there an explanation why you didn't end up in Hampstead?

HF   I think it also has to do with awareness of social bonds and of the kinds of communities that have a relationship to a particular place. This was very much true of Salford, because although to outsiders it appeared just part of the anonymous industrial conurbation that spreads across much of north-west England, in fact people identified very strongly with it as somewhere separate. There were long established kinship and friendship networks there, which often went back several generations. When I worked as a clinician among Salford people, I soon realised that one had to try and make use of these networks, rather than to see them as isolated individuals, which is perhaps what a traditional psychiatric training might convey. I became clinically committed to many patients, some of whom I looked after for more than 20 years. I think that one of the contributions psychiatry can make to medicine as a whole is a longitudinal view of illness, rather than focusing on episodes.

Then secondly, becoming involved in research, particularly with the case register, I was aware that it would take many years to produce information of value – which was indeed what happened.

GW   You were at The Maudsley Hospital between 1958 and 1960. What were your impressions of that experience?

HF   I came almost directly from the Army, with an interval of a locum for one month at Prestwich, a very large mental hospital, north of Manchester, where I later returned as a consultant. In fact, Prestwich was like the Army in some ways, and when I first encountered the Medical Superintendent, my instinct was to salute him!

I suppose one could describe going to The Maudsley as like being thrown into an ice-cold bath intellectually, because it was so totally different from anything I'd experienced before. It brought tremendous stress, but at the same time intellectual excitement and comradeship. For the first few months, I shared the residential accommodation at Bethlem with Michael Rutter, and I think we gave each other a certain amount of support with this new experience. My first job was with Felix Post, and what I particularly learnt from him, which I have valued ever since, was the need for the most rigorous attention to the details of patients' clinical states and histories. He demanded very high standards from that point of view. It was exciting to experience the interactions of so many outstanding people, concentrated together and engaged from time to time in bruising disputes on both theoretical and practical aspects of psychiatry.

As well as Felix Post, the people who impressed me particularly were C. P. Blacker, Willy Hoffer, Bob Hobson, Elliot Slater, the forensic pioneers Peter Scott and Trevor Gibbens, and David Stafford-Clark, who could always be relied on to liven up any occasion at which he was present. On the other hand, there were also some extremely mediocre figures, who contributed very little.

The down-side of this intellectual excitement, though, was the paranoid atmosphere of the institution, and what I felt were the destructive influences which emanated from Aubrey Lewis. He and I had a rather adversarial relationship, and I left after two years because I felt that under his leadership, the institution was completely out of touch with important developments that were going on outside, particularly in the social and community fields.

GW *How did this adversarial relationship develop?*

HF Maybe he sensed that I reacted against what seemed to me his preoccupation with unimportant details, and a tendency to favour activities which had no clinical relevance. Whereas if you were concerned, as I was increasingly, with the way that services were organised for populations, you received no sympathy or support. In spite of being at one of the world's leading postgraduate institutions, I had to organise my training in social psychiatry entirely myself, finding out where innovative work was being done and arranging visits to these places. These issues were never mentioned at the Maudsley then; it was only later, when Douglas Bennett arrived, that there was any change. Of course, Aubrey had started the Social Psychiatry Research Unit, but I don't recall the everyday activities of the Maudsley being in any way influenced by what that unit was investigating.

The reactions to Aubrey recorded in this series of interviews seem to follow a bimodal distribution. People either saw him largely as benign, helpful, and kind or as hostile, destructive, and sinister; I was definitely in the second group, much as I admired his intellectual qualities. (Incidentally, I found his lectures very boring). He made some people's careers, but destroyed other people's, unless they got away.

After I'd been there for a while, I felt that I would like to go into social research, and after speaking to Maurice Carstairs, I requested an interview with Aubrey about that. He said 'Give me some indication of your capacity in this respect'. I had heard that there were some interesting service developments going on at Oldham in Lancashire, so I contacted Arthur Pool, who was the consultant responsible for them, and a largely forgotten pioneer now. I took a week's leave and went up to observe how the service ran, as well as going through all the records I could find, trying to construct some sort of data from them. Then I wrote a long report about it and gave it to Aubrey. The only thing he ever said to me about it subsequently was 'Thank you very much'; that was the last I heard of it from him.

However, I then sent the report to *The Lancet*, who accepted it, and I was in the perhaps unusual position of having an original, single-authored paper published there as a registrar. Though Aubrey didn't respond to it, Sir George Godber wrote to me from the Ministry of Health, as soon as he read the paper, and took a close interest from then on in the work that I was doing. So perhaps it's not surprising that he's my main medical hero. Having no idea how important he was, I invited him to visit the Bethlem Day Hospital, and he replied very graciously that it was difficult for him to get away from the Ministry!

As you will have gathered, I never had the chance of going into a research post, but in my second year, I had been registrar at Bethlem Day Hospital. This was a very powerful experience, because it was so much more involved with real life than the ivory tower atmosphere of the Maudsley itself. I was left largely on my own there, to develop my own interests, and took advantage of that. I had also tried to get a research project going for a thesis, on social networks. This was then a completely new field, and I had help with it from George Brown, who had just arrived at the MRC Unit, and Lily Stein, who was a statistician and the sister of Jacob Bronowski. Aubrey gave me some encouragement at first, but it was eventually abandoned, for reasons which I've completely forgotten – I suppose I have repressed them. However, I keep coming back to this subject because I believe it's an important borderland between psychiatry and sociology, which is still scientifically neglected.

After the Bethlem Day Hospital, I was the first registrar of the in-patient psychotherapy unit, which Bob Hobson had started. Ironically, though, what impressed me most during that time was our first use of antidepressants – both imipramine and phenelzine. We were fairly sceptical about them, because the only drugs available up to then had been amphetamine, which did little real good to people with major depression. I was extremely surprised when the first patient on whom I had tried imipramine told me after two weeks that he had begun to feel better; he had a chronic depression which had failed to respond to ECT or psychotherapy. Soon after, I admitted a woman in a manic state who had been intractably depressed for several years, until she started taking phenelzine. When, a few years later, the MRC antidepressant trial concluded that phenelzine was no different from placebo, I agreed with Will Sargant that the nation's combined academic brain-power had made a fundamental mistake.

I decided to leave at the end of my second year, and was appointed a Senior Registrar at Oxford. There was then no university department of psychiatry and I was based at Littlemore Hospital. Leaving the Maudsley turned out to be almost as much of a life event as arriving there, since even a very active provincial mental hospital – and Littlemore had some outstanding people then – was so very different from Denmark Hill.

Perhaps I should add that in the same year that my *Lancet* paper appeared, I had one in the *BMJ*, jointly with Don Kendrick – a clinical psychologist at the Maudsley – which reported the first case in this country of a phobia treated by behaviour therapy. This was of a lady with fear of cats and it was picked up by most of the national newspapers, the BBC, and *Time*; there was even a cartoon about it in the *Daily Mail*. So 1960 was something of an *annus mirabilis* for me.

GW   *What do you have to say about developing services, and the development of psychiatry during the '60s.*

HF   I was fortunate in that I became a consultant when I was 31, and I think it's very useful to have an independent command when one still has all the energy of youth. I had a very rapid rise through the ranks in psychiatry, which I started in the Army. My first experience of it, though, was as a locum at Wakefield, immediately before the Army. The neuroleptic era was just beginning then, but this mental hospital was quite Hogarthian in many ways, and some of the staff seemed to me as peculiar as the patients. When I first arrived there, on a misty January night, it was like the opening of a Hammer film.

GW *Was your career good fortune or good strategic planning?*

HF It wasn't strategic planning at all, because I certainly had no game plan when I began. When I came to Salford, I found that I had enormous responsibilities in an extremely backward mental hospital, though at least it wasn't geographically remote from the catchment area, like most of the London ones. I also had duties in two general hospitals, in each of which there was an embryonic psychiatric department. But most importantly, I had an involvement with the local authority, and that was really where the strength came from – such strength as there was at that time.

GW *What was the relationship between the local authorities and mental health services at that time, in contrast to the present?*

HF In most parts of the country, it was very bad. You will remember that this was when the Medical Officers of Health were responsible for mental health, but nine out of ten of them had no interest in it. They just provided a skeleton service of mental welfare officers for compulsory admissions, and little else.

But there were a number of exceptions, and one of them was certainly Salford. This was due to two people. Firstly, the MOH – Dr Lance Burn – a great public health innovator, who never received any public recognition. The other was Mervyn Susser, who had a joint appointment between the local authority and the Department of Social Medicine at Manchester University. He subsequently became, of course, the very distinguished Professor of Psychiatric Epidemiology at Columbia, but at that time, his considerable energies were going into both service development and research in Salford. In fact, it was largely through his influence that the rather unique job to which I was appointed was created. The epidemiological work that was started then – both for psychiatric illness and mental handicap – was really innovative, though it was all done with virtually no financial support.

GW *Can you tell me a bit more about your working life as a clinician, because this is something that tends to be rather neglected. People spend their life working very hard with patients and it's too often undervalued.*

HF That's very true. I think in the professional stakes, you get very little credit indeed for the quality and extent of your clinical work, which tends to be known to a fairly limited number of people. Some well-known psychiatrists have been rather poor clinicians, who never carried much of a case-load. Looking back, I find it hard to understand how I got through what I did at that time, dealing with huge numbers of patients at three hospitals, with a very high rate of referral and turnover. There were very few junior medical staff, and those we had were not always of a high quality; there were also very few supporting staff of other kinds. What I had to do was to try and create a more responsive service, primarily through integrating such resources as were available. I also cut out the conflicts and horse-trading that had been going on until then between the different bodies involved in mental health services, which had absorbed much of their energies. For the first five years, I was the only person through whom all these lines of communication passed; then I was joined in Salford by Michael Tarsh, and we had a very happy professional partnership for over 20 years.

I should add a word about E. W. Anderson, who was Professor of Psychiatry at Manchester when I was a student and when I returned as a consultant, since a couple of people have spoken very positively of him in their interviews. As students, we never had any contact with him at all. As a consultant in the region, I regarded him as a disaster. He may well have been very good at giving a small number of postgraduates a thorough training in psychopathology. However, what was needed for more than four million people in the region was a large number of trained professionals, since even the relatively few consultant and senior registrar posts that were established weren't all filled. Yet the University Department was producing only handfuls of psychiatrists and PSWs, until Neil Kessel came in 1965 – a situation for which I believe Anderson was largely responsible.

GW *The President of the College has recently highlighted the idea of a 'personal physician' relationship between consultant and patient, and this is attractive; you mention the word 'quality', and going back to your work in Salford, what do you think the quality of the service offered was then, under the restrictions that you've just described?*

HF   You have to consider what we offered in relation to the alternatives that then existed; one must avoid being ahistorical. For almost the whole of the country at that time, the only psychiatric service provided was in mental hospitals, and the general quality then both of clinical care and of accommodation for patients in them was extremely variable, but on the whole pretty bad.

At that time, the psychiatric profession here was very small, compared with today, and the greater part of it consisted of doctors who had grown up in mental hospitals under the apprenticeship tradition. There was very little alternative to that, as the Universities and teaching hospitals provided only very few places indeed for those who wanted to train in psychiatry. So whatever we provided has to be seen in comparison with what patients' experience would have been in a large, very overcrowded mental hospital, where the average professional quality of the staff was, to be quite frank, rather dismal. I wasn't anti-mental hospital in general – a large part of my responsibilities were in a mental hospital, and I felt that what I had to do was use its resources, such as they were, in the best possible way.

The first thing I did was to take responsibility for every patient who came from an address in Salford – whether an acute admission, a chronic schizophrenic, or a case of senile dementia. This was the 'Dutchess County' principle, which I had first seen when I went to America, a few months earlier, and met Ernest Gruenberg. The second change was to set up a system of screening before admission, so that people didn't just arrive in the mental hospital – sometimes on a Section Order, sometimes not – but usually out of the blue, and without any sort of organised relationship with those who were working outside. In this, I had to depend primarily on the mental welfare officers, because there really was no-one else at that time, apart from a minority of the GPs who were keen to co-operate. I was very fortunate that Salford had more mental health social workers, and these of much better quality than any other authority in the North of England. Indeed, the city compared favourably then with almost any other part of the country in this respect.

The working principle was that we would use what we had in the most flexible way, so that people could be treated as in-patients, if they needed it, but so far as possible as out-patients or day patients. This may not seem very exciting now, but it was fairly revolutionary at the time. We had no special building for a day hospital, just one room in a child welfare clinic, with one untrained staff member (who was actually superb); otherwise, people came daily into hospital wards. There was one hostel and a weekly social club, run by volunteers, with a mental welfare officer always present. That was all.

GW Do you look back at that period of service development with satisfaction?

HF Yes, for one thing, there was a great feeling of camaraderie and of optimism, in spite of the enormous difficulties. This is the overwhelming difference from today. We knew that there was a huge amount more that we wanted to do, if we had the resources, but at least things were getting slightly better all the time. Now, it seems to be the opposite.

In Salford, there was a very high level of morale, which allowed us to do far more with the resources available than might have been expected. We did see rapid changes, for instance in the reduction in numbers of long-stay in-patients, and of those coming in under orders, with corresponding increases in out-patients, day patients, and people seen at home. Psychiatric home visits were done together with a mental welfare officer in a large proportion of cases, and together with the GP in rather fewer. Today, with our rather greater sophistication, these sort of numerical changes are treated with some scepticism, but it did represent a real difference from the way things had been up to then, and most patients and families seemed to welcome it.

You have to remember that at that time, Prestwich Hospital, where the mental hospital part of our service moved in the early 1970s, had well over 3,000 patients. You say things are the same now, but these vast numbers were then being looked after by a handful of professional staff, and many patients were there for very long periods. Situations like that no longer exist, and this is a very significant change – though perhaps in some ways the pendulum has swung too far.

GW What do you regard as the most significant developments, looking at your career in Salford in the '60s and '70s?

HF When I started, all we had in the general hospitals was an out-patient service, and it was a poor, fragmented one; it had no accommodation of its own, there were virtually no supporting staff, and a few beds had just been grudgingly allocated to psychiatry in a medical ward. It was agreed that we were to get a whole ward of our own in Hope Hospital, but that took more than ten years from the time I arrived. In circumstances like that, patience isn't just a virtue; it's a necessity.

After six years, we had a day hospital, a purpose-built out-patient clinic of our own, proper facilities for physical treatment, and four social workers jointly appointed with the local authority, covering both the mental and general hospitals. So there was the basis then for multidisciplinary teams. In the mental hospital, we had our own wards and unit office, which was an enormous change from the previous system, where everything was run in a hierarchical way from the Medical Superintendent's Office. Most important, I think, we had very close functional relationships with the hostels, day centres, social clubs, and domiciliary work which were being provided mainly by the local authority. All the pieces then fitted together into an integrated whole – and that was something you would have found in very few places indeed elsewhere. Visitors were often astonished by it.

There's a tendency now to devalue the kind of administration that was practised at that time, but in fact, we had a superb administrator in the Salford Hospitals, even before the 1974 reorganisation, and a superb Matron at Prestwich Hospital. They, and many other non-medical staff, were keen to do the maximum possible within our resources – not the minimum, as is often the case today.

GW   What about relationships with other disciplines, and the growth of these disciplines within mental health?

HF   When I started, they hardly existed at all. The first clinical psychologist arrived after I did. There was one social worker in the general hospital, and one or two in the mental hospital – not just for Salford, but for other areas as well. Occupational therapy was also in its infancy, and the community social workers were all untrained, although many of them had great personal qualities. So there was no tradition of multidisciplinary team working; that was one of the achievements of our efforts in the '60s. Another thing I did from the beginning was to respect the mental welfare officers as professional colleagues, and deal with them on that basis. In most places, at that time, they were treated as very lowly members of the MOH's service, which was run in a rigidly bureaucratic way.

GW   How do you think this developed towards the latter part of your career?

HF   Well unfortunately, the Seebohm Report brought the creation of generic social services, in which psychiatric social workers were absorbed into unified social services – a disaster for psychiatry. Lord Seebohm himself, in my interview for this series, admitted that his Committee really hadn't seriously thought about mental health. They just assumed that it was the same as everything else. Unfortunately, when the generic social services were created in 1971, it was immediately clear that mental health had a very low priority in their activities. This was partly because the Chief Officers nearly all came from child care, and they had to observe statutory responsibilities for children and certain other groups. On the other hand, mental health work was still almost entirely optional, and the relatively few experienced and trained mental health social workers tended to get fairly rapidly moved into administrative or teaching positions.

We certainly found in Salford then that there was a dramatic fall in the quality of work actually being done with patients, particularly with the severely ill and disabled. We also found that dealing with the enormous bureaucracy that had been spawned by the reorganisation meant the loss of the easy, informal working relationships that we'd had with the previous mental health department. There was also a deliberate destruction of specialisation nationally, so that specialised training in mental health work only remained in a very few places. The result was that we now encountered a shifting population of social workers, most of whom had very little knowledge of mental health work and not much more interest in it. The idea that generic area teams would devote much of their efforts to mental health work never happened in practice.

Even so, it was possible in Salford, for some years, to preserve an island of special experience in mental health work, within the generic social services, and such a situation had become fairly unusual by then. But things just weren't the same, and as Kathleen Jones rightly pointed out, the 'integration' of social work meant the disintegration of co-ordinated mental health services, where these had developed. There was certainly a need for change – the mental welfare officers were miserably paid and rarely given any respect as professionals – but it could have been done in a more constructive way.

GW   *There is an inevitable growth in professional autonomy and we've seen that in social work, in psychology, and in other professions. What can psychiatrists learn from this development?*

HF   The growth of autonomy in other professions has been largely at the expense of what was regarded as the 'imperialism' of medical psychiatrists, but I think one has to remember that psychiatry itself was, with great difficulty, establishing itself then as a recognised profession, with good standards of training and competence. Quite frankly, until the 1950s, most doctors working in psychiatry weren't very capable of getting on in any other kind of medicine, and it was from that very low level that a largely new profession had to be created. The fact that in Britain today, psychiatrists are one of the largest and best trained body of specialists is a tremendous achievement – one of the most important developments that's occurred in my professional lifetime. It's also a great achievement for our College.

GW   *Looking back then, did you miss the clinical part of your life or is it something that you've just put behind you?*

HF   I would find it intolerable to work in the conditions of the NHS today. Having devoted virtually the whole of my professional lifetime to the NHS, I'm extremely sad to see what has been going on, particularly in the last couple of years. I think this is the negation of the principles which went into the establishment of the service and indeed, which kept it going for years in the face of enormous difficulties and shortages. Re-reading Aneurin Bevan's speeches about the NHS from 1946–48, as I have been doing for my historical studies, I find it very sad that all the idealism and brave hopes of that time should have ended in the squalid commercialism that is ruining the service today. The NHS was one of the best things that ever happened in Britain.

I find that the shift in the philosophy of the service is, with a widespread loss of idealism and commitment, the most disturbing change of all. It derives mainly from the domination by managers and accountants, who seem to have no personal concern with the objectives of a Health Service, but of course, it's also part of a general cultural shift away from the liberalism and sense of community of the post-war period.

GW   *Where are we going as a profession? It sounds as if we're moving away from health services, and the other end of the spectrum seems to be the private sector.*

HF   There is indeed a considerable shift in that direction, and I personally regard it as a disastrous one. I've travelled abroad a great deal, and seen a lot of health services in many parts of the world. I always used to come back here feeling that we had one of the best systems that was possible, in dealing with the realities of life. What it still needed was for us to give a rather greater proportion of the national resources to health than we had been doing, and so bring ourselves more into line with similar industrialised countries. But that never happened.

In spite of that, the achievements of the NHS, given its very limited resources, were incredible. One of the main reasons, of course, was its extremely low administrative costs, and this is something that has been completely thrown away with the changes of recent years. To describe them as 'reforms' is a perversion of the language. Costing every activity and negotiating between every purchaser and provider is extremely expensive, and all the money to pay for that is deducted from what could have been spent on the care of patients. In any case, most of the money quantities used are largely meaningless. Trusts are the negation of all the work that had been done towards integration of care for communities over more than 40 years.

GW   *Looking at it from a global perspective, do you have any views about the development of mental health services; you had a special interest in Europe, of course, but you've travelled widely.*

HF   I've spent quite a bit of time in developing countries, mainly for WHO. One of the biggest problems that one finds in nearly all these situations is the absence of an administrative structure that is capable of making changes, should there be a political will to make them in their health services – and that's not present very often. This was something which we did have in this country, to a remarkable extent; it was a legacy of the Victorian Civil Service reforms, which created a devoted cadre of public servants, to which we owe a great deal. One soon becomes very much aware of the lack of this in other places.

Another frequent problem, particularly in Europe, is the division between private and public health services, which often results in very unfortunate discontinuities of care, for instance, between mental hospital in-patient care and private out-patient treatment. Again, we had largely escaped this through the NHS.

Thirdly, I felt there was a genuine devotion by NHS staff to serving the health needs of people as a whole in this country, which one simply didn't find in many other places.

Politically, health usually comes fairly low in the pecking order, so that Health Ministers rarely carry a great deal of political weight, and this is often a big obstacle to changing things for the better.

The longest spell I had overseas was three months in the West Indies, mainly in Grenada, for WHO, at the end of 1970. My assignment was to start a general hospital psychiatric unit, but as most of the essential supplies weren't there when I arrived, I spent a good deal of time in the mental hospital, where most of the patients hadn't been seen by a psychiatrist for several years. The hospital had been built by the French as a fort in 1779, and a few nineteenth-century wooden buildings had been added to that. The cooking, such as it was, was done in huge cauldrons over wood fires, underground. There was a very limited range of drugs available and the nursing staff was almost totally untrained – in fact, they were politically appointed, like all public service workers. At the general hospital, there was just one trained sister, who had arrived back from England; with her help, I started giving ECT, using some fairly primitive apparatus, and I believe we were able to do quite a bit of good. It was, of course, a great experience for my family, though we had none of the comforts that tourists in the Caribbean usually expect. I soon became aware that everything I did had political implications, and there were in fact some rather nasty riots while we were there. Unfortunately, the psychiatric unit, which became well established under a locally-born psychiatrist who had trained at Edinburgh, came to an end during the subsequent troubles in Grenada.

GW   When one thinks of mental health services, one's drawn to the American experience, the Italian experience, Greece, Romania, and so on . . . Where would you place the UK internationally in terms of mental health services?

HF   We're still very near the top from many points of view, including the number of well trained psychiatrists that are available to people in general – not just to a privileged minority. I am concerned, though, that we may be losing this high world ranking. Firstly, through the consistent underfunding of health services for a good many years now, with a complete failure even to keep up with inflation. Secondly, through the loss of clinical autonomy, which has resulted from the newly dominant position of managers and accountants that I mentioned. Thirdly, through the ever-widening gulf between Health and Social Services. The co-ordination which was achieved earlier in many parts of the country has been lost, and there often seems to be an innate hostility coming from Social Services to psychiatry. What is the point of Ministers constantly talking about the importance of collaboration, when Social Services can unilaterally withdraw all the social workers from a child psychiatry clinic or mental health service? That is what has happened in a number of places – it would have been unthinkable in the 1970s.

Another worrying trend is of some developments in nursing, including a new curriculum which, as in social work, seems to start from a confrontational attitude towards medicine, rather than a co-operative one.

GW   Can you say something about your involvement with MIND?

HF   That's a long and unhappy story. Very briefly, I became involved with NAMH, as it then was, soon after starting work in psychiatry, and was delighted to be asked to become Editor of their journal, which was then called *Mental Health*, in 1964. I continued doing that until the early '70s. During this time, NAMH was a mainstream voluntary organisation in the British model, and there was a significant involvement of professionals in it, together with volunteers, particularly in the local associations. There was a small, devoted headquarters staff, but things changed in the early '70s, partly because of the cultural revolution of 1968 and the subsequent growth of anti-psychiatry. I ceased to be one of their consultants, as did the others, when there was a new Director in 1973; that was not of my own doing. Subsequently, most of the other psychiatrists who had been associated with the organisation parted company with it.

However, I came back to MIND in the early '80s, when it seemed that some of those difficulties might have passed, and I was, in fact, Vice-Chairman for several years until 1987. By then, the organisation had completely changed its orientation, at least at the national level. It seemed to see its role as being a confrontational, antagonistic one to the mental health professions, particularly to psychiatry. Indeed, it took on board many of the tenets of anti-psychiatry, particularly those with a political, Marxist flavour.

I stayed on with the organisation for some time as a member of the Council, trying to preserve some link with psychiatry, but eventually felt this was impossible. By then, some extremely strident and hostile complaints were being made by leading people in MIND against psychiatry, which really made co-operative relationships unworkable. This is not to suggest that the excellent work of local associations in providing practical services should be discounted in any way, but there has now been, for some years, a considerable problem about the central organisation of MIND. Until there is some significant change there, I don't think it's going to be possible for psychiatry to re-establish the kind of co-operation that used to exist with them.

GW   I see, like you, quite a difference between the activities of the central and the local branches of MIND, but I'm still concerned about the lack of dialogue with MIND. Should we take MIND more seriously?

HF   I can assure you this is not through lack of trying. Repeated efforts have been made, both in public and behind the scenes, to try and get that dialogue going, and up to now it hasn't proved possible. The basic problem is that MIND is dominated at present by people who simply do not accept the legitimacy of what psychiatrists do. For instance, they describe anyone who has experienced psychiatric treatment as a 'survivor' and ban terms like 'mental illness' or 'psychiatric disorder'. Until that situation changes, I don't seem much grounds for hope.

One of the main difficulties comes from the activities of those who describe themselves as 'users' representatives'. When you ask them what evidence they have that they are in fact representative of the millions of users of mental health services, they don't reply. My view is that they are totally *un*representative, but unfortunately, they have taken a very prominent position, not only within MIND, but also in a number of other organisations.

I had a much happier experience of a voluntary organisation with the North West Fellowship for Schizophrenia, which is now called *Making Space*. That was a model for how an enthusiastic voluntary organisation can very constructively add to what the statutory services offer. I was one of their medical consultants until I moved to London.

Outside psychiatry, I've had quite a big involvement with environmental organisations. I was on the Regional Committee of the National Trust and the Manchester Historic Buildings Panel, and was Vice-Chairman of the Manchester Heritage Trust. I also started a campaign to save the world's first railway station – Liverpool Road in Manchester; this was taken over by other people, and was eventually successful.

GW *The next area that I want to tackle is your experience of editing and you mentioned that this began in 1964 with 'Mental Health'. How did you take on that position?*

HF I suppose I should say my very first editorial role actually was with the *Oxford Guardian*, which was the journal of the Oxford University Liberal Club. I also became Secretary of the Club later, and worked with people like Robin Day and Jeremy Thorpe. But the editorship of *Mental Health* came about largely through the influence of Harvey Flack. I don't know if many people will remember him now, but he founded the magazine *Family Doctor* and associated publications for the BMA; for many years, these were extremely important in health education. I got to know him when I started writing some pieces for *Family Doctor*, and he felt I would be a suitable editor for *Mental Health*, when Roger Tredgold retired from that job at the end of 1963.

I think one of the things I learnt from him was the importance of keeping the goal of communication with one's audience always in the forefront, whether that was a lay audience, as in *Family Doctor*, a wholly professional one, as in psychiatry, or a mixed audience, which *Mental Health* was designed for.

GW *You have been involved with a large number of journals, and have edited a number of books.*

HF I started editing books in the early 1960s and the first two were done jointly with a hospital administrator at the Maudsley, James Farndale, who later became a university teacher. Although they've long been out of print, those two books are still in use by people studying the organisation of mental health services.

Since then, editing books has become something of a habit. The two I am most pleased with both appeared in 1991 – *Community Psychiatry* with Douglas Bennett and *150 Years of British Psychiatry* with German Berrios. I have very much valued my experience of collaborating with both of them. Probably my biggest project was producing *Mental Health & the Environment*, in 1985. This appears as an edited book, though in fact, I wrote a good deal of what appears under some other people's names. It was then, and as far as I know is still, the only book in print on the subject. I am now preparing a second version, together with Stephen Stansfeld.

My journal editing, as I say, began seriously in 1964. *Mental Health* was a bit like a parish magazine when I started, but I did make very substantial changes to it, both in its content and its presentation. We found, though, that the readership for a quarterly journal like that, purely about mental health, but not for any one profession, was relatively limited. That situation has remained unchanged ever since.

I started getting involved with other journals, firstly by writing for them; my first paper was in the *Journal of the RAMC* in 1958. Later, I was invited onto some editorial boards and I wrote a good deal – anonymously – for

The Lancet at one time. I also started doing book reviews for the lay press and for non-psychiatric learned journals. It's a very good way of making oneself read useful material. Before coming to this journal, I was Deputy Editor of the *International Journal of Social Psychiatry*. It was run and owned by Joshua Bierer – one of the most colourful characters of post-war British psychiatry, who established the first day hospital here, in 1948 – but not an easy person to work with.

GW   *Was there a grand plan?*

HF   Absolutely not. As I said at the beginning, my interests had always been more in the arts than the sciences, so writing and editing were the kind of activities that followed from that.

GW   *In a word, communication?*

HF   One aspect is that I like things to be expressed in a way that's both accurate and readable. That's why I've always tried to wage war on unnecessary jargon, which is such a virus in scientific literature. Perhaps it's a bit of an obsessional disorder, but I spend an enormous amount of time improving other people's English.

Here, I should say something about my involvement with the Society of Clinical Psychiatrists – known as the 'Oedipal Group'. John Howells described some of the background to it in my interview with him.

It all sprang, in my view, from a failure in 1948 to adapt the old medical administration of mental hospitals to the role of consultants, who were then being appointed. In fact, an NHS consultant's rights and responsibilities were completely at odds with the powers of a medical superintendent, but there was a typically British compromise which fudged things on both sides. Supporters of the superintendent system pointed to examples of outstanding individuals like T. P. Rees and George Bell, but in fact, these were very atypical exceptions.

When in 1959 the Mental Health Act introduced the statutory role of the Responsible Medical Officer, the superintendent's role became even more anomalous – as it was also in relation to the lay Administrator. However, many superintendents were fighting in the last ditch to preserve the status quo.

I strongly supported the SCP from the beginning, because I was convinced that the medical superintendent system was obsolete and a bar to the kind of progress I wanted to see. The SCP was also lobbying on behalf of a College for us, whereas many of the 'leaders' of our profession were actively sabotaging the effort. They really wanted to be physicians, and were highly ambivalent about their role as psychiatrists.

The SCP eventually asked me to edit their *Newsletter*, which was produced by a Roneo duplicator in a mental hospital OT Department. I developed this as well as I could, but it clearly needed to be brought out in a more attractive way; on the other hand, the Society had practically no money to pay for it.

After some looking around, I got agreement from Astra Pharmaceuticals that they would take it on, and distribute it free to all psychiatrists in the British Isles. Believing that there was nothing to lose, I gave this publication a very grandiose title *The British Journal of Clinical & Social Psychiatry*. Apart from my very helpful NHS secretary, I ran the entire thing single-handed, and it was published quarterly for about three years. Unfortunately, Astra then left the

CNS field, because zimelidine had to be withdrawn, and while I was wondering what to do next about it, I became editor of the *British Journal*. On balance, I think it wasn't at all a bad publication, and quite a few people were glad to get published in it, because the yellow journal was then very much smaller than it is now.

GW *What about the balance between clinical art and clinical science. Did you have a view or have you now got a view about the balance between these two, about which there is sometimes tension?*

HF That's quite true. In the case of the *British Journal of Psychiatry*, one always has to remember that it has two different audiences, as all general medical journals have. On the one hand, the majority of readers are clinicians who basically want to read things which are interesting to them and which will be helpful to them in doing their jobs. Secondly, there are the hard scientists, who are interested in publishing and reading original scientific data. Much of what they produce will be intelligible only to a very limited number of people in the psychiatric profession, but the scientific standing of the Journal, particularly in international terms, depends almost entirely on that kind of paper. The journal also has a very important role now in keeping all the different sub-specialities in touch with each other. It would be very bad for psychiatry as a whole if they only read their specialist publications.

As part of this role, I have expanded the number of specialist referees on our list to over 1,500, and this number will probably keep on growing. One of the most important things an editor has to do is to be constantly looking for new reviewers, while pruning the list of those who are unable or unwilling to go on doing the job. Peer review is the life-blood of scientific publishing, but unfortunately, some of our colleagues are not willing to play their part in it.

GW *Do you regard your editorship of the British Journal of Psychiatry as being the culmination of your editorial career?*

HF Well, who knows!

GW *How have you achieved the goals that you had when you started as Editor of the British Journal of Psychiatry?*

HF I didn't start with a clearly formulated set of goals, though I had some ideas of the kind of changes I would like to make, and most of them have been accomplished. One project I have particularly enjoyed doing is the series called *The Current Literature*, in which several people comment on a paper published elsewhere. That was an idea that only occurred to me after several years in the editorial chair.

GW *Are there any other changes or achievements that you would pinpoint in your editorship of the Journal?*

HF When I arrived, the College was still evolving out of the old and much smaller RMPA and, quite frankly, its administrative and financial structure was simply not up to the job. My predecessor, John Crammer, had tried to make some sense of the publishing finances, but had been defeated by the then College bureaucracy. After a few months, I came to the conclusion that we lacked the capacity to run and develop the *Journal* in the way that was needed, and thought we would have to accept one of the many offers of partnership that were coming from commercial publishers. Almost at the last moment, Mike Pare, who was then Treasurer, suggested that we should seek help from the RSM, which had just reorganised its publishing activities. The result was that Howard Croft, who had become Managing Director of the RSM's publications, was appointed our business adviser. From then on, we never looked back. We were able to reduce costs steadily, while enormously increasing the output of printed material, and at the same time contribute substantially to the College's finances. When new senior appointments were made, including that of David Jago as Publications Manager, everything began to get on to a really efficient footing. An important development of the last few years has been computerisation of much of the editorial activity; this has already improved things greatly, but it is by no means finished.

Another thing I did early on was to introduce the section of Brief Reports. Not only because I thought this was a useful addition to the *Journal* contents, but also because I hoped it would provide an opportunity for younger colleagues particularly to get into print, and I think it has been successful in that way. I was also strongly committed from the beginning to starting a supplement programme, but I had to fight a hard battle, first of all to get the principle accepted, and then to defend the actual content of what was produced in some of the early supplements.

GW   *There's no such thing as a free supplement, and as you say, there's been controversy over some of them. What do you have to say about the economics of running a journal and the tension that there is between publishing and disseminating information in the best way and the fact that there is a cost attached to that?*

HF   The objectives of the Supplement Programme were basically two. The first, and I say that deliberately, was to have an extra opportunity of publishing useful scientific information for which there would not otherwise be space in the *Journal*. The second was to bring in extra income. Now, my taking-up the editorial chair coincided with a drastic curtailment by the Government of the money that pharmaceutical companies could spend on promotion, including advertising in journals. This resulted overnight in a loss of about £70,000 worth of revenue per annum; that was the situation I faced on the first day. It was equivalent to double that sum in today's money. At the same time, the subscription price had not been increased for several years, so that income from that source had been falling steadily in real terms. It was extremely important from the College's point of view to find some way of generating extra revenue, because the College is basically a poor organisation and the profits from publications have been one of its most important incomes. Now, there are a limited number of sources from which one can get money to support publications. One is official bodies like universities, Government departments, research councils, WHO, etc. The second possible source is charitable foundations, and the third is the pharmaceutical industry.

Obviously, from the practical point of view, the third of those is the most important. Pharmaceutical companies are not in fact malicious and corrupt organisations, as some people seem to think, but they have a need to sell their products, or they won't have the money to develop new and better drugs, among other things. One of the most important ways to do this is to communicate information relevant to their products – but not necessarily *about* their products – to the largest number of psychiatrists. Therefore, some supplements have consisted of groups of papers in which some, but only some, are related to a particular drug. I've never been able to understand why some colleagues have objected so violently to papers of this kind being published with the help of a company. If you pursue that argument logically, you would exclude any mention of any treatment method from the *Journal*, because you could argue that eventually, some commercial organisation would thereby profit from it. Yet information about treatment methods is one of the things that readers want most of all.

My experience with the pharmaceutical industry is that they operate to a very high ethical standard. I have *never* been exposed to anything that I could regard as unethical pressure from any company. Indeed, it's not in their interests to have inaccurate information published or unhelpful data suppressed, because sooner or later the truth will come out, and they would suffer more than they would benefit from any pressure like that.

GW   Pursuing the economic theme, my sense of you is that you have, to a certain extent, seen the Journal as subsidising the College; the College is a poor organisation, it needs the funds. Do you see this as desirable, and what are the consequences for the College if, say, the Journal didn't have an aggressive economic policy?

HF   If making a profit was our primary consideration, we would do things entirely differently. We would put out a journal that was a fraction of its present size, as many commercial publishers do. We give very good value indeed for money, and my principal objective has always been the dissemination of information, in which financial considerations are secondary. But we have to live in the real world, and the fact is that the profits from publications, which increasingly in recent years have come from books and not just from the *Journal*, are an essential part of the College's income. The College is very fortunate to own such a publication, which has outstanding international recognition and which is, at the same time, very profitable. No other British College has anything comparable, I believe, particularly not the older ones. It's probably not sufficiently recognised here just how much the *Journal* is read and highly respected all over the world.

GW   I wanted to highlight the book programme because this is another area of growth. Where do you see this programme going?

HF   For many years, the books were just an occasional off-shoot of the *Journal*. They came out at irregular intervals and there were very few of them. I felt from the beginning that this was something which ought to be developed, both in quantity and quality, and also that we needed to put it on a sounder financial footing. As you know, the programme has grown enormously in its scope, but one of my main objectives has been to keep all our books at a price which is affordable for members, and particularly for younger colleagues. We have, in fact, been able to do this quite successfully by looking for help towards the costs of publication, from a variety of sources. This has meant that we have kept the price of most of our books far below those charged by commercial publishers.

Apart from these general developments, for a couple of years now, we've been preparing a major new series called *College Seminars*, which are specifically designed for trainees. Although they are not, in any direct sense, Membership textbooks, we hope that those who make use of them will get most of the information they need for the examination, and that established clinicians will also find them very useful for updating their knowledge. Publication of the series began this spring.

In spite of a lot of effort, I have not been able to improve the psychotherapy content of the *Journal* as much as I had hoped. There's a widespread misconception that it's unfriendly to this kind of paper, which is entirely untrue; the problem is that we receive very few worthwhile submissions. With Bob Hinshelwood, Editor of the *British Journal of Psychotherapy*, we have been running a prize competition this year for original papers, and I hope this may give a permanent boost to the *Journal*'s coverage of the issue. A frequent problem, though, is that many psychotherapists write in language that is unintelligible to anyone else.

There's one other important area which we're just beginning to go into, and which you, as my successor, will have the responsibility for. That is Continuing Medical Education, for which a whole new series of publications are going to be necessary in the next few years. I believe this will provide a great new opportunity for the College – not only in the British Isles, but throughout Europe.

Another thing I did was to be the founding Editor of *Current Opinion in Psychiatry*, which is one of a series of journals, established with the aim of helping clinicians and scientists to cope with the ever-growing flood of publications. As you know, it summarises the literature of the previous 12 months on a series of topics within psychiatry, also providing an annotated reference list, which is available on disk as well as in the hard copy. This has been very successful, as a result of special arrangements between the publishers and the College. I am also retiring from this post, and will be succeeded by Gethin Morgan.

GW   *Are you going to continue your editorial life; do you have any plans?*

HF   I have connections with it, in the sense of being a book reviewer, referee, or Editorial Board Member for a number of journals. I'm working on at least one other edited historical book at present with German Berrios, and I also act as a freelance editor; I think I bring a fairly unusual combination of skills to that kind of work.

GW   *You've written or edited 12 books in the 1980s. Is that something that's going to continue?*

HF   I would like to, but to my shame, I've never written a single-author book up to now, whereas my wife produces them all the time. I think that's something that needs attention. In the later 1960s, I was pressed by several publishers to write a book on community psychiatry. I made several starts, and tried bringing in collaborators, but we were all much too involved in day-to-day work. It needed a sabbatical year, but I had no chance of anything like that.

GW   *You have a number of late-life achievements, so I'm sure that you are going to realise that ambition. You obtained your DM from Oxford in 1988; and you are currently doing a PhD, which, no doubt, will come to fruition in due course too.*

HF   The hoped-for PhD that you mention is on medical history, and this really takes me back to my academic starting-point in the arts. It's concerned with the evolution of mental health policy in this country in the post-war period, because I think there's a great deal that is still unknown about that. However, my research in the Public Record Office and the interviews I've done so far teach me that it's going to be extremely difficult to unravel the whole story.

GW   Do you have a hypothesis?

HF   I believe that this policy was largely the result of a decision by a small number of key people in the Ministry of Health, who in the mid-1950s came to feel that the existing mental hospital system was obsolete. They were influenced a good deal by the example of tuberculosis, where what had been a huge demand for hospital in-patient care disappeared almost overnight, with the development of the antibiotics. As a result, they felt the future lay in a system based in general hospitals, and this then got merged into the hospital plans which began in the early 1960s. I should add that I think one of the key people in that process was my main medical hero, Sir George Godber.

GW   Tell us about Sir George Godber, why is he your hero?

HF   He was Chief Medical Officer at the Ministry of Health, and then DHSS, for 14 years from the early 1960s. One of my own interviews was with him a few years ago, but I think his modesty concealed the essential part he played in the development of the NHS, including the mental health services. His work and his influence represented what I have always felt to be the true ethical and ideological basis of the National Health Service – that its commitment was to the health needs of the people as a whole, and that other considerations such as private profit should be excluded so far as possible.

GW   Another late-life achievement was your Professorship in the Department of Sociology & Anthropology at the University at Salford. Rightly or wrongly, when I think of you I think of someone who has been a sceptic about academia, and so there is an irony in your Chair. Yet, I think that this is something that you are very proud of. Can you say something about the Chair and what it means to you?

HF   Well, I've never been very respectable from an academic point of view. I think I've always been a bit of a maverick in that sense. At the same time, I have great respect for scholarship and for scrupulous academic and scientific work. I was involved in Salford with the origins of the University; it was first of all a Technical College, then a College of Advanced Technology, and finally, a University.

At first, I was concerned in the sociological activities there, because my medical interests always had a strong flavour of that kind. Then, in the late 1960s, we started a joint organisation between the incipient University and Salford Hospitals to form a postgraduate medical institute. At that time, postgraduate medical education in the north-west of England was in a fairly terrible state, so that Salford clinicians really filled the gap that the established medical school wasn't providing for. It seemed possible at that time that a medical school might be established as part of the new University of Salford, but in the end that idea was dropped, and the Manchester school was expanded instead.

In 1974, Salford University provisionally offered me a Chair as Director of the Postgraduate Medical Institute, which was comparable to those in Exeter and Bradford. However, it was dependent on the agreement of Manchester

University, and they refused to give this, so that the appointment never happened. It was obviously a great disappointment. I continued being involved with Salford University, though, doing some teaching in environmental sciences, and also postgraduate supervision and teaching in the Sociology Department, and it was as a consequence of that, rather to my surprise, that they made the offer of this appointment to me in 1986.

GW *I was asking you whether you felt proud about it.*

HF Yes. I was proud to receive this recognition, particularly from an Institution that I'd been intimately concerned with for so many years, whilst remaining basically a clinician. But at the same time, I was an honorary member of the Psychiatric Department of Manchester University, because my general hospital became a teaching hospital for Manchester in the early 1970s. We had no university staff in adult psychiatry at the Salford campus of the medical school, so that all the teaching had to be done by NHS clinicians. We tried to give it a flavour of our own, and I think our students mostly did pretty well. I once took all six of them on a domiciliary visit – which the patient and relatives greatly enjoyed.

I should add that within a few days of hearing of my appointment at Salford, I was told that I had been made a Visiting Fellow of Green College, Oxford. Shortly before that, I had been enormously lucky in being given a four-month sabbatical there, through the generosity of Sir John Walter and the Nuffield Provincial Hospitals Trust. It was the longest break from clinical responsibilities that I had had since starting work in the NHS, more than 30 years earlier. It was wonderful to be able to get on with some writing, though I continued my editorial duties as usual.

I am also very proud of the fact that my wife was made a Professor towards the end of last year, at the new Middlesex University.

GW *I want to turn now to some of your research activities. You've published a number of papers on a variety of themes; what were your main interests?*

HF I think they all stem basically from clinical necessities. Most of the papers I published in the earlier period were about the organisation of services. Obviously, they should have had some evaluative data attached to them, but the fact is that, at that time, nobody knew how to evaluate services. Not only the methods, but even the thinking were at a fairly primitive stage, and I had no money at all to carry out any formal research activities then. So to a large extent, they had to be descriptive, but I think they had a value for that period – and perhaps historically – because what we did in Salford was to create a model for the later national programme, and this was embodied in *Better Services for the Mentally Ill* in 1975. That may seem rather an extravagant statement, but I think you'll find that the principles of what emerged at that time in the national plan were being carried out in Salford in the 1960s, as I described in a number of publications.

From this service interest, two main strands developed: one was epidemiology and the other psychopharmacology, particularly the treatment of schizophrenia. The second one related specially to the use of depot drugs, which I think is an interesting story. The services which I developed in the early '60s particularly focused on schizophrenia, because I thought that this was the single most important problem in psychiatry, and I still think that's so. What happened then was that patients would be admitted, improve in hospital on medication, go out, stop taking the tablets, and relapse. Towards the end of 1966, though, I heard about the first depot drug – fluphenazine enanthate – and started using it. I soon felt that this was one of the most important things that had happened in psychiatry for a long time. Through this interest, I got to know Gerry Daniel, who was then Medical Director of Squibb, and he was the biggest source of support and encouragement that I had. With that help, I began to do some research, which had to be fairly simple because the resources available were minute, but what I focused on was a comparison of schizophrenic patients before and after depot treatment, in terms of the time they spent in hospital. Obviously, this is a very crude and sometimes misleading measure of morbidity, but it was the only form of reasonably hard data that was available. In fact, when patients were switched from oral to depot treatment, it was possible to show dramatic reductions in their need for hospital care, which were comparable to those that occurred when lithium was introduced for patients with recurrent bipolar disorder.

Today, this kind of study seems methodologically simplistic, but its objective was a practical one – to show that using depot neuroleptics in the framework of a comprehensive service could reduce relapses and the need for long hospital stays. The fact that each patient was his or her own control meant that the results were not contaminated by the enormous variability of schizophrenics in their need for medication – which we have no means of predicting early in the illness. I did the early studies together with Donald Johnson, who was then starting in psychiatry, and went on to have an outstanding research career of his own that has always been firmly rooted in clinical needs. For a long time, Squibb did more to promote education and research in this area than any official body, but unfortunately, their interest eventually moved to other areas of medicine.

In America, NIMH carried out a huge and expensive comparison of oral versus depot fluphenazine in the 1970s, which showed no significant difference. However, they had made a basic methodological error, in that the conditions under which patients took oral medication in the trial bore no relation to those of real life – they were under intensive supervision, which came to an end as soon as the research did. You will find the same contamination in a number of American studies. Unfortunately, those who do important research there are so drawn into what one might call entrepreneurial activities that they soon tend to lose touch with actual patients. All this was discussed at a meeting which NIMH arranged in Italy in 1977, when I and Donald Johnson both presented our work. However, for reasons which I could never discover, the proceedings of that meeting were never published.

The Salford epidemiological work was started by Mervyn Susser, who then went to America in 1966. It resulted in the establishment of a case register, which was modelled on the Camberwell one, but was actually more comprehensive in the data it collected. This has continued ever since, and I used it particularly to do some population-based studies in schizophrenia. The basic problem with the register, though, was that it had just enough money to collect the data, which were of a very high standard, but practically no resources to make use of them. So unfortunately, this superb database has never really been exploited to the extent that it deserved, and it failed to get the general support of clinicians, because it wasn't clearly helping them in their everyday work.

GW   Do you think that you got the balance right in your output of clinical work, literary efforts, administration and research?

HF   It's gone through different phases. The 1960s were mostly devoted to developing an integrated clinical service and seeing an enormous number of patients. It was very gruelling, routine work, with little support. In the 1970s, I had a great deal of managerial involvement. I was elected Chairman of the Medical Executive for the Salford Hospitals, and with the 1974 reorganisation, became a member of the Area Management Team. That was an important part of my work for the next five years, but unfortunately, suffering from feelings of omnipotence, I agreed to continue all my clinical commitments at the same time. The result was that I did neither the administrative nor the clinical work as well as I should have done, because there was simply far too much of each. One of my administrative colleagues in management was Duncan Nicol, who has since become head of the NHS Management Executive.

Through learning that lesson, I decided to retire from the NHS at the beginning of 1988, and give virtually all my time to the Editorship. Before that move, I had been supported nobly by my colleagues in Salford, particularly Michael Tarsh and Som Soni. At the Regional level, I was elected Chairman of the Psychiatric Sub-committee of the Regional Medical Committee. The parent body was totally ineffective, but our Sub-committee did provide a meeting-place and collective voice for colleagues from every District, and in representing their views, I didn't always make myself popular with the RHA. Three objectives that I set were to start training arrangements in the north-west for child psychotherapists, to start similar arrangements for nurse therapists, and to get more consultants appointed in mental handicap. None of these were achieved while I was still Chairman, but two of them have been subsequently. I could never understand why the RHA didn't seem to want us to discuss anything important, but I have since discovered in my historical research that at the national level, the same thing happened with the Standing Mental Health Advisory Committee. Administrative bodies don't like professionals getting too closely involved in their activities.

GW   Putting it all together, could you identify a singular success, and also an area where you perhaps didn't devote sufficient energy, or you wish you had developed further in your career.

HF   When I was 31, I made the decision to go for a consultant job in which I had to work tremendously hard, and this meant that I never had time to establish a basis of major original research to my name. That's something I've suffered from since, both professionally and in terms of my own self-esteem. The thing I'm proudest of is the service work I did in the 1960s, but I discovered that in terms of professional advancement, it counts for practically nothing.

GW   You say that with some feeling, but is there a sense of resentment about this, about how clinicians seem to be perceived by Establishment figures: clinicians are hard-working committed serious people, who have got something to say and give, but they're in the back-water, neglected, cannon fodder, the private soldiers, so to speak.

HF   It's a very fundamental problem, not only in medicine, but in other professions too, that those who are effective practitioners don't benefit much in terms of esteem from their colleagues. What I resented very much personally was the fact that the work that I and many other people were doing in the north-west of England wasn't really recognised on a national scale. When Ministers from the Department of Health, and other official bodies looked for advice, they generally turned to people who actually had very little clinical experience; some of them in fact had never worked in the National Health Service outside a teaching hospital. I think that's an unfortunate aspect of British life, but it also happens in other countries, to varying extents.

GW *It's a formidable problem. I remember that in your manifesto for the editorship, you made a point of standing out for the consultant in the 'sticks' and you've hinted at the importance of an editor knowing the readership, or putting it another way, knowing who the electorate are. I wonder, linking it up with professional development, whether or not psychiatry as a profession has got more to learn about professional development and advocacy: that to a degree, one might blame those in the 'sticks' for not shouting out louder.*

HF Those who are deeply involved in the hurly-burly of carrying large clinical commitments often have neither the time nor the energy to devote to blowing their own trumpets. But of course, to some extent, it's a question of personality and choice; people make a decision either to devote themselves primarily to the care of patients or to what one might describe broadly as 'politicking'. It's not easy to combine both these activities successfully, and very hard indeed to combine both with research and academic work also.

GW *I think that there are some other professions close to us who have been more fortunate in their use of politicking and while I hear what you say and I agree with it, looking to the future, maybe all the management training that the senior registrars are having will be effective in making sure that whatever resources there are are kept within psychiatry and mental health.*

HF I think the worst thing that happened from that point of view was the total failure of psychiatry to respond to the ideological challenge of the late 1960s, when anti-psychiatry developed from the political movements of that period. The ideas of R. D. Laing particularly were taken up then by the media, and to some extent, by political groups, which resulted in a wholesale attack on the whole legitimacy of psychiatry as a professional activity. There was virtually no response to this from the psychiatric profession. Of course, the RMPA was a fairly small organisation at the time, but it did nothing whatever to try and counter what I felt was a very sinister movement, that could be very harmful to patients. I myself did enter the battle, in whatever way I could, but hardly anybody else did. Since then, I have got involved in many similar scraps, for instance, in the correspondence columns of the serious newspapers. I look over my shoulder, figuratively, to see who else has joined the battle on our side, but the answer often is no-one.

GW *And so to conclude?*

HF In almost ten years that I have been Editor, the total profits on publications amount to nearly £1 million in today's money. Combined with the scientific quality of the publications, I think that's quite a significant achievement. I haven't mentioned the *Psychiatric Bulletin*, though I was joint editor of it with Alan Kerr for a short time, before moving on. I have encouraged the development of this other journal as much as I could, and I believe the result is greatly appreciated by most College members. It has now become an important journal of administrative and social psychiatry in its own right, as well as a record of the College's activities and views.

I was also keen to start a Trainee Editor Scheme, and this finally happened last year. It has worked very well with our first two appointees – Tom Fahy and Tim Rogers – and I hope this will be a regular arrangement now.

Finally, I would like to acknowledge the tremendous help and support I have enjoyed during my time as Editor. Firstly, from the College staff, particularly David Jago, Ralph Footring, Judy Ashworth, and Elaine Millen; secondly, from my Associate and Assistant Editors, and thirdly, from all those colleagues who have helped as invited authors, as referees, or in giving advice. The job could never have been done without them all.

Index

Compiled by Stanley Thorley